EMDR Therapy has been acclaimed by [specialists, and academicians . . .

"It's been a mere 25 years since Francine Shapiro's momentous discovery of the most effective and practical approach to trauma healing yet found. In that time, EMDR has gone from a private insight to a scientifically validated and world-recognized therapy for PTSD and other trauma-based disorders. EMDR has already brought unnecessary inner suffering to an end in millions of trauma victims. It is my conviction that the EMDR therapy modality will in due course be hailed as one of the great health discoveries of our time—in its consequentiality on par with penicillin, the polio vaccine, and oral rehydration."

—ROLF C. CARRIERE, former UNICEF Country Director in Asia, currently Senior Adviser to Nonviolent Peaceforce

"Thanks to EMDR we are now able to help people to an extent that I never dreamed of some years ago. Dr. Shapiro's work has proven invaluable to clinicians around the world in helping people following trauma."

—ATLE DYREGROV, PhD, Center for Crisis Psychology, Norway, and United Nations Consultant to UNICEF and UNHCR

"EMDR is a proven therapy. Traumatized individuals have used this method to heal fractured souls. Francine Shapiro has made an enduring contribution to the field of psychotherapy."

—JEFFREY K. ZEIG, PhD, Director of the Milton H. Erickson Foundation

"EMDR has become a lifesaving process for battered women who are attempting to heal. Francine Shapiro has literally given new life to these valiant trauma survivors and everyone who has experienced the psychological pain from abuse or knows someone who has should know about EMDR!"

—LENORE WALKER, EdD, ABPP, Diplomate in Clinical Psychology, Executive Director, Domestic Violence Institute

"People often have 'stuck issues' such as phobias, or attitudes about themselves, or tendencies to 'freeze' on the verge of doing something they would really like to do. These stuck issues persist even with a clear understanding of their senselessness and quite often even after many years of otherwise productive psychotherapy. EMDR leads to the rapid resolution of chronic psychological problems like these and has helped my patients resolve issues which had previously seemed unrelenting."

—SANDRA SHAPIRO, PhD, Board Member, National Institute for the Psychotherapies, Associate Professor of Psychology Emeritus, City University of New York

"EMDR is by far the most effective and efficient treatment we have ever used with dissociative episodes, intrusive memories, and nightmares with Vietnam combat veterans."

—Howard Lipke, PhD, former Director of the Stress Disorder Treatment Unit,
North Chicago Veterans Administration Medical Center

"EMDR is the most powerful tool I've encountered for treating posttraumatic stress. In the hands of a competent and compassionate therapist, it gives people the means to heal themselves."

—Steven Silver, PhD, former Director of the PTSD unit,
Veterans Administration Medical Center, Coatesville, Pennsylvania

"During the last 40 years, I have been working with emergency services personnel, who have been stressed by the traumatic events they handle in the workplace. For many, EMDR has been one of the most effective therapeutic interventions available."

—Jeffrey T. Mitchell, PhD, Clinical Professor of Emergency Health
Services at the University of Maryland, Baltimore County, and Cofounder
and President Emeritus, International Critical Incident Stress Foundation

"At least 50 percent of people using illegal drugs are using them to block some sort of trauma or abuse and they are not very responsive to traditional treatments, but EMDR is very effective."

—Alan Hassard, Clinical Psychologist,
Plymouth, England, quoted by Jerome Burne in *Harper's*

"EMDR provides a proven approach to address the trauma that can interfere with healthy grief and mourning following the loss of a loved one."

—Therese A. Rando, PhD, BCETS, BCBT,
Founder and Executive Director, Institute for the Study and Treatment of Loss

"EMDR is a valuable addition to our therapeutic arsenal. It is not a panacea, but it has tremendous power in addressing the sequelae of trauma and a wide variety of psychological problems."

—Richard P. Kluft, MD, Clinical Professor
of Psychiatry, Temple University School of Medicine

"EMDR quickly opens new windows on reality, allowing people to see solutions within themselves that they never knew were there. And it's a therapy where the client is very much in charge, which can be particularly meaningful when people are recovering from having their power taken away by abuse and violation."

—Laura S. Brown, PhD, ABPP,
Clinical Professor of Psychology, University of Washington

"EMDR has bridged the mind-body connection and moved psychotherapy into the 21st century."

—RONALD DOCTOR, PhD, Professor of Psychology,
California State University at Northridge

"EMDR is one of the most powerful and integrative methods I have learned in my professional career."

—JOHN C. NORCROSS, PhD, ABPP,
Distinguished Professor of Psychology, University of Scranton

"Dr. Shapiro's current book belongs in the library of all thoughtful, progressive therapists as well as in the hands of their patients."

—CATHERINE G. FINE, PhD, Temple University, School of Medicine

"The history of psychology will one day acknowledge EMDR as one of the most important psychological innovations of the 20th century. This book is a must-read for the professional therapist who treats trauma victims and for the general public who are victims of trauma and the relatives and friends of victims. EMDR offers hope and light to the despair and darkness of traumatic injury."

—CURTIS C. ROUANZOIN, PhD, former Chair of the
Graduate Department of Psychology at Hope International
University, and Clinical Psychologist specializing in PTSD

lauded in the news media . . .

"Where traditional therapies may take years, EMDR takes only a few sessions."

—*Stars and Stripes*

"EMDR, which to newcomers sounds implausible and way too good to be true, may become the psychological wonder cure of the nineties, the non-pharmaceutical equivalent of Prozac."

—*New York Magazine*

"One of the hottest trends in clinical psychology."

—*Newsweek*

"EMDR . . . is at about the same place that gravity was before Newtonian physics: It's here, and it works, whether we understand it or not."

—*Natural Health*

"EMDR therapy has emerged as a procedure to be reckoned with in psychology. . . . Almost a million have been treated . . . research appears to support the remarkable claims made."

—*Washington Post*

"EMDR provides a way for people to free themselves from destructive memories and it seems to work, even in cases where years of conventional therapy have failed."

—*20/20*, ABC News

"A mainline therapy busily accumulating research on its efficacy, it is also a therapy that makes room for the soul."

—*Common Boundary*

and celebrated by the patients themselves . . .

"The treatment made me look deep—very deep—into my own existence. I'm more attentive to my feelings. Now I treasure each and every moment of my life."

—RICHARD WEBSTER, mine fire victim, quoted in *Family Therapy Networker*

"Now, when I talk about what happened to me, it's definitely reality, but the fear's not there anymore. . . . It's astounding. I've been given a portion of my life back."

—EMILY G., victim of abduction and brutal rape, quoted in *American Health*

"Within two or three of four sessions, we had resolved issues that I'd been discussing for four or five years with other people."

—ERIC SMITH, Vietnam veteran suffering from PTSD, quoted on *20/20*, ABC News

"In four, hour-long EMDR sessions I was able to get at issues that years with other therapists couldn't touch."

—SHERRY MORGAN, rape trauma survivor, quoted in *Orange County Register*

EMDR

The Breakthrough Therapy
for Overcoming Anxiety,
Stress, and Trauma

FRANCINE SHAPIRO, PHD
AND MARGOT SILK FORREST

BASIC BOOKS
New York

Published by Basic Books,

An imprint of Perseus Books, a division of PBG Publishing, LLC, a subsidiary of Hachette Book Group, Inc.

Designed by Jeff Williams

A CIP catalog record for this book is available from the Library of Congress.

Library of Congress Cataloging-in-Publication Data

Shapiro, Francine.
    EMDR: The breakthrough therapy for overcoming anxiety, stress,
and trauma / Francine Shapiro and Margot Silk Forrest.—1st ed.
        p. cm.
    Includes index.
    ISBN-13 978-0-465-04300-2 ISBN-10 0-465-04300-3 (cloth)
    ISBN-13 978-0-465-04301-9 ISBN-10 0-465-04301-1 (paper)
    1. Eye movement desensitization and reprocessing—Popular works.
    I. Forrest, Margot Silk. II. Title.

RC489.E98S53 1997
616.85'210651—dc21
96–46586

ISBN 978-0-465-09674-9 (2016 edition)
ISBN 978-0-465-09675-6 (ebook)

LSC-C

10 9 8 7 6 5 4 3

Dedicated to the
EMDR FACILITATORS, CLINICIANS, AND CLIENTS
who had the vision and courage to attempt something new
and to share their experiences of it

and to the memory of
RON MARTINEZ,
an inspiring human being with quadriplegia who died of cancer.
His life affirmed for us all that it's not what happens to you that
matters, but how you deal with it.

AUTHOR AND PUBLISHER DISCLAIMER

This book is NOT a training manual. It does not contain complete information regarding the clinician's use of EMDR therapy. It should be used as a basic overview of clinical applications of EMDR. Actual treatment should be provided by a well-chosen, licensed, and EMDR-trained clinician.

Although the therapy is called *Eye Movement Desensitization and Reprocessing* (EMDR therapy), directed eye movements are only one form of stimulation used as a part of its complex methodology. The protocols and procedures that comprise the overall EMDR methodology are necessary for comprehensive therapeutic effectiveness as well as client safety. There have been reports of harm caused by people who have attempted self-use of the eye movements, or by clinicians who have not received appropriate training and have used the stimulation without the procedures and protocols that comprise the *entire* EMDR therapy approach.

Laypeople should not attempt to use the eye movements on their own except as instructed by a licensed, EMDR-trained clinician. A client should make sure that his or her prospective clinician has taken an EMDR Regional Association–approved training course (see Appendix A). Numerous clinicians desiring to learn EMDR therapy have mistakenly taken training in various so-called eye-movement techniques or workshops given by people insufficiently schooled and experienced in the methodology. The therapeutic effects demonstrated in this book should not be expected to occur unless the entire EMDR approach is used, and used appropriately, by a licensed and experienced EMDR-trained clinician.

The first-person pronouns throughout the book refer to Francine Shapiro, PhD, the originator and developer of EMDR therapy.

Author and Publisher Disclaimer

Most of the names and some of the external circumstances of a number of the clients in this book have been changed to protect their confidentiality. Every effort has been made to present the symptoms and therapeutic efforts as they actually occurred.

In order to avoid sexism without the stylistic awkwardness of phrases such as "he or she," the personal pronouns have been alternated throughout the book.

CONTENTS

ACKNOWLEDGMENTS

This book was a labor of long duration and many contributors. The content is based on the experiences of hundreds of people, and I hope it has done them justice. Special thanks go to the clients who willingly shared their stories in the hopes that others might be helped. I also wish to gratefully acknowledge the special contributions of the following clinicians: Judy Albert, David Blore, Jac Carlson, Cathy Davis, Nancy Davis, Ron Doctor, Jean Eastman, Sandra Foster, Chad Glang, David Grand, Lew Hamburger, Ad de Jongh, Tim Kaufman, Robert Kitchen, Laura Knutson, Deany Laliotis, Steven Lazrove, Andrew Leeds, Jennifer Lendl, Patti Levin, Howard Lipke, Joan Lovett, Marilyn Luber, Pavel Lushin, John Marquis, David McCann, Daniel Merlis, Gerald Murphy, A. J. Popky, David Price, Gerald Puk, Gary Quinn, Therese Rando, Graciela Rodriquez, Susan Rogers, Curt Rouanzoin, Beverly Schoninger, Elan Shapiro, Jocelyne Shiromoto, Steven Silver, Roger Solomon, Pablo Solvey, Robert Tinker, Sheryll Thompson, Linda Vanderlaan, Rosemary Vienot, Silke Vogelmann-Sine, Donald Weston, Geoffrey White, David Wilson, Sandra Wilson, Carol York, William Zangwill, and Joan Zweben.

As the developer of EMDR, I offer my gratitude to Margot Silk Forrest for her extraordinary writing talents which allowed the stories of suffering and transformation that are described in this book to come alive so vividly. Special thanks to Robbie Dunton for her tireless support. As usual, I couldn't have written this book—or accomplished any creative work throughout the year—without her having freed my time and my mind for the task. Many thanks to Robert B. Welch, Steven Lazrove, and Silvia Hines for their special editing efforts, and to MaryAnn Gutoff for her technical assistance. My thanks also to Barb Hensley, Ad de Jong, Susan Brown, and David van den Berg for their research assistance in this latest edition. Writing a book and bringing it to the public is a herculean task. Its success depends upon the input and assistance of many, including an entire publishing staff. For her extraordinary flexibility and skill, my gratitude goes to Quynh Do, my editor at Basic Books. My appreciation to my agent Suzanne Gluck for her multi-faceted talents and support. My unending gratitude to all of my friends and colleagues who have joined with me through the years and helped to share the vision. And finally, a special acknowledgment to my parents, Danny and Shirley Shapiro, and to Bob Welch, my husband and oasis.

—F. S.

I want to add my heartfelt thanks to my many friends and the courageous staff of *The Healing Woman Foundation*, all of whom supported me with patience and love during the writing of this book.

—M. S. F.

Introduction

IN THE EIGHTEEN YEARS since this book was written, many things have changed, and Eye Movement Desensitization and Reprocessing, or EMDR, therapy is now widely accepted as a research-supported, effective treatment for trauma and other adverse life experiences. Yet the primary guiding principles of EMDR therapy have remained the same. It is worthwhile here to review those principles and to answer some questions.

Trauma Comes in Many Forms

Most of us are used to thinking of trauma only as those big events that appear in the newspapers. War veterans, survivors of natural catastrophes and terrorist attacks, these are the sufferers of trauma in the popular imagination. But, in fact, by dictionary definition, trauma is *any event that has had a lasting negative effect*. We all know people who have lost jobs, loved ones, even possessions and who have truly suffered as a result. When you lose your peace of mind, or if you never had it, there can be serious physical and psychological consequences no matter what the cause. Regardless of the "triggers," the causes are generally found in earlier life experiences. We call these experiences *traumas*.

Trauma Can Be Healed

Anxiety, stress, guilt, rage, and fear, regardless of the cause, are extremely unhealthy if they are long-lasting. Fortunately, the body uses a process similar to digestion in order to resolve upsetting experiences. Just as the digestive system extracts nutrients from the food we eat, so the mind's information processing system, when functioning properly, extracts useful information from our experiences. What we learn from this information allows us to move forward. When the memories of upsetting experiences are processed, the related emotions, beliefs, body responses, and thoughts are transformed, becoming healthy and adaptive. Sometimes, though, negative experiences remain in memory unresolved, leaving a residue of emotion to dominate our daily lives. The system becomes "stuck"—as if it was choking on trauma—and often requires assistance in order to get moving smoothly again. This is where EMDR therapy comes in.

Therapy for the Body, Therapy for the Mind

Most people think that therapy involves only talking about problems. However, one aspect of EMDR therapy is that you do not have to talk in detail about a trauma for it to be digested by your own information processing system. Basically this involves what some have called *bottom-up* instead of *top-down* processing.[1] In other words, rather than trying to talk through the problem, the processing occurs on a physiological level and allows new associations, insights, and emotions to emerge spontaneously. EMDR therapy involves a very specific set of procedures to help this "digestive" function in the brain, which neurobiologists refer to as *information processing*.

EMDR therapy is guided by the Adaptive Information Processing model, which identifies negative life experiences stored in the brain as central to mental health problems.[2] A number of neurobiologists and memory researchers point out that major traumas and other disturbing life experiences are stored in the wrong form of memory.[3] Instead of being stored in memory where they can be remembered without pain, they are stored in memory where they hold the emotions and body sensations that were part of the initial event. Because these memories are not able to connect with other, more helpful information, they remain isolated from other life experiences in our memory networks. For example, even though we can look at things rationally where other people are concerned, and know they aren't to blame for certain things, we can't view ourselves in the same way. We may recognize that a victim of rape should not be blamed for the actions of the rapist, yet, placed in the same circumstance ourselves, feel somehow at fault. Basically, no matter how intelligent or spiritual or experienced or educated we are, the memories can simply be stored in the wrong form of memory. We didn't cause it—we are suffering from it.

The memory system is in the brain, and the brain is part of the body. Most of us recognize that if our body is cut it will begin to heal unless there is a block, such as a splinter. We are willing to enter into surgery because we know our body will close and heal the wounds, just as it's supposed to do. But for some reason, we don't think of "mental problems" in the same way. Traumatic memories are located in the brain, and since the brain is part of the body, it can and should heal in the same way. Although we expect the physical bruises of crime victims to heal in a matter of weeks, we believe that healing psychological wounds may take years. This is not necessarily so. In reality, the brain can heal at the same rate as the rest of the body.

In many ways EMDR therapy is like having your arm set by a doctor. Both conditions are physical and both need assistance to prepare, align, and stimulate the body's own healing mechanism. EMDR therapists are trained to work with the information processing system in order to access the troubling experiences. Once accessed, these experiences need to be addressed to bring the client to full health.

Who Needs EMDR Therapy?

EMDR therapy has been used with combat veterans, firefighters, policemen, emergency service workers, and missionaries—all trained to help others and to "tough it out." They came for help because they realized that they did not need to treat the mind differently from the body. We all need help sometimes, and sometimes it's hard to find the right *kind* of help.

But there are many forms of therapy—so saying, "I tried therapy and it doesn't work" is like saying, "I tasted a fruit and didn't like it, so I'm not going to eat any fruit." There are hundreds of thousands of licensed mental health clinicians in the United States alone. There are hundreds of techniques and many different types of therapies. Psychodynamic therapists alone may follow the principles and practices of many different, well-respected therapists, such as Freud, Jung, Horney, Adler, or a dozen others. Therapists who practice Cognitive Behavioral Therapy (CBT) may be more focused on behavior or cognition and may draw from a variety of techniques, depending on their own training and life experience. EMDR is a distinct form of therapy and has principles and practices that are different from these and other approaches. While EMDR integrates aspects of other therapies, it also gives the client a different experience. The purpose of this book is to provide examples of those experiences so that you and your loved ones can be sure you are receiving EMDR therapy, and not someone's distorted version of it.

Unfortunately, what has changed in the years since *EMDR* was first published is that more people are affected by trauma than ever before. These may be both what we can call *large "T"* and *small "t"* events. Large "T" traumas are those experiences that are necessary to diagnose posttraumatic stress disorder (PTSD). Large "T" events are technically called *Criterion A* events and include natural disasters, combat, accidents, catastrophic illnesses, and the loss of a loved one. However, while these kinds of events are necessary to officially diagnose PTSD for many people, research now supports the Adaptive Information Processing model guiding EMDR therapy and indicates that general adverse life experiences can result in even more PTSD symptoms than major trauma can.[4] Small "t" events are those more prevalent experiences that make us feel unsafe, unloved, or without control or hope. These can be humiliations, failures, or losses of any kind. For children, the events can include being bullied or excluded or even falling off their bicycle. Events that can seem unimportant to an adult can be devastating to children and can have lasting effects. In fact, a Kaiser Permanente study that evaluated 9, 508 participants reported that adverse childhood experiences were associated with a wide range of mental health disorders and several leading causes of death in adults.[5] Given the current state of the world, pressures and uncertainties have compounded the daily problems that many adults face, and many more people are in need of help than ever before. Fortunately, help is available to a greater degree than ever before.

When this book was first published, there were 20,000 clinicians trained in EMDR and about one million people had been treated. EMDR was as well supported by research as any other treatment approach, but unknown in many circles, and suspect in others. Today, hundreds of thousands of clinicians have been trained worldwide, and millions of people have been successfully treated.

Does EMDR Work?

EMDR is recognized as an effective trauma therapy by numerous organizations worldwide. For instance, in 2009, the International Society for Traumatic Stress Studies[6] declared that EMDR therapy's effectiveness was supported by research. In 2002, the Israeli National Council of Mental Health designated EMDR as one of three preferred trauma treatments for terrorist victims.[7] In 2010, the U.S. Department of Defense and Department of Veteran Affairs issued new guidelines putting EMDR into the category of therapies with the highest level of evidence and recommending it for treatment of PTSD.[8] Most recently, in 2013, the World Health Organization reported that trauma-focused CBT and EMDR are the only psychotherapies recommended for children, adolescents, and adults with PTSD.[9] The report also noted the differences between the two forms of treatment: "Like CBT with a trauma focus, EMDR aims to reduce subjective distress and strengthen adaptive cognitions related to the traumatic event. Unlike CBT with a trauma focus, EMDR does not involve (a) detailed descriptions of the event, (b) direct challenging of beliefs, (c) extended exposure, or (d) homework." These differences will be evident in the cases described throughout this book.

The many organizations recommending EMDR therapy based their decisions on the large number of research studies that support it as an effective and long-lasting treatment. Research has shown that about five hours of EMDR treatment eliminates PTSD in 84 to 100 percent of civilians with a single trauma experience, including rape, accident, or disaster.[10] When civilians experience multiple traumas, more treatment is needed. Research indicates that about eight to twelve hours of treatment can result in 77 to 80 percent elimination of multiple-trauma PTSD in civilians. A study funded by Kaiser Permanente reported that 80 percent of multiple-trauma victims and 100 percent of single-trauma victims had PTSD eliminated in an average of six fifty-minute sessions. However, it should not be assumed that all symptoms can be handled for everyone in that amount of time. Everyone is different in their biological, psychological, and environmental makeup. Nevertheless, these research studies offer clinicians and clients a guide as to what to expect in clinical practice. (A list of all the published EMDR studies mentioned in this introduction is included in Appendix B.)

Given the uncertainties of our time, with many men and women facing combat, we are thankful that EMDR is a treatment that works well with soldiers. A randomized* study that evaluated a full course of EMDR treatment with combat veterans reported that after twelve sessions, 78 percent of the Vietnam combat veterans in the study no longer had PTSD.[11] The fact that there were zero dropouts, unlike studies of other treatments that generally have about a 30 percent dropout rate, can be attributed to several factors: (1) EMDR therapy results in a rapid decrease in emotional disturbance that occurs even in the first session, (2) there is no need to talk about the memory in detail, and (3) it eliminates fear, anger, guilt, and sleep problems.[12] A 2007 study of sixty-three active-duty personnel with PTSD reported that after trauma treatment, the emotional disturbance was basically "eliminated and a new more positive perspective had developed." The average treatment time was four EMDR sessions—eight sessions if they had been wounded in action.[13] Positive research reports include a field study of a Veterans Administration (VA) program and several articles reporting positive treatment effects with veterans from World War II, the Korean War, and Desert Storm and current active military personnel (see Appendices B and C). Overall, these results mean that no matter how long their symptoms have lasted, veterans and their families can be healed of the ravages of pain. Chapter 3 describes a case in detail. These results also mean that those who serve in daily combat on our city streets such as the emergency service workers, firefighters, police, and others can also be healed.

Regardless of how tough a person might be, the bottom line is that the memories of disturbing experiences can be stored in the wrong form of memory. The intrusive thoughts, dreams, disturbing emotions, and sensations are all products of a physical problem that can be helped without resorting to drugs or alcohol to mask the pain. In fact, a National Institute of Mental Health (NIMH) study reported that EMDR was superior to Prozac in treating trauma.[14] After people were taken off the medication, their symptoms returned, while those treated with EMDR therapy kept getting better. These findings emphasize why the World Health Organization did not recommend any drugs for the treatment of PTSD. They also underscore the

---

*Participants are assigned to treatment conditions in a random manner so as to minimize differences between the groups (e.g., treatment is not chosen because of time, location, or to suit the characteristics of the person).

Adaptive Information Processing model principle that targeting and reprocessing the trauma is preferable to merely treating the symptoms.

What Is the Difference Between EMDR Therapy and Exposure Therapy?

There are several cognitive behavioral therapies for PTSD that use exposure; however, the one most commonly recommended for PTSD is prolonged exposure (PE). The therapist asks the client to hold the disturbing experience in mind, identify and "feel the feelings" that arise, and describe it all to the clinician in detail for an hour to ninety minutes at a time, saying things like "I feel the pain; I see the blood." The client is not allowed to let the mind move away from the experience, because that is considered "avoidance" and is thought to make people worse. The session is audio taped and the client is expected to listen to it each night until the next session. In addition, the client is also supposed to go to physical locations they find disturbing as a result of the trauma experience. This might be the area where the client was raped, or the location of the car accident. They are instructed to stay in the area for about one hour each day, until the disturbance goes away.

In contrast, EMDR therapists ask clients to concentrate on a disturbing part of the memory, and then let their minds move to "whatever comes up" during sets of eye movements or other forms of bilateral stimulation. The client may spend only a short period of time on the disturbing memory itself. While there may be a certain amount of distress, there is generally a decline at the end of the first session,[15] and new insights and understandings tend to emerge. A Harvard researcher[16] has proposed that the same neurobiological processes that occur during rapid eye movement (REM) or dream sleep cause this tendency. REM state is known for processing experiences, learning skills, and reducing emotional disturbance. It is easy to recognize the similarities between REM and EMDR, as EMDR therapy produces the same effects. In fact, one of the guiding principles of EMDR therapy involves stimulating the natural information processing tendencies of the brain, while also not restricting or dictating the client's reactions. The EMDR clinician is trained to help guide the processing according to consistent procedures and protocols. All of these characteristics of EMDR therapy are explored in the chapters of this book.

How Important Are the Eye Movements?

EMDR is not simply "eye movement therapy." It is a complex approach to psychotherapy that is listed in psychology encyclopedias[17] along with psychodynamic therapy, cognitive therapy, family therapy, and so forth. It combines aspects and procedures that are found in the different therapies in order to address the whole person. That is, rather than concentrating on any one specific part of the clinical picture, EMDR therapy addresses the emotions, thoughts, physical sensations, attitudes, behaviors, and more. In doing so, people are then able to feel joy and love, to bond, connect, and feel good about themselves. All the procedures and protocols are combined to achieve comprehensive success as defined by a decrease in symptoms and an enhanced ability to function in life. Of course, I want to underscore that all forms of psychotherapy have their place. However, each form of therapy offers people a different experience, during which they may achieve different goals. Whether or not you have had previous therapy, reading this book will show you specifically what EMDR has to offer.

Unfortunately, in 1987 I included the words "eye movement" in the name of the therapy. However, in 1990, after EMDR had already achieved name recognition, I discovered that other forms of stimulation could also achieve success. When blind people came in for treatment and could not move their eyes, we found that hand taps and audio tones could work as well. Many neurobiologists have argued that the taps and tones work on the same principle as the eye movement, by causing an "orienting" or "interest" response in the brain that fosters the processing. Others say that the different stimuli affect the "visuo-spatial template of working memory." Still others have supported the notion I discuss in Chapter 6 of this book, that EMDR links into the same processes that occur during REM or dream sleep.[18] Basically, there are several research-supported theories for why EMDR therapy works,[19] and there is a strong likelihood that all are correct and come into play at different times in the therapy process. However, there is not enough known in the area of brain physiology and neurobiology to know for sure. That is the case for any form of therapy. We know something works because we can observe the outcomes, but we don't know *why* it works. No one can explain on a neurobiological level why, for example, family therapy works. We don't even know exactly why most medications work.

For many years, the eye movement component was considered controversial because of research that was considered flawed in the 2000 International Society for the Study of Traumatic Stress Practice Guidelines.[20] At this point, however, more than thirty randomized controlled studies have supported the effects of the eye movements, and a meta-analysis published in 2013 has confirmed the effects,[21] such as decreases in negative emotions and imagery. The eye movements also promote the connection with new associations necessary for information processing to occur.[22] Moreover, numerous randomized studies have demonstrated effects such as increased memory retrieval and recognition of true information.[23]

Again, though, EMDR is much more than eye movements. It is a combination of standardized procedures and protocols guided by certain principles. Anyone who uses only eye movements is *not* using EMDR.

When Should EMDR Be Used?

EMDR practice is guided by the Adaptive Information Processing model. Just like psychodynamic and behavior therapies, EMDR's principles are separate from particular neurobiological mechanisms. The purpose of any psychotherapy model is to explain clinical effects, predict successful outcomes with certain types of problems, and guide clinical practice. In accordance with its information processing model, EMDR therapy addresses the experiences that have contributed to the problems. While some problems may have a biological foundation, such as certain forms of depression, most others are based on or influenced by experiences. For instance, in Chapter 4, the impact of an extremely insensitive statement by an authority figure appeared to have had a lasting and devastating effect on a woman until she received therapy.

While most of the EMDR research has concentrated on PTSD, many other uses have been described in clinical journals. One published article reported that five of seven people who came into therapy believing there was something horribly wrong with their appearance discovered that it was based upon the emotional impact of an inappropriate insult.[24] They were successfully treated with EMDR within three sessions. Our views of ourselves are based on our previous experiences. Anyone who feels unlovable, useless, a failure, or guilty can find out in a short time if they can be helped by EMDR therapy. Whether these kinds of problems involve you or a loved one, help may be just a few weeks away. (A list of problems that have been described in professional articles appears in Appendix C.)

It is important to remember that good therapy is an interaction between client, therapist, and method. If you don't find the right therapist, you will not receive good therapy (see Appendix A). It is important for people to be informed, and for consumers to make sure that the therapist they choose has experience and special training in their particular complaint. For instance, if you are struggling with alcohol or drug problems, you should see an EMDR therapist specially trained in the field of substance abuse. Therapists will know when and how to use EMDR if they have appropriate experience and training. In other words, EMDR should always be integrated into the wisdom of field.

In addition to being qualified to address your particular problems, it is also important that you make sure that your therapist has been well trained in EMDR. Make sure that the therapist has finished a program certified by the EMDR International Association, the EMDR Europe Association, EMDR Iberoamérica, or EMDR Asia* and, preferably, is a member so that he or she is keeping up with all the latest developments (see Appendix A). Also investigate whether your therapist is using EMDR as a "technique" or as an "approach." In other words, some clinicians may be using EMDR only if they feel that something is "stuck," instead of using it systematically to address the entire clinical picture.

To receive the most thorough EMDR therapy, your clinician should teach you a self-control technique, such as the "safe place" exercise, before beginning any direct processing with eye movements or other stimulation. This and other techniques will help you to deal with your feelings and emotions while therapy is taking place.[25] The clinician should also take a thorough history in order to identify the (1) earlier events that set the foundation for the problem, (2) the present situations that cause the disturbance, and (3) the skills and behaviors necessary for the future. You may not know what the earlier events are, but a skilled clinician will help you identify them by using a variety of techniques she or he would have learned in the EMDR training and from my professional textbook. If your clinician has not taken a certified training and read the text,[26] this person would not be a good choice as an EMDR clinician.

---

* http ://www.emdria.org, emdr-europe.org, emdriberoamerica.org, emdrasia-assoc.org

EMDR therapy is not a good choice for everyone. If you are not willing to be in touch with your feelings and don't want to learn the techniques to help you do so, or if you have a problem that is purely biological, EMDR is not for you. Those problems that are purely caused by imbalances that only medications can address will not be changed by EMDR. However, some forms of depression are caused by experiences that have left the person feeling helpless and hopeless. An example of this is described in Chapter 12. Given how long it takes for medications to take effect, trying a few sessions of EMDR may indicate that the medication is unnecessary.[27]

The amount of EMDR therapy you will need depends upon many factors, including your readiness to deal with emotions and your personal history. Those people with long histories of childhood abuse will not be treated completely in only a few sessions. While the PTSD research indicates that three EMDR sessions will complete treatment on a single trauma, more traumas need more treatment. It may not be important to address each traumatic experience, especially since the positive treatment effects can generalize to similar events, but more therapy will be necessary. We also need to be aware of the difference between reducing the obvious suffering of a particular disorder and coming into full health. Comprehensive EMDR treatment involves addressing those experiences that contributed to both problems and achievement. At the end of therapy, success would be defined by a person who can love, bond, feel secure, and find joy in living. (Guidelines for choosing a clinician are in Appendix A.)

Why I Wrote the Book

The chapters in this book describe real people who wanted their stories told in order to help others find their way. In addition to chapters that cover the evolution and structure of EMDR therapy, each of the chapters describes a different type of problem and shows what caused it, and how it was treated. These are not the only types of problems that can be dealt with by EMDR treatment, but millions of people are struggling needlessly with these kinds of common symptoms. The goal is to give you a good understanding of who can be helped, where problems come from, and what EMDR treatment looks like. In addition, Chapter 12 of this book deals with the frontiers of EMDR therapy, and its "global reach." This includes a description of the work done by the nonprofit Trauma Recovery/EMDR Humanitarian

Assistance Programs (HAP)* to help underserved populations in the U.S. and around the world. The basic belief that many of us hold is that violence begets violence, and trauma begets more suffering. We believe that unhealed traumas cascade into the next generation, whether from one family member to the next, or through the anger that fuels much of the ethnopolitical warfare throughout the globe.[28] If, after receiving EMDR therapy, you believe it has helped you, please consider helping to make the treatment available to suffering people worldwide. (Information about HAP and its accomplishments can be found in Appendix A.)

My hope in writing this book is that people will recognize themselves or a loved one in its pages, and see that help is available. I also want this book to illustrate what good EMDR therapy looks like so that clients can be informed consumers and make sure their own treatment stays on track. Most clients should be ready for processing within a few sessions. It doesn't take months or years to see if EMDR therapy is appropriate for you or a loved one. Maybe things you think can't change, actually can. It may not take that long to find out.

---

* http://www.emdrhap.org

1

The Journey of Discovery

Freedom is what you do with what's been done to you.

—JEAN-PAUL SARTRE

LINDA CRAMPTON TURNED and, deep in thought, headed slowly back toward her bedroom to finish dressing. At that moment, the blast from the two-and-a-half-ton car bomb at the Alfred P. Murrah Federal Building a block away picked Linda up, hurling her through her living room and dining room, and flung her against the far wall of her kitchen, where she landed, unconscious, on the tile floor. Then, with astounding force, the backdraft of the bomb sucked out the contents of her kitchen cupboards, yanked the microwave from the wall, and dropped them all on top of her. It was 9:02 a.m., April 19, 1995, in Oklahoma City.

When Linda came to a few minutes later, her apartment had been leveled. Twisted steel reached like crabbed fingers from the concrete walls. Splinters of glass from the large plate-glass windows jutted from every surface and were embedded in Linda's skin. Though she was bleeding from hundreds of tiny cuts, Linda suffered no serious harm. Not physically, at least.

Linda climbed over the debris to what was left of her front door. She was determined to find her neighbor, Anna, an elderly woman who was like a mother to her. The hallway looked like a war zone. It was dark with the smoke of cars burning on the street below. People were screaming and moaning. Blood and broken glass were everywhere. Linda started banging on Anna's door, pushing it, kicking it with her bare feet, pounding it with her fists. When she got the door open, her friend was standing there covered with glass, bits of it sticking out of her face.

Together they made their way to the stairwell and crept slowly down seventeen flights of stairs with the forty other shocked and bloody residents who had been home at the time of the blast: about a quarter of those who lived in the Regency Towers. One of them was Linda's upstairs neighbor, Aren Almon, whose pixie-faced infant daughter, Baylee, was in day care at the Murrah building. Linda knew them well, had stroked Baylee's hair the day before when they rode in the elevator together.

When they reached street level, no one could get the door to open, so they went down one more floor to the garage. The blast had bent and jammed the overhead garage door but left a narrow opening at the bottom. They lay down and rolled under it. Outside, it was even smokier, and there were hundreds of people, crying, running, wailing. Linda and Anna turned to their right (away from the Murrah building), stumbled along for about half a block, then sat down in the middle of the street. Someone had wrapped a towel around Linda to staunch her bleeding. She was shaking from head to foot and sobbing. Later, a doctor, seeing the saturated towel, came over to check her wounds. "You're okay," he told her. "You're going to be okay. Just stay right here."

Linda was not okay. This became increasingly obvious to her family, friends, and colleagues as the weeks went by. At first, Linda had been housed in a motel with other evacuees; then she was moved to the home of a close friend. She could not function independently. She couldn't remember what day or week it was. She had to be reminded to eat, take a shower, brush her teeth, and go to bed. She started losing weight at the rate of four pounds a week. Every night she woke up screaming, crying, wet, and scared. She slept most of the day and ground her teeth until they were worn down to the gums; her grinding could be heard from two rooms away. Her dentist fitted her with teeth guards to prevent her from destroying her jawbone.

After a while, Linda went back to her job as a corporate sales representative, but she was on "automatic pilot," and when she got to work, she sat at her desk and cried. She had forgotten how to work. Linda had no memory of the bombing or her frightening escape from the skyscraper with Anna. It was as if her mind had gotten stuck at 9:01 a.m., April 19. The last thing she remembered clearly was getting her taxes in at the last moment. By the end of eight weeks, she was down to eighty-five pounds.

On June 12, Linda was in her office talking to her boss and long-time friend, Bob Harraldsen. She couldn't take in much of what he was saying, but she did catch the word bomb.

"What bomb?" Linda asked.

"Linda, I think the bomb has really affected you," Bob said.

He's lying to me, Linda thought. Why is he lying to me? There was no bomb! She started screaming and throwing things, destroying her office in the process.

Linda's boss and coworkers had known from the first time they saw her after the bombing that something was seriously wrong, but Linda had kept refuting their impressions. "I'm fine, I'm fine," she would say. "It's no big deal."

When Linda finally calmed down, her boss took her aside. "I think you need some help," he said.

"No," Linda replied. "I just need to go home for a while and rest. That's all."

"Linda," Bob said, "You haven't been in your apartment for two months, since this happened."

With Linda sobbing, Bob drove her to Project Heartland, an organization set up to help bombing victims. On the way, Linda made him promise that he would not let anyone put her into a hospital. She had grown up in an orphanage and wanted nothing more to do with institutions of any type.

The people at Project Heartland felt Linda's case was too serious for them to handle. They referred her to a mental health clinic in the suburbs, where Bob took her that day. The psychiatrist there examined Linda, an anorexic-looking woman who was now in hysterics and shaking uncontrollably. She listened to Bob's story and assessed the situation. "We need to put you in the hospital," the doctor finally said. "We need to get you on some medication. It's that serious." Linda cringed back wailing "noooo" long and loud. Protectively, Bob took her by the arm and drew her toward the door. The psychiatrist took one quick step to intervene but stopped when she saw Bob's face. As a last-ditch effort, she told them to go to a place called the EMDR Free Clinic.

⁓

Linda Crampton came under the care of an out-of-state psychotherapist, one member of a team of thirty-six Eye Movement Desensitization and

Reprocessing (EMDR) psychotherapists who had flown to Oklahoma City at their own expense to help the bombing victims. Although EMDR was a comparatively new form of therapy at that time, it had already proved itself effective in treating trauma victims quickly and thoroughly.

"Please don't hospitalize me," Linda begged her EMDR therapist. "Just help me."

A year later, Linda described her first EMDR treatment as "the weirdest thing I had ever experienced, with the exception of the bomb." As a prelude to the first session, Linda received the standard screening and preparation for EMDR. Then she was asked to bring a specific aspect of the bombing to mind while following with her eyes the back-and-forth rhythm of the therapist's hand as it moved across her field of vision (a component of EMDR treatment).

"I remember crying a lot," she said, "and thinking I was watching something happen. It was like someone had sat me in a room and showed a video of everything that happened to me that day. I started remembering everything. I remembered the actual bomb. And I realized it was now June."

EMDR had jump-started Linda's own healing process. Each person's response is unique; Linda's "video" played for ninety minutes and covered every moment of the bombing and her escape. When she left the session, Bob was waiting for her. "My God," he said. "You're back." Then they both started crying.

That evening, Linda called her daughter and told her what had happened.

"Mother, oh my God!" her daughter said. "You sound like my mother again."

After her first EMDR treatment, Linda's nightmares about the bombing stopped, and she was able to go back to work. After her second treatment, she stopped grinding her teeth. After her third, she felt fully back to normal.

༄

Amazing as this case may sound, it is typical of the reports from the thousands of psychotherapists currently trained in EMDR and the millions of people who have been helped by it. EMDR is a complex and powerful psychotherapy that integrates many of the most successful elements of a wide range of therapeutic approaches. In addition, it uses eye movements or other forms of rhythmical stimulation, such as hand taps or tones, in a way that seems to assist the brain's information-processing system to proceed at a rapid rate.

It is a measure of how radical EMDR's results are that it became the subject of a lively and sometimes bitter controversy played out in the popular press, in professional journals, and on the Internet. The phrase heard most often from skeptics was, "It's too good to be true." Of course, controversy is to be expected with most dramatic innovations. As a matter of fact, one interlocutor[1] on a Veterans Affairs Medical Center Internet forum described the similarities between the rise of EMDR and the acceptance of para-aminosalicylic acid (PAS) as an effective treatment of tuberculosis. Initially, PAS was considered suspect because the drug was a derivative of the lowly aspirin. Controversy reigned for years. A chronicler of that resistance explained that "perhaps the majority of doctors and patients remained skeptical of the cure until they had seen it happen with their own eyes. The awe of tuberculosis, the ageless leviathan of terror, was so great and the prevailing despair so ingrained, it would take a decade of convincing before [the treatment was] generally accepted into medical practice."[2] Likewise, skeptics of EMDR therapy questioned how the eye-movement component or, for that matter, any single method could possibly have such a powerful effect. Yet if we substitute the term *posttraumatic stress disorder* for *tuberculosis* in the preceding quote, we have the story of EMDR. Fortunately, the decade of proof of EMDR's effectiveness was marked by the initial publication of this book.

One of the benefits of having a chorus of concerned skeptics is that it drives proponents to produce an extraordinary amount of evidence to back up their claims. As a result, there are now more than thirty randomized controlled studies supporting the effectiveness of EMDR.[3] Multiple studies[4] indicate that 84 to 90 percent of the people using EMDR—victims of rape, natural disaster, the loss of a child, catastrophic illness, or other traumas—have recovered from posttraumatic stress in only five hours of treatment. Before EMDR, that success rate was unheard-of. Other psychological methods for healing trauma generally use many more sessions or assign homework or do both.[5] Nonetheless, extraordinary claims demanded extraordinary proof. The ongoing research supports EMDR's efficacy; however, as in any psychological approach, further studies are needed to expand on these findings. Meanwhile, people's stories keep coming in.

Many of EMDR's successes have already been chronicled by reporters throughout the world. The method has received media attention in many newspapers and magazines, including the *Washington Post*, the *Los Angeles Times*, *New York* magazine, and *Newsweek*, and there has been local TV coverage around the globe. As gratifying as the extensive media coverage has been, however, some reports have been more accurate than others.[6] Consequently, many people have mistakenly come to think of EMDR as a therapy that uses only eye movements. That is far from true.

In its unique combination of elements, EMDR focuses not just on a person's troubling feelings, but on the thoughts, physical sensations, and behaviors related to those feelings as well. For example, suppose a child's dog was killed when it nosed open the screen door, dashed into the street, and was hit by a car. The result may be that the boy feels sad and angry at the loss of his dog. He may also think the accident was his fault ("I should have fastened the latch"). He may have a physical sensation of tightness in his chest, and he may start obsessively checking the latches on all the doors in the house day and night.

With EMDR, we expect all those aspects of the boy's grief to heal and to heal relatively rapidly. His feelings would evolve from sorrow to acceptance; his guilty thoughts would change to "I am not to blame" or the realization that nobody is perfect; the tightness around his heart would disappear; and his obsessive behavior would stop. No longer does someone in pain have to wait months to see if therapy is working. Most people are able to see some change occur after every session. This way, the therapist is accountable to the client.

Many people who use EMDR find that it reactivates some aspect of their traumatic memory as the first step in its resolution. Individual EMDR sessions can be hard work, therefore, but once they are over, health can emerge; the person no longer has to fight off feelings of despair, guilt, or anger or to guard constantly against destructive urges. Much of what we consider to be mental disorder is the result of the way information is stored in the brain. Healing begins when we unlock this information and allow it to emerge. I regard this healing process as an activation of the person's innate ability to heal psychologically, just as his body heals itself when he is physically wounded. A self-healing system like this makes sense: We are all biologically and emotionally geared for survival and mental equilibrium.

EMDR therapy seems to have a direct biological effect on the nervous system, and because we all share the same nervous system, the results of certain experiences are fairly predictable. What Linda went through in Oklahoma

City could have happened to any of us. Although each of us has unique characteristics, any of us could have developed the devastating symptoms she did. Fortunately, in most cases the effects of trauma are reversible. Through competent treatment with EMDR, even suffering that has gone on for decades can be relieved. Just as Linda was able to find relief after the bombing, World War II combat veterans and adult survivors of child abuse have used EMDR therapy and found peace.

One of the most exciting aspects of EMDR is seeing how many people are helped and what a high success rate is achieved. EMDR's success is not limited to people who have experienced a diagnosable trauma. The human mind is miraculously complex, and sometimes what seems to be the most innocuous event can leave an indelible mark on a person's psyche and behavior. Almost every kind of suffering that we define and label a disorder—almost every type of psychological complaint—can be traced to earlier life experiences, which can also be healed. EMDR accesses the memories of these experiences but does not dwell on them and does not, as traditional therapy can, last for years. It is a focused, present-oriented therapy that makes use of some of the most recent research in the areas of neurophysiology. Its other advantage over some other forms of therapy is that it does not rely on pills to effect rapid psychological change. That means that when used appropriately, there are no long-lasting debilitating side effects and relapses are not expected, as can often occur when medication is stopped.

Because EMDR is so powerful, it should never be used except with a licensed, EMDR-trained therapist. One important reason for this book is to discourage the small cottage industry of "eye-movement therapies" that has sprung up owing to the media attention: Therapies that do not use the principles, protocols, and procedures we use in EMDR. Often the therapists have not been trained in the methodology, and in fact, they may not even be licensed clinicians. It is important that prospective clients make sure that they are being treated responsibly with EMDR and that they know what to expect from the therapy. For example, it is vital for people to understand that EMDR may be surprisingly rapid but that it is not simple.

One of my goals in writing this book is to describe EMDR in action so that readers can see for themselves how—and how well—it works when used properly. The stories contained herein are of men, women, and children who have used EMDR to recover from, among other things, the horrors of war, medical trauma, abandonment, panic and phobias, the death of a child, rape, and drug addiction. All of them have given permission for their stories to be told so that others can be helped. All of the cases in this book are true; none is a composite. The therapists you will read about have been trained in EMDR and are using it properly. By reading these stories, you will get enough of an understanding to help you pick the right person to work with and to make sure your own therapy stays on track. There is information at the back of this book about how to find an EMDR-trained therapist.[7]

⌘

That EMDR appears to so powerfully and successfully combine the physiological with the psychological has made many people stop and examine their views about health, healing, and the interaction of the body and the mind. For me, the need to do this came in 1979, when I was diagnosed with cancer.

Having cancer—especially in the late 1970s, when it was more frequently fatal—changes one's life on many different levels. After surgery and radiation, the doctors told me, "Well, it appears to be gone, but some patients get it back. We don't know who and we don't know how. Good luck." I was shocked. Here I was, living in one of the most technologically advanced cultures on earth, but we were still in the Dark Ages about our own bodies. I knew there must be something I could do to improve my odds.

I started reading everything I could find about illness and discovered that people were beginning to talk about stress as the instigator of or a contributor to disease, especially cancer. But other than Norman Cousins's prescription for laughter,[8] *Getting Well Again* by Simonton and Creighton,[9] and some unpublished treatises on nutrition, nothing I read offered any practical advice on what a person could do. I felt there had to be helpful information out there. Why wasn't it available? When I learned that the type of colitis my younger sister had died from at age nine was now considered stress-related, my shock turned to determination. I dedicated myself to finding whatever information was available on body-mind interaction and healing and getting it out to the public, where it belonged.

This was the start of my nearly twenty-year journey to what has now become known as EMDR therapy. In the beginning, I was not focused on finding an answer in psychology. I was looking for anything, from any discipline that could help people heal from serious illness. This included ways to use the mind or the body to cope with stress so we wouldn't damage our health in the first place. My search took me cross-country and into dozens of workshops, seminars, and training programs. As the journey unfolded, it brought me into contact with myriad forms of psychotherapy. Ultimately, I ended up with a doctorate in clinical psychology, working as a Senior Research Fellow at the Mental Research Institute in Palo Alto, California, one of the birthplaces of family therapy and brief therapy. But that came later.

The seed of EMDR sprouted one sunny afternoon in 1987, when I took a break to ramble around a small lake. It was spring. Ducks were paddling by, and bright blankets full of mothers and babies were laid out on wide green lawns. As I walked along, an odd thing happened. I had been thinking about something disturbing; I don't even remember what it was, just one of those nagging negative thoughts that the mind keeps chewing over (without digesting) until we forcibly stop it. The odd thing was that my nagging thought had disappeared. On its own. When I brought it back to mind, I found that its negative emotional charge was gone. I must confess that one of my college heroes was Mr. Spock on *Star Trek*. Like him, I had always considered emotions a challenge, but I had never noticed such a quick shift of thoughts and feelings before. Because I had been using myself as a laboratory for mind-body investigation for eight years, this change definitely captured my interest.

I started to pay careful attention as I walked along. I noticed that when a disturbing thought entered my mind, my eyes spontaneously started moving back and forth. They were making rapid repetitive movements on a diagonal from lower left to upper right. At the same time, I noticed that my disturbing thought had shifted from consciousness, and when I brought it back to mind, it no longer bothered me as much. I was intrigued. I tried doing it deliberately. I thought about something else that was causing me mild anxiety, and this time I did the rapid eye movements intentionally. That thought went away, too. And when I brought it back, its negative emotional charge was gone.

In the days that followed, the process continued to work for me, so I asked others to try it: friends, acquaintances, interested students. Although these people were not in need of psychotherapy, they could each identify some disturbing thought to experiment on. The process seemed to work for them, too, although most needed help in getting their eyes to move consistently. I started holding my index finger in a casual upward-pointing gesture and asked them to follow its quick diagonal movement while thinking about whatever was making them anxious.

At that point, although I joked about "flicking" the anxiety out, I was thinking of this technique as a form of desensitization, a procedure used in behavioral therapy to reduce a person's anxiety about something specific. As I tried my new method with more and more people, I noticed that although the eye movements did indeed cause a desensitization effect, most people did not get rid of their anxiety completely. The diagonal eye movements alone were not enough to ensure success. I learned that I had to ask the person to change the focus of his attention (to a different aspect of the thing he was anxious about) or lead his eyes in a different way, perhaps horizontally, or faster, or slower. The more I experimented, the more I found the need to come up with alternatives to jump-start the positive effect when it became stalled.

In other words, as I worked with the first seventy people, I discovered that I had to develop a procedure around the effect of the eye movements to resolve the anxiety consistently. Over time, the method came to include important elements of all the major schools of psychotherapy: psychodynamic (based on Freud's work), behavioral, cognitive, systems, and body-oriented. Every person I worked with gave me new insight into the clinical application and helped me refine it further. I simply kept altering the procedures through trial and error to improve the results. Because the changes in a person's images, thoughts, and feelings came about—or didn't—so rapidly (usually within one session), it was relatively straightforward to fine-tune it into a comprehensive approach.

For instance, in its simplest form, the client and I would identify something that was mildly disturbing, such as a fight with a neighbor. I would ask the person to concentrate on the fight, have her think of the most upsetting part of it, then start leading the eye movements. I would hold two fingers about twelve inches from the person's face, then move my hand rhythmically back and forth across her field of vision. Without moving her head, the person would track this movement with her eyes. This would continue without stopping for a certain amount of time (say, one minute), which I called a *set*; then we would stop and talk about what was happening. If her anxiety about the fight hadn't changed much, I would ask the person to concentrate on a different aspect of it, such as what the person said, and we would do another set. When it worked, the result was a rapid change from set to set. I quickly learned what worked best and what not to do.

With gratifying regularity, people reported that their thoughts had changed for the better or their disturbing mental images had disappeared completely, along with the anxiety that had accompanied them. It was often an intensely emotional experience, and I noticed repeatedly how important it was to do the appropriate preparation with a person and use it with good clinical skills in a proper setting. Unexpected memories frequently came up as the procedures quickly got people to look at the root of the problem, not just its leaves and branches.

For example, during that time one woman asked me to use the procedures to treat her phobia about leaving the country. She started with a mental image of herself arriving at the airport of a foreign country and wandering around, feeling desolate and abandoned. As we did the procedures, a new mental image came to mind: herself at age six, waving goodbye to her parents at a train station. The memory was quite upsetting to her. If I had worked with her earlier, before I had fine-tuned the procedures, she might have ended up in more distress than she had started with. But using some of the variations I had refined, we kept at it until her anxiety about this memory was completely defused and her thoughts about traveling abroad had shifted from "I can't do it" to "I can travel comfortably." When I followed up with this woman a month later, she was busy planning a trip to Greece.

More traditional psychotherapies certainly could have helped this woman. However, psychoanalysis might have taken years to unearth that pivotal childhood memory with no effect on her behavior; cognitive therapy might have changed her negative belief about herself but had no effect on her emotions; and behavioral therapy might have lessened her level of emotional distress but not enhanced her self-respect. The rapid change in her emotions (no more anxiety) and her behavior (traveling abroad), along with the recognition of the reasons for her distress and a radical change in how she viewed herself and her abilities, are results typical of EMDR.

The stories in this book will show you that even the most tenacious emotional problems can change. In these pages, you may see yourself, a neighbor, a family member, or a friend. We all feel fear, pain, despair, guilt, or unrelenting anger when certain experiences and pressures converge. The message here is that we do not need to be trapped by these feelings.

Most people come into therapy because they know something is wrong. There is an "I" that feels locked up and knows that there is a better way.

But over the years I have come to see clearly that this "I" is intrinsically healthy. EMDR therapy can remove the block that is preventing the natural movement toward health. It can release you into the present you always wanted for yourself, a present where you can feel free and in control. EMDR has taken thousands of people further than they've dreamed possible. Even some Olympic athletes have used it—to achieve peak performance.

There are so many people who have tried psychotherapy and are still suffering, and so many others who never have bothered to try because they feel their problems are hopeless. Now there is a reason to hope. EMDR is not a panacea, but it may be able to unlock your innate, physiological healing system and allow you to change at a rate and in a way you never thought possible.

This book makes the inside stories of EMDR therapy available to everyone. Ironically, although my bout with cancer led me to search for mind-body methods of healing to bring to the general public, I ended up creating one. This book is a culmination of that journey.

2

Laying the Foundation

If you have built castles in the air, your work need not be lost;
that is where they should be. Now put the foundations under them.

—HENRY DAVID THOREAU

WHAT DO WE MEAN by the word *trauma*? Is it traumatic to be in a near-fatal car accident? To see a person robbed and beaten? To be locked out of your car in a storm? To find out you need surgery? When psychotherapists talk about trauma, they are generally referring to events that would be upsetting to nearly everyone and that involve a reaction of fear, helplessness, or terror. Unfortunately, many people (and some psychotherapists!) mistakenly believe that events are somehow unimportant if they do not meet this standard. But many events can be disturbing because of their personal significance, such as overhearing a passing remark that you are unattractive, getting a failing grade in school, or having a pet run away. Although in some types of conventional psychotherapy, there may be a struggle to distinguish between the two types of trauma, this separation is irrelevant in EMDR. Because EMDR therapy focuses on personal experience, it downplays what the therapist thinks of the event and, instead, deals directly with how the experience has affected the client.

Experiences of all sorts play an important role in our inner life. But for now, let's clarify and distinguish what we can call big "T" trauma—which the psychology community recognizes as a cause of posttraumatic stress disorder (PTSD)—and what in EMDR we refer to as small "t" trauma. Big "T" trauma includes events that a person perceives as life-threatening: combat; crimes such as rape, kidnapping, and assault; and natural disasters such as earthquakes, tornadoes, fires, and floods. These events are so stressful they can overwhelm our ordinary capacity to cope.[1] They result in intense fear, extreme feelings of helplessness, and a crushing loss of control.

The symptoms of PTSD span two classes of simultaneous, and diametrically opposed, behaviors. In one type, the traumatized person cannot get away from his trauma: He is forced to relive the original event through intrusive symptoms such as flashbacks, nightmares, panic attacks, and obsessive thoughts. In the other, he can't get near it: He is compelled to insulate himself from reminders of the trauma through avoidance symptoms such as social isolation, emotional numbing, and substance abuse. Trauma victims also have physiological reactions, such as insomnia, hypervigilance, and the tendency to be easily startled by any reminder of the event, such as a particular sound or touch.

Small "t" trauma, on the other hand, occurs in the innocuous but upsetting adverse experiences that daily life sends our way. It can result in some of the same feelings as big "T" trauma and have far-reaching consequences. This fact was brought home to me in the early days of EMDR by Paul, a man who had been diagnosed with AIDS and wanted to pursue some alternative methods of healing but found his efforts sabotaged by his belief, "I can't go after and get what I want." Paul had no memory to explain why he felt that way, but he remembered always believing it and felt it had held him back his whole life. He came in for help when he recognized this belief might prevent him from living his last days to the fullest.

Because Paul had no memory of where this negative belief came from, I asked him to hold the belief in mind during the procedure. After one set of eye movements, he said he felt a strange sensation running down his arm. I asked him to pay attention both to the belief and to the physical sensation. After a few more sets, Paul said that it was as if a veil was peeled back and he saw an image of himself at age four. He was playing with a ball at the top of the stairs. His mother called out to him not to go down the stairs. But the ball fell, and Paul chased after it, then tripped and fell on his arm. His mother came running after him and, grabbing him by the arm, started spanking him for—in Paul's mind—going after what he wanted. The processing experience liberated Paul, and as he explored alternatives for healing, he also expanded in his personal and professional relationships. Before he died, he called to tell me that he had embraced life with more freedom in his final years than he had in all the time previously. He had stopped holding back.

Clearly, Paul's mother was not guilty of abuse. This is the type of experience that children have hundreds of times while growing up. But these types of experiences, just like big "T" trauma, can take up residence in the mind and govern our behavior for decades. Although less dramatic experiences like these do not meet the clinical definition of trauma, they certainly meet the dictionary definition: "an emotional shock that creates substantial and lasting psychological damage; something that severely jars the mind or emotions."

This undercurrent was exactly what I had seen consistently in the seventy volunteers with whom I first used EMDR. Many had started with a current negative feeling and associated their way back to its historical source. So I knew EMDR worked with small "t" trauma. Would it work with big "T" trauma? This was the question that spurred me to do a formal, randomized controlled study of EMDR. I selected as the participants people who were the predominant victims of PTSD in today's world: combat veterans and rape or molestation survivors. Before starting the study, however, I needed to do a test run of EMDR with someone suffering from a major traumatic event to make sure it could work. In search of a willing subject, I went to a number of counselors looking for volunteers. One of them was willing to try it himself.

Doug was a well-adjusted and successful forty-three-year-old who said he had one particular memory from his days as an infantryman in Vietnam that still really distressed him. The memory was this: One day Doug and another soldier were unloading litter after litter of American corpses from a helicopter flown in from the front lines. As the men were laying out the dead and mutilated bodies side by side on the ground, Doug noticed that rigor mortis had set in for the one they were holding. Using the black humor that so often arises in desperate situations, he joked, "We can use this one as a coffee table." The other soldier turned to Doug and said, "Hey, that's his son sitting over there." As he spoke, Doug saw that one of the wounded men was looking at him in horror, his face wracked with pain. Suddenly, Doug felt that for all his bravado, he was the most insensitive, unfeeling person on the planet. It was a watershed experience that shook him to the core, and it continued to haunt him for the next twenty years. No matter how many clients Doug helped as a counselor, whenever that memory came up (and it came up often), he was flooded with feelings that he said made him near catatonic with shame and grief.

In the course of the procedure, I asked Doug to hold the scene in mind and follow my finger with his eyes. As Doug's eyes tracked the rapid sweeps of my hand, the anguish on his face intensified, then relaxed. At the end of the second set of eye movements, he said, "I can still see the scene, but when the guy talks, there's no sound coming out of his mouth." We continued the sets. Then Doug reported that the scene had shrunk to the size of "a paint chip," and somehow it looked as if it was underwater, "blurry and silent." Then he added, almost as if to himself, "The war is over. I can tell everybody to go home now."

This type of metamorphosis of the traumatic scene—the softening of the painful images and sensory details—became something I would hear about frequently from clients using EMDR. Later, when I asked Doug to think of Vietnam so I could see whether the upsetting scene would reappear, what came to his mind was a memory of the first time he had flown over the country. With eyes closed and a slight smile, he told me, "It looked like a garden paradise." This was the first time in twenty years that Doug had recalled anything but the horrors of Vietnam.

In November 1987, I set to work designing a controlled study, in which one group of randomly selected trauma subjects would receive EMDR treatment, and the other, the control group, would receive a treatment not expected to have as significant an effect. I decided to talk to the members of the control group as if we were doing traditional "talk" therapy. These people would concentrate on the traumatic event and tell me about it in detail. Then I would interrupt them with the same questions (such as "How are you feeling now?") asked the same number of times as in the EMDR sets of eye movements. Unfortunately, talk therapy has been shown to have about as much success in treating PTSD as a sugar pill, so using it as a comparison in a controlled study seemed an appropriate way to test whether EMDR could systematically, consistently, and quickly relieve the subjects' specific symptoms.

Measurement is at the heart of all scientific research. If you aren't measuring the right thing or if you're using the wrong yardstick, your results will be useless. To see whether EMDR relieved the symptoms of PTSD, I knew I would have to measure three aspects of the disorder. The first was how disturbing the traumatic memory felt to the subject before, during, and immediately after EMDR treatment, with follow-ups one month and three months later. Without long-term positive results, no treatment for trauma can be considered successful. Any positive results immediately after treatment could simply be a placebo effect, in which the client's belief in the effectiveness of the treatment produces mild and temporary relief from his symptoms.

Deciding to measure something as intangible as a person's disturbing feelings is one thing; figuring out how to do it is another, and it is something researchers argue about. For my part, I decided to use a scale called *Subjective Units of Disturbance* (SUD), a widely accepted tool developed in the late 1960s by Joseph Wolpe, a psychiatrist and renowned figure in behavioral therapy.[2] To use the SUD, the subject thinks of a memory and rates how disturbing it feels on a scale from 0 to 10, in which 0 is neutral, or no disturbance, and 10 is the greatest disturbance imaginable. For example, in my study, I might ask a combat veteran to remember a time he was ambushed by a Viet Cong soldier. Even though the incident happened twenty years ago, it could still be upsetting, and the subject might rate it at 8, 9, or 10. After EMDR treatment, the subject's SUD level should go down to 0 or 1, meaning that he could bring the ambush to mind and it no longer upset him.[3]

The second element I needed to measure in my study was whether the negative "lessons" my subjects had learned about themselves from their trauma still held sway over them. My reading of the psychiatric literature showed that negative self-beliefs were a big problem for PTSD victims. Rape victims, for example, often had thoughts like "I'm worthless," "I should have done something," or "I'm damaged goods." If EMDR worked, I postulated, that negative lesson would change to a positive one, such as "I'm fine," "I did the best I could," or "I'm a good person." It was the strength of this positive lesson that I chose to measure.

The scale I developed, and continue to use today, called for my subjects to rate how true their positive belief felt to them on a scale from 1 to 7, in which 1 means completely false and 7 means completely true. I also asked them to give me their gut-level response rather than tell me the way they thought they should feel. I called this measurement the *Validity of Cognition* (VOC) Scale. In general, people start EMDR treatment with a VOC of 4 or less. After doing EMDR, clients should report an increase in how true their positive cognition (belief) feels; unless the VOC is at 6 or 7, the disturbing memory is not fully resolved.

We all learn lessons from our past experiences. The question is, did we learn the right lessons? For instance, almost everyone has been humiliated sometime in grade school. Did we learn that we were inept and useless, or did we learn that we were spunky and tenacious? If we are stuck in the past, negative self-beliefs rule our life in the present and continue to cause us incalculable harm. The VOC Scale, which rates the person's preferred, positive belief, tells how well the right, or healthy, lessons have been learned, both before and after treatment.

The third and final measurement I decided to take in my study was the frequency with which the person's posttraumatic symptoms occurred, such as the number of nightmares or intrusive thoughts the person had per week. As I did with the SUD and VOC ratings, I recorded this information before EMDR treatment and at the one-month and three-month follow-up sessions. To prevent inaccurate reporting by the subjects—in other words, to make sure they didn't tell me what they thought I wanted to hear—I sought confirmation of any changes by talking with the subject's therapist, spouse, or other family members.

My twenty-two subjects ranged in age from eleven to fifty-three, with the youngest being a sixth-grader who was still terrified of her molester, even though she knew he was in prison. Their occupations were varied: There were blue- and white-collar workers, artists, therapists, and an unemployed Vietnam War veteran living in the woods. The most recent trauma any of these people had suffered had occurred one year earlier; the most distant, forty-seven years previously. The amount of psychotherapy they had had for their traumas ranged from very little (two months) to a very nearly unconscionable amount (twenty-five years); the average time was six years. The subjects' symptoms included flashbacks (up to six a week), intrusive thoughts (averaging six a week, but one subject reported as many as six a day), sleep disturbances (four times a week on average), and intimacy problems.

When the results were in, they were invigorating. Almost without exception, those treated with EMDR successfully resolved their traumatic memory in one session; the thought of it no longer disturbed them. In addition, they made huge leaps in the way they felt about themselves. My subjects shed their deep-rooted denial, fear, guilt, shame, and anger literally before my eyes and replaced these emotions with self-esteem, confidence, forgiveness, and acceptance. Measured by the frequent SUD ratings I took and the subjects' comments, the changes took place so rapidly, I could *see* them. It was like watching free association at turbo speed.

Of course there were glitches, but even these turned out to be useful because they told me more about how EMDR worked. For example, an eleven-year-old girl who had been molested over a long period of time had been having frequent flashbacks, especially during school hours, when she said she would see her teacher's face "turn into someone who would hurt me." The same thing would happen to the faces of people she passed on the street. She would freeze, seeing "some weird guy who wants to kidnap a kid." She was too frightened, however, to conjure up the face of the man who had molested her to focus on during the treatment. I asked her to picture the man's shirt and pants the way they had been at his trial and just imagine or pretend to see his face. In this way I was able to get around her fear, and the treatment worked. This case taught me that it was not necessary for the client to have an exact image of the traumatic event to achieve positive results with EMDR.

One combat veteran, Tony, worked on the memory of his wife having him committed to a mental institution after he returned from Vietnam. His negative cognition was "I'm not in control." He started with an SUD level of distress of 8 (out of a possible 10) and worked through the memory in successive sets of eye movements until he reached an SUD of 0, meaning he no longer felt any distress when he thought of the event.

This result was excellent, of course, but Tony still did not believe in his positive cognition, "I can be comfortably in control." When I asked him what prevented the statement from being a 7 on the VOC Scale (completely true), he replied, "I'm not worthy to be comfortably in control." When I asked him where this new negative belief came from, he told me about a failed sexual experience he had with someone he cared deeply about. We repeated the procedure on this new memory, which in turn led to another memory of having failed to get a batch of plasma back to his medical unit in Vietnam in time to save two men. Using the procedure on that memory got Tony in touch with the problems he had with authority, which stemmed from never being able to please his father. After we finished using EMDR on this feeling of being "a failure," Tony was able to go back to the first memory and reach a VOC of 7 on the statement, "I can be comfortably in control."

Tony's experience proved fairly typical. Many subjects reported that their picture of the initial trauma had switched to a different upsetting event. It became clear that a number of factors and intertwined events could underlie the obvious problem. My session with Tony lasted ninety minutes, the longest of any during the study. Most of the sessions lasted less than fifty minutes. Nothing in the literature on treating posttraumatic stress (which uniformly described it as long-lasting and difficult to cure) could have prepared me for the swiftness or the magnitude of the healing I saw taking place. Not only was it touching to watch these changes, it was like looking through a window into the workings of the mind.

A transcript from part of an EMDR session best illustrates this process. Jonas was a Vietnam War veteran whom I had already treated for a number of combat-related traumatic experiences. The problem he wanted to focus on in this session was his relationship with an incompetent coworker. Although incompetence in a coworker is bound to be annoying to anyone, Jonas reacted with so much anger and anxiety it became impossible for him to work.

During the part of the session that follows, I ask Jonas to visualize the target (in this case, the incompetent coworker's face) and to hold it in mind while he gets in touch with the distressing feelings he has about the man. At this point, we begin the eye movements. Note that with each set of eye movements, new information emerges, and the client's perspective evolves to a healthier state. At the end of each set, I ask Jonas, "What do you get now?" He replies by telling me his dominant thought, feeling, or mental image, which gives me a reading on the new information. You will also see how I use the 0–10 SUD Scale to help Jonas identify the intensity of his distressing feelings.

In later chapters, I present EMDR sessions in detail, but at its simplest, a session works like this:

FS: Let's start with seeing this guy you consider to be incompetent at work. When you think of him, what words describe the negative belief you have about yourself?

JONAS: I'm helpless.

FS: What would you rather believe?

JONAS: I am in control.

FS: How true do those words feel, from 1 (completely false) to 7 (completely true)?

JONAS: 3.5

FS: When you hold the words "I'm helpless" and the picture of him together in your mind, what emotion do you feel?

JONAS: Anxiety, anger.

FS: From 0 to 10, where 0 is neutral and 10 is the worst feeling you can think of, how does it feel, now?

JONAS: 7.

FS: Where do you feel it in your body?

JONAS: In my stomach.

FS: Just think the words "I'm helpless," look at him and see his face, and feel how incompetent he is. Concentrate on the feeling and follow my fingers with your eyes.

At this point we start a set of eye movements. During the set, Jonas says nothing, but I can see from his face that he is beginning to work through the situation with his coworker.

FS: Good. Blank it out and take a deep breath. What do you get now?

JONAS: I don't know. I guess it feels a little bit better. Before coming in today I worked through some of the things, and at least on an intellectual level I realized . . . well, it's work, and you know I'm going to be late on the schedule and people are going to be upset at it, but that's always going to be true. I mean in the computer business someone is always late. So I started making some connections with that.

FS: Right. When you bring up his face now and get into the sense of his incompetence, from 0 to 10, where is it?

JONAS: Probably a 5.

FS: Hold that. [We start another set of eye movements.] Good.

Next, Jonas follows a chain of association around what he calls "acceptance."

JONAS: One thing that comes up is part of the reason it's frustrating is that because of my boss's situation, he can't evaluate the other guy's ability. I guess it feels a little better in that other people can. I mean there are other people that see it and are frustrated by it. But I guess it's like I need everybody to realize what's going on. And since my boss can't recognize it, and agree to it, I guess it gets back to me needing to be competent and having other people feel I'm competent.

FS: Think of all of that. [Another set of eye movements.] Good.

JONAS: Slowly but surely, I'm starting to have periods where I realize I don't need other people's acceptance. I have a lot of people's acceptance, and those are probably the ones that are important. It's difficult right now 'cause my boss is one of them that I probably don't have, but that's his problem, not mine. [Jonas laughs.]

Notice that Jonas is coming to his own realizations rapidly, without my directing him.

FS: Okay. Think of that. [Another set.] Good.

JONAS: I guess that I've got enough of his acceptance. I've got as much as I need. I mean he needs me really badly right now, so certainly my job isn't in danger. So I've probably got as much as I need.

FS: Okay. Think of that. [Another set.] Good.

JONAS: Ah . . . the thing that occurs to me is that probably in the next couple of months the pressure's going to let up on the project, and by that time he'll be able to see.

FS: Okay. Hold that one. [Another set.] Good.

JONAS: About the same.

At this point I bring Jonas back to the original target.

FS: Okay. Now what happens when you go back to the guy's face that you feel is incompetent? What do you get now?

JONAS: It bothers me. I know I'm going to be frustrated by him in the future, but I think I'm going to be less likely to lose sight of what's going on.

Note that Jonas's level of anxiety has dropped but is still bothersome. During the next set, the eye movements stimulate other memories associated with "incompetence." Here we discover the impact of Jonas's Vietnam combat experience: In Vietnam, if someone was incompetent, it meant people might die.

FS: Just see him again and feel the incompetence. [Another set.] Good.

JONAS: The thing that came to mind is in this case the stakes aren't high. I mean, assuming I'm right and he is incompetent in this area and he gets in and screws everything up. So what? [He laughs.] I mean we can turn it around.

FS: Really. Hold that one. [Another set.] Good.

JONAS: Um, it's just nice to know, it's nice to think about the stakes and realize that it's just a bunch of computers and obviously the issue is that people aren't dying. That you can't reverse.

FS: So if you bring up this picture again, what do you get?

JONAS: Um, it's sort of comical!

FS: Yes.

JONAS: I mean he's a very bright guy. He's a very capable guy. It's just that when I look at the kinds of errors he makes, they're comical and they're the same ones we all made when we first tried this stuff out. You know you found a problem, you solved a little bitty piece of the problem. There's this giant problem out there but you went, "Yeah! Great, I solved it," 'cause it was the only thing you could find. [Jonas laughs.] And so you're so excited you found it, you pretended that was the whole thing. And other people are seeing it as well, and they've been handling it better than I have. I think they've always been at the chuckling level. You know, "Well, what do you want him to do at the level he's at?" They just handle it better, but they all see it as well, and I think it's sort of cute that he thinks he can solve the world.

FS: Okay. Think of that. [Another set.] Good.

JONAS: About the same.

FS: Great.

JONAS: Yeah, it feels good. It's nice to not be lost in the frustration and anger, and that's where I was last week. I was losing it, and I felt like there was nothing I could do about it. I tried to sort of detach myself, but I couldn't.

This part of the session, including the nine short sets of eye movements, took only five minutes, yet it had a significant impact. Jonas not only changed the way he felt and thought about his coworker; he changed his behavior toward him, too. When I saw Jonas five years later and asked him about it, he was matter-of-fact. "It was good to realize it wasn't Vietnam," he told me.

The problem many trauma victims face is that the upsetting experience from their past (including the feelings, beliefs, physical sensations, and behaviors) is "stuck" in their nervous system. Like a puppet master, this old experience governs the person's reactions to present-day situations. In Jonas's case, the intensity of his anger at his coworker came from the experiences he had had in Vietnam. EMDR sessions such as this one showed me clearly that earlier traumatic experiences somehow were linked to the present, an observation that helped me refine the EMDR protocols we will explore in later chapters.

తా

In the winter and spring of 1988, I conducted one-month and three-month follow-up sessions with each of the twenty-two subjects I had treated with EMDR. It was at this critical juncture that I would see whether the positive effects of EMDR had lasted and whether my subjects would report any changes in their symptoms.

The first subject I interviewed was a Vietnam War veteran who had endured twenty-one years of flashbacks and recurrent nightmares. He now reported only one nightmare since his treatment. Although the dream was about a knife-wielding intruder creeping into his bunker, he told me it had "no power to it." He also told me he had recognized his own face on the assailant and realized that "the person cutting my throat was me." He never had the dream again.

Another subject, a therapist who was abused as a child, had a lifelong history of one or two violent dreams a week; we had targeted one of the dreams during the treatment session. He told me that on the night following EMDR, he had one of his usual nightmares in which he was being chased by samurai enemies trying to kill him. This time, however, he suddenly stopped running, turned to his pursuers without fear, and "ritually bowed" to them. They returned his bow, and then they all "joined forces" and went off together. The therapist's wife confirmed that he no longer thrashed around at night and was more relaxed in general. I learned through experiences like this what a powerful target dream imagery can be. Since then, whenever a client reports a disturbing recurrent nightmare, it becomes one of the first things we address.

Tony, the Vietnam veteran who had three different traumatic experiences come up during his EMDR session, reported that his daily panic attacks were gone. He'd had only one attack during the first month after treatment. He said he no longer had flashbacks or dove for cover when planes flew overhead and, he added with a grin, he had been able to gain and maintain an erection for the first time in three years.

The mother of the girl who had been molested told me that her daughter no longer woke up screaming in the middle of the night and was doing well at school. (Several years later, I heard that her molester had been released from prison and the girl, now a teenager, had unexpectedly run into him in the grocery store. "Who let you out?" she huffed.) Another subject reported that his daily headaches had ceased.

It was during these follow-up interviews that I learned that EMDR could bring about some sort of generalization effect. One of the subjects had worked on a specific memory of having been molested by her father. During the follow-up, when I asked her to bring the memory to mind, her fear and anxiety were gone, but she felt some anger and indignation toward him. Then I asked her to bring to mind another time he had molested her. Although we had not targeted this specific memory with EMDR, she reported very little fear and anxiety about it; instead, she experienced a similar admixture of anger and indignation. This generalization effect meant that every frightening memory did not have to be targeted separately: The positive effects of EMDR would extend to similar events. It was something I would see again and again with EMDR.

For the most part, these follow-up interviews showed spectacular results. The subjects' anxiety about their trauma had remained low, and their positive sense of self stayed high. Also, the symptoms they cited when they entered the study had been relieved, a fact that I was able to confirm with a therapist or family member in all but four cases. (In those four cases, I was unable to contact an outside person to verify the change.)

There was one notable exception. Marie, a rape victim, showed a sharp increase in her anxiety level: Her SUDs (which had started at 8 out of 10) jumped from a score of 0 immediately after EMDR to 4 at the one-month follow-up. When I asked her to tell me about it, Marie said she had recently heard through friends that the rapist was still in the area, and she was scared that he would rape her again, as he had threatened to. She no longer had intrusive thoughts about him and felt more detached and in control, but she said she considered her current level of anxiety "very realistic" given the situation. This was one of the first indications I had that EMDR would not desensitize a person's negative feelings if they were appropriate to the situation. This is important: There are times when it makes perfect sense—and is completely adaptive—to feel afraid or angry. Marie's remaining level of anxiety about her rapist ensured that she would pay attention to locking her doors and would not walk alone at night.

These kinds of rapid and adaptive responses seemed to mean that in some way EMDR was tapping into the person's physiological system so that innate wisdom and health could spring forth. Not only were the negative emotions defused; something more was going on. My subjects seemed to see their past suffering in the context of their whole lives, recognizing that their painful memory was a small (though perhaps sad) part of the whole. The meaning had changed, for example, from "this happened because I'm a loser" to "I did the best I could. I was just a kid." They were not just at peace with their trauma; they were at peace with themselves.

This healing process came from within. I was a guide, a facilitator, and a witness, but I hadn't caused my subjects to change. I hadn't talked them through their fears or analyzed their dreams. I hadn't repeatedly questioned their persistent, irrational, and negative beliefs. I hadn't suggested the insights they had come up with. In fact, my subjects' insights had followed their own logical (and emotionally healthy) train of thought, moving, for example, from "I was to blame," to "I was very young," through "I did the best I could," and finally to "it wasn't my fault. I am fine as I am."

What was happening was clear: People were healing themselves with the help of EMDR. The results of my study were published in 1989 in both the *Journal of Traumatic Stress* and the *Journal of Behavior Therapy and Experimental Psychiatry*.[4] Now, years later, more than thirty objective, independent, randomized controlled studies of hundreds of subjects have been completed, confirming my original findings.[5]

Why does EMDR work so rapidly? There is no doubt that it is a complex therapy and that many factors contribute to the effect. What exactly do the eye movements do? The truth is, we still don't know for sure. Despite more than thirty randomized controlled studies demonstrating the positive effects of the eye movements (see Appendix B), scientists do not yet know enough about the complexity of brain processes to definitely confirm any theories.

My earliest theory was based on the work of Ivan Pavlov.[6] In 1927 Pavlov conjectured that there was an excitatory-inhibitory balance in the brain that maintained normal functioning. If something caused an imbalance to occur (as when something caused overexcitation), a neural pathology—a kink in the wiring, so to speak—resulted. According to Pavlov, the way to return to normal functioning and cure a "neurosis" was to restore the balance be-tween excitation and inhibition. Although few people speak of neuroses anymore—that is outdated language in the field of psychology—I consid-ered whether Pavlov's theory might apply to EMDR. Perhaps trauma causes an overexcitation to the nervous system, and perhaps the eye movements cause an inhibitory (or relaxation) effect that counterbalances it.

This theory might account for what happens in rapid eye movement (REM) sleep, also. Rapid eye movements occur during dream states, and there is some evidence that dreams are a way of working through life expe-riences.[7] Perhaps when upsetting memories come up in dreams, rapid eye movements bring about a relaxation effect to allow processing of the experi-ences. Going a step further, perhaps the effect is due to what Joseph Wolpe called "reciprocal inhibition," the factor responsible for the anxiety-relieving results of his systematic desensitization treatment.[8] Systematic desensitiza-tion consists of conditioning a client out of his fear (fear of flying, for exam-ple) by teaching him to do deep muscle relaxation first in the presence of a mild version of his object of fear (such as a drawing of an airplane), then progressively moving to more potent versions (imagining going to the air-port), and arriving eventually at a full-strength version (imagining being on a plane). The theory is that deep muscle relaxation inhibits low-level anxiety, and as low levels are treated, the whole hierarchy of fears drops down in in-tensity. After enough treatment is given, imagining being on a plane is also viewed with low anxiety so that it can be desensitized as well.

I theorized at the time that perhaps the eye movements in dreaming re-ciprocally inhibited the distress. If the person's disturbance was mild enough (as in the everyday worries of life), perhaps the eye movements of sleep would offset them. That might be one explanation for the experience of go-ing to sleep upset about something but feeling better about it or understand-ing it more clearly in the morning. If the disturbance is too severe, however, perhaps it offsets the effect of the eye movements. Maybe this was the reason that combat veterans woke up in the middle of nightmares instead of com-pleting them.

There were a lot of "maybes" to my original REM theory, but I contin-ued to develop it. Unfortunately, researchers at the time had decided that the eye movements in sleep merely represented the dreamer scanning the dream environment.[9] It wasn't until 1994 that other studies declared that the amount of REM was connected to the intensity of the negative emotion in the person's dream.[10] Before that, the psychology community did not support my theory and did not like my application of Pavlov's theory.

It is interesting, however, that two teams of psychiatrists (one in Australia and another in England) subsequently came up with similar theories, also based on Pavlov's work, to account for EMDR's success.[11] These authors conjectured that a reflex has developed through evolution that allows mammals to observe danger. The resulting excitation, they say, causes the animal to fight or flee. They suggest that the eye movements in EMDR trigger an associated innate mechanism that inhibits that response. The result is a rapid psychological reorientation that brings about a sense of safety. However, further research will be needed to test these hypotheses.

Another theory, suggested to me in 1987, was offered by a neurobiologist who had been studying memory in rats by applying repetitive low-voltage current to electrodes implanted in their brains.[12] He said that this current caused a change in synaptic potential (the electrical charge in the space between receptors in the brain) that was directly related to memory processing. He thought the eye movements might be doing the same thing. It made sense to me at the time, and it still does. The neuronal bursts of the rapid eye movements (like a low-voltage current) could be causing an inhibitory effect in the place where the traumatic memory is stored, thereby reversing the neural pathology. It is possible that the same thing occurs in REM sleep. Still other researchers believe that the eye movements tax the limited capacity of working memory, which decreases imagery vividness and emotions (see Appendix B).

In the coming chapters, I explore many of the more recent theories, but they, too, are just that: theories. The definitive issues are still unresolved by research, and it will be years before neurobiological procedures are precise enough to provide those answers. However, the lack of a proven explanation should not stand in the way of people using EMDR therapy. Scientific discoveries are often made and used before they are understood. After all, it took forty years to understand why penicillin works, but not knowing why it worked did not stop physicians from using it or patients from being cured by it during that period.

〜

Even if I cannot offer a conclusive explanation for why EMDR therapy works, I can describe what appears to be happening during EMDR. I have developed a theory I call the Adaptive Information Processing model.[13] Like most models, it is simply a working hypothesis; however, it does seem to correspond to what neurobiologists know about brain physiology. In later chapters, I explore the application of this model to clinical practice and look at some of the research that supports it.

It appears that within each of us there is an information-processing system that is designed to process upsetting events so that we can maintain a state of mental health. When something unpleasant happens, we think about it, talk about it, and dream about it until it doesn't bother us anymore. At this stage, we can say it has arrived at an "adaptive resolution." We have learned whatever was useful about the experience (such as the danger of walking in dark alleys) and stored it in our brain with the appropriate emotion so it can guide us in the future. We have also discarded what is useless, such as the negative emotions, physical sensations, and self-beliefs that stemmed from the event.

When something traumatic happens to us, however, this innate processing system can break down. Our perceptions of the terrible event (what we saw, heard, felt, and so on) may be stuck in our nervous system in the same form as when we experienced them. These unprocessed perceptions can be expressed as the nightmares, flashbacks, and intrusive thoughts of PTSD. In EMDR we ask the person to think of the traumatic event, and then we stimulate the person's information-processing system so that the traumatic experience can be appropriately processed, or "digested." As this "digestion" process takes place, insights arise, the needed associations are made, whatever is useful is learned, and the appropriate emotions take over.

With EMDR, this information-processing system can work quickly. It can progress at the same rate of speed seen in the body after physical trauma. If someone is raped, her body may go into shock, bleed, or shake. But with the appropriate medical care, the body may repair its wounds in days or weeks. Why do we think that the mind should take longer to heal? It is affected by the physiological state of the brain, and the brain, too, is part of the body. One of the things I think EMDR does is to reconnect the stored event with the physical information-processing system of the brain. Then, through the natural healing process, trauma is digested, and the mental wounds can be healed, perhaps as rapidly as those of the body.

Because the success of EMDR is not limited to healing major trauma, this Adaptive Information Processing model can guide therapists in helping people with many other problems. Two of the first questions I ask clients are, "What are you doing that you don't want to do?" and "What are you prevented from doing?" The answers to these questions help the clinician to home in on the causes of present-day despair or "disease." Unless a psychological complaint is caused by purely organic or chemical factors (as with brain damage or some forms of schizophrenia), it is probably based on the person's history. Earlier life experiences, many of which took place in childhood, long before we had any choice, appear clinically to be one of the primary reasons for certain kinds of depression, phobias, anxiety, stress, low self-esteem, relationship difficulties, and addictions. In the following chapters, I demonstrate that many of these issues can be quickly resolved through EMDR.

Although most of the clients discussed in this book have experienced major traumas, the same healing principles apply to all of us. One of my purposes in writing this book is to demystify the why, what, and how of therapy. After reading these stories, you will be able to see why symptoms occur and what happens when they change. Most important, you should be able to see that, regardless of how predictable and understandable symptoms may be, beneath them all is a unique individual who can blossom forth. This book allows us to investigate the universal fabric of the mind as well as to celebrate the triumph of the individual.

3

The Spirit and the Sword:
Combat's Tragic Legacy

We honor our warriors because they are brave and because by seeing
death on the battlefield they come to respect the greatness of life.

—WINNEBAGO ELDER

SOME OF THE most dramatic early successes using EMDR unfolded with
Vietnam War veterans who continued to suffer from PTSD fifteen years after
returning home. When I first walked into a VA outreach center in 1988, I
was shocked to discover how many men were still deeply wounded by the
war: Nearly one out of every three people (men and women) who served
there developed full-blown PTSD. At that time, more than twenty years after
the truce was signed, half of them still had symptoms.[1]

It is important to realize that the symptoms of psychological disorders,
including PTSD, are extensions of behaviors we have all experienced. If you
have a fight with someone who is important to you, for example, you may
find yourself thinking about the fight when you don't want to. A mental image of the scene, your anger, anxiety or fear, or what was said might pop up
while you're at the office or might come to mind because of something you
see on TV. After a while, however, the fight usually stops bothering you and
you don't think of it any longer. In people with PTSD, these intrusive, disturbing thoughts can persist for years. They are not resolved with the simple
passage of time. People with PTSD can wake up screaming from the same
nightmare month after month, even year after year. Imagine having to relive

the moment of a bomb blast or a good friend's death over and over. It's as if the brain is stuck in a state of shock and replays the same scene at unexpected times whether you are awake or asleep. In some instances, the person has full-blown flashbacks in which his feelings are so intense he thinks or feels that he is reliving the event.

For these men and women, the trauma of combat got locked in their nervous systems and was triggered almost daily by loud sounds, recurring dreams, physical pain, and the daily pressures of life. Their heads echoed with bombs exploding overhead, friends blown to bits in front of them, calls for help they couldn't answer, and the faces of people they had killed. These soldiers were still stepping on land mines in a war that the rest of the nation had all but forgotten.

The psychological impact of combat has been known to physicians for a long time. In 1871, Jacob Mendes Da Costa did a study of Civil War veterans who complained of heart pain yet showed no evidence of cardiac disease.[2] He termed their condition *irritable heart*, but he could find no way to treat it successfully. After World War I, this clinical phenomenon was known as soldier's heart or shell shock, the latter term coined to describe the psychological results of concussion caused by artillery shells.

By World War II, psychiatrists had identified the long-term emotional distress seen in war veterans as combat neurosis. For many, the name reflected the Freudian belief that childhood events or physiological predisposition was the real cause of the client's suffering; war had merely brought it to light. Until the 1970s, many mental health experts continued to believe that a normal personality could undergo any amount or type of war stress without a problem. This line of thinking stigmatized any expression of the trauma. If veterans talked of their pain, they were regarded as weak or abnormal. Generations of warriors died with their psychological wounds unrevealed.

Some, however, could not remain silent. Their condition was more commonly known as battle fatigue, and by the end of World War II, thousands of psychologically damaged veterans were inpatients in VA hospitals. Even decades later, World War II and Korean War veterans were coming into the VA hospitals still in pain from remembered trauma. Retirement seems to trigger the same feelings of isolation and lack of control that they experienced in combat, and with those feelings come the haunting mental images of the battlefield.

Although this condition was identified, the position taken by many professionals was to minimize the effects of combat. In 1968, when the Vietnam War was in full swing, combat trauma was considered so rare that the American Psychiatric Association dropped any mention of stress disorders from the newest edition of its official diagnostic manuals.[3] But shortly after that manual was published, record numbers of American soldiers started showing up at veterans centers emotionally shattered from duty in Vietnam. This war seemed to be affecting a much higher percentage of men and women in the service than previous wars had. Part of the reason may have been the younger age of the troops: The majority of U.S. soldiers in Vietnam were only eighteen or nineteen years old. Another contributing factor may have been the chaotic political situation in Vietnam and the lack of clear goals, as compared to the patriotic goals of World War II. In addition, the homecoming given to Vietnam veterans bore no resemblance to the ticker tape parades that welcomed back Americans fighting in previous wars. The boys who fought in Vietnam returned home to a civilian society in which many despised them. Some were literally cursed and spat on by the crowds that rallied with antiwar signs to meet them. These scenes could still reduce some of the veterans to tears as they recounted them to me years later.

It took another twelve years and the 1980 revision of the official psychiatric diagnostic manual before the suffering of Vietnam veterans was formally recognized and labeled as PTSD. Almost a million men and women who served in Vietnam have been diagnosed with PTSD at some point after returning from the war. Of those, half were found to be still suffering from the disorder twenty years later.[4] An additional 11 percent (nearly four hundred thousand) had some symptoms of PTSD, such as intrusive thoughts, nightmares, and flashbacks.

The fact that a psychological condition was both officially recognized and widespread, however, does not mean it was fully understood. Even in the late 1980s, the question of how best to treat PTSD was guaranteed to raise hackles in the world of psychotherapy. The only thing that everyone agreed on was that it was very hard to cure. Few clients walked away from the consulting room or the hospital symptom-free.

Of course, controversy among the different schools of psychology is nothing new. The various types of therapists did what they knew how to do best, even though the rate of cure was disappointingly low. Psychodynamic therapists told traumatized veterans they needed to "talk it out" and so gain mastery over their past. Behavioral therapists told them that talking was a waste of time; all they needed was to be deconditioned out of the old, inappropriate, and automatic combat responses they were having to present-day civilian stimuli. Meanwhile, cognitive therapists were targeting the veterans' negative beliefs about themselves and trying to teach them how to think differently about their trauma. Pharmacotherapists wrote out prescriptions for antianxiety and antidepressant drugs.

None of these approaches completely solved the problem. Thousands of Vietnam veterans had been trying all known forms of therapy for two decades, and for many, no form of therapy had made much of a dent in the suffering. According to some directors of PTSD treatment centers, it got harder every year to see any change.

∽

When I met Eric Smith, he was a clean-cut, soft-spoken, and polite computer programmer about to turn forty. He was also an ex-Vietnam War infantryman now in his twentieth year of a hellish battle with recurring nightmares, severe depression, insomnia, alcohol and drug abuse, obsessive thoughts, and relentless guilt. He later became a symbol for me of the thousands of men and women who were still locked in Vietnam's grip. When I first met him, the suffering of this wonderful man deeply touched my heart.

Eric had been nineteen, one year out of high school and living at home in Santa Barbara, California, on the morning he stepped out of his uneventful life and into a maelstrom that would take him halfway around the world. President Lyndon B. Johnson had agreed to Commanding General William Westmoreland's request to increase U.S. troop levels in Vietnam to 542,000 by the end of the year. Escalation of the Vietnam conflict had begun in earnest. In June of 1967, Eric was called on to be part of that escalation.

Eric did not panic when he received his draft notice; his family doctor had assured him that his broken eardrum and his ulcer would earn him 4-F status. To his surprise, Eric not only passed the physical examination but found himself a few hours later on a plane headed to boot camp in Fort Bliss, Texas. He had no change of clothes, no toothbrush, no razor. He hadn't even had time to call his mother and tell her he wouldn't be home for dinner.

Seven months later, in January of 1968, Private First Class Eric Smith of the 199th Light Infantry stepped off a troop transport into the steamy climate of Saigon. The infamous Tet offensive was to begin a few weeks later, on January 31. Eric knew nothing about Vietnam and nothing about the war. "I was just a little kid with orders," he told me. "When the Army said, 'You're going to Vietnam,' I just went along with the program. I didn't have a lot of alternatives. When I got there I thought, yes, it's terrible, but I gotta do what I gotta do—put in my time and get out."

Shortly after his arrival, Eric was sent back home on emergency leave. His father, with whom he'd always had a difficult relationship, had been diagnosed with advanced lung cancer. Three weeks later, he died. Three days after that, Eric found himself back in Vietnam. When he stepped off the plane, a sergeant grabbed him and said, "Your old man is dead. Let's get on with Vietnam."

Eric's first big firefight took place about a month after he arrived in the country. His company had pulled back to a riverbed when Eric suddenly realized his buddy Paul was not with them. Eric jumped up and started back for him: Paul was the one man in the platoon who had taken pity on Eric as a scared recruit and had shown him the ropes. Then the lieutenant screamed, "Nobody's going back there! Stay where you are." Later, they found Paul dead. Eric carefully zipped his friend into a body bag, hoisted him over his shoulder, and carried him to the helicopter.

The hell did not end there. One night out on ambush, Eric had to call in an air strike to defend his company from mortar shelling, a strike that might have wiped out a village of women and children. He never got a body count—his company moved out the next day—but he was haunted by the thought of it. Another night, he saw his buddies murder a Viet Cong prisoner by pretending to let him escape so they could level him with M16 fire. Eric was also ordered to select and train a green recruit to replace himself as point man (taking lead in a patrol to watch out for danger) while he went on R and R (rest and relaxation). The boy was killed his first morning out. Finally, while on a three-man patrol in September 1968, Eric was blown eight feet in the air and fifteen feet backward when he stepped on a booby-trapped grenade. Shrapnel tore into the skull of the man walking point and ripped open the chest and belly of the soldier behind him, killing them both. The grenade blew Eric's legs to bloody ribbons. It won him a Purple Heart and put him in a wheelchair. At the time, the Army doctors told him he would never recover full use of his legs.

After six months in a military hospital in Japan, Eric was sent home. He started an intensive two years, which eventually grew to ten, of successful physical therapy to regain the use of his legs. He decided to go to college. He got married. He had two children. He found a decent job working for the computer industry. It wasn't Eric's body that refused to heal; it was his mind, his heart, and his soul.

Eric had recurring nightmares. He began to drink and soon became an alcoholic. He took up skydiving and spent entire weekends on an adrenaline high at the drop zone, reliving the intense fear of combat. A high-risk sport like this had a strong unconscious appeal for Eric because the adrenaline release it produced blocked all other thoughts and feelings. It also gave him an activity into which he could funnel his agitation. Veterans with PTSD are often unknowingly driven to behaviors that mirror their combat experience and worsen their present suffering. They may avoid intimate relationships and distance themselves from their families, or they may have violent outbursts of anger, which sometimes culminate in their beating their wife or children. The pain from Vietnam is locked in their nervous systems, as is the intense anger that allowed them to kill. They often hate how they act, but they can't understand it and they can't control it.

Inside his head, Eric replayed violent scenes from Vietnam: the same five scenes twenty times a day, day after day without rest. He thought he was crazy. He decided he had been a coward in combat, that he'd made all the wrong decisions, that he should have died back there in the jungle. He blamed himself for the deaths he had witnessed. He was sure that he could have prevented them if he'd been a better soldier.

Eric's obsessive thoughts included a harrowing fantasy in which he saw his young daughter and son killed while he stood by, powerless to stop the brutality. He also envisioned being in happy situations, such as meeting the mayor, where he would suddenly break out in violence, horrifying others and humiliating himself. Both of these scenarios replayed themselves over and over in his mind, as if they were stuck in a satanic feedback loop. He used marijuana, LSD, and cocaine to escape his incessant thoughts, but it didn't work. He slept little and was often too depressed to get out of bed in the morning, eat breakfast, and get dressed.

Occasionally, Eric asked his physicians about his problems. They looked at him kindly and said, "War is hell and Vietnam was tough, but you're fine." He learned to stop asking. One day, nine years after being evacuated from combat, Eric was sitting in a bar with some skydiving buddies when someone mentioned Vietnam. Eric turned and walked out of the room, refusing to talk about it.

About a year later, Eric woke up screaming one night when he was hospitalized after a skydiving accident. His pelvis was broken and he had a bolt through one leg; his body was strapped and suspended in the bed exactly as it had been for six long months after his devastating grenade wound. The hospital sent a psychiatrist to talk to Eric. The man listened to Eric's story and then said, "War is hell. You're all right. There's no problem. Just grab your bootstraps and pull a little harder."

Eric stuck it out for several more years. He and his wife separated, then divorced. She got custody of their son and daughter. Eric shut down emotionally more and more; he dropped his friends for acquaintances who only wanted to surf, fly, or skydive with him. He didn't want anyone to get close. He didn't want anyone to see what was going on inside.

～

It is one of the heartbreaking symptoms of veterans with PTSD to avoid any reminder of the trauma, which cuts them off from others, even from their fellow veterans who might be able to help. This means they also get cut off from any positive memories connected with combat, like the companionship and bonding with other soldiers. They may use alcohol or drugs to dull their pain and avoid thinking about Vietnam. They may also restrict what they do and where they go to avoid being triggered. Some veterans can't walk city streets, shop in malls, or go to sports events because the crowds and the chaotic background noise bring up old fears and trigger terrifying flashbacks. In a flashback, the sights, sounds, smells, physical sensations, and emotions from the time of the original event come back so forcefully that the veteran believes he is back in Vietnam. For example, he may hit the ground when he hears a car backfire or a plane overhead. The reaction is reflexive, like a knee-jerk response; there is no control.

Flashbacks and other intrusive symptoms are part of an automatic physiological response to old stimuli; their presence is a hallmark of PTSD. This hair-trigger sensitivity makes the veteran with PTSD susceptible to many stimuli. Even the most benign action, like a friend's gentle hand on the shoulder, can set off an immediate physical response of fear, anxiety, or pain. These symptoms point clearly to a traumatic event locked in the nervous system. Because the event has not been worked through, it continues to spark, causing old images, feelings, and fears to emerge repeatedly.

∽

By 1985, Eric knew he had to see someone about his pain. He went to a local veterans outreach center and started meeting other veterans, hearing their stories, and painfully telling his own. It brought him a lifeline. To his astonishment, he found that he was just like the other Vietnam veterans. They had different lifestyles, but all of them had the same symptoms and the same problems.

After this discovery, Eric began what would turn out to be two full years of weekly one-on-one psychotherapy. Eric's counselor, himself a veteran who had served in Eric's unit, knew the territory of Eric's nightmares. Eric also attended formal group therapy, where he joined other veterans in dissecting their experiences in Vietnam. He began to see that he had been a competent soldier after all, had indeed made good decisions under fire. He also came to accept that all the lives he felt so guilty about taking were taken in self-defense. War was hell, Eric admitted to himself, and he had had no choice about entering its gates. He forgave himself intellectually; however, he could not forgive himself emotionally. Traditional therapy was not enough.

∽

Many of the nearly one million Vietnam veterans suffering the symptoms of PTSD sought treatment, as Eric did, through the Department of Veterans Affairs. The VA had offered these men and women individual therapy, group therapy, and even inpatient treatment (which could include extensive psychodynamic therapy, behavioral therapy, group therapy, pharmacotherapy, and more) for decades. Unfortunately, little controlled research had been done on any of these treatments, and what research there was had shown few positive results. The only clear finding was that PTSD was highly resistant to placebo effects according to drug studies,[5] a fact that suggests there is a physiological aspect to PTSD that must be addressed before victims can heal. Until EMDR came along, none of the controlled research on

PTSD treatments with combat veterans had shown a success rate of more than 30 percent.[6]

Even though group therapy was offered throughout the VA system, there was no controlled research on its effectiveness. Personal testimony from veterans, however, indicated that group sessions brought relief by showing them that they were not alone. However, the talking and the insights that occur in group therapy may have no effect on the symptoms themselves. Knowledge alone is apparently not enough. Although a veteran in group therapy may be able to forgive others for acting as they did in combat, often he is emotionally unable to forgive himself. The irony is that the source of these veterans' suffering generally is their own nobility. The fact that they consider themselves evil and worthless because of what they did in Vietnam is poignant; clearly, if these men really were as terrible as their obsessive thoughts make them think they are, they wouldn't feel bad about anything they had done in the war. They certainly wouldn't still be suffering after all these years. They can see that irony concerning others, but they often cannot see it concerning themselves.

〜

Regardless of how clearly Eric understood that he was not crazy, his feelings about Vietnam did not change. His nightmares, obsessive thoughts, and flashbacks continued. By the winter of 1987, nineteen years after he returned from Vietnam, Eric found himself dangerously close to suicide. He was on a ski trip in Salt Lake City, alone in his sixth-story hotel room. It was eleven o'clock at night. He was writing in his journal, as his counselor had suggested, trying to recall the elusive details surrounding one of his worst, most obsessive memories of combat. As soon as he started writing, the whole event unfolded before him. "Again, I took responsibility for the deaths," he later told me. "I just couldn't handle that. I thought, 'I've taken lives. I don't deserve to live.'"

Eric got up and started toward the window, planning to jump. Then, for some reason he will never know, he stopped, sat down on the floor, and reached for the phone. He dialed 0 and said in tears, "Please give me the police. I'm in trouble."

Eric was taken first to an emergency room and then committed to the psychiatric ward of the local hospital. There he spent three chilling days, watching the other patients and wondering if he, too, was truly insane. When he returned home, he applied for admission to an intensive ninety-day PTSD inpatient program, which accepted veterans considered to have the greatest potential for full recovery. Most of the counselors and several of the doctors at the highly respected program were Vietnam veterans. Their success rate was not high—only 15 percent—but it was higher than that of any other treatment for veterans at the time.

After three months of intensive residential treatment, however, nothing had changed for Eric. He was still severely depressed and still having obsessive thoughts about the same five events in Vietnam. He returned to the veterans outreach center in San Jose, California, sitting in on group therapy and trying to keep a positive outlook. In reality, Eric had lost all hope. Even the antidepressants that had worked earlier offered him no relief.

∽

Research has shown that the amount of trauma that a person has suffered, the number of tours of duty he has served, and the magnitude of the stressors he has experienced all contribute to the severity of PTSD.[7]

In addition, traumatic events from childhood can make a person more vulnerable to PTSD. (In Eric's case, his troubled relationship with his father and his father's sudden death may have put him at extreme risk for PTSD.)

∽

One night in group therapy, the counselor told the men about my work and mentioned that I was looking for Vietnam veterans with obsessive thoughts to try my method. Most of the men refused. They didn't want to work with a woman. They didn't want to work with anyone who wasn't a Vietnam veteran, who hadn't been there. They also didn't want to try another "experimental" treatment; they had felt like pawns and guinea pigs since the war began. Not Eric. He didn't care. As far as he was concerned, I could have been a man, a woman, a veteran, a civilian, or a new life form from an alien star. He had given up expecting much in the way of results, but he was willing to try anything.

Eric and I started working together in March 1988, twenty years after he first set foot on Vietnamese soil. In the first of what would be five ninety-minute EMDR sessions spread over the next nine weeks, I asked Eric to tell me about his obsessive thoughts. In a quiet voice, he began describing the war that was still being fought twenty times a day inside his head.

"I feel like I have a sick attraction to these thoughts, like someone who rushes to the scene of a car crash. I'm caught in a loop. I can't stand it." As Eric spoke, he turned his head and stared out the window, swallowing repeatedly. "I see scenes from Vietnam, situations where I can't decide if I did the right thing or not." As Eric gave me the details, what leaped out was his terrible guilt about two specific combat situations in which he felt responsible for the deaths. I decided we would use EMDR on these two events first and see where it led.

"Let's start with the incident with the prisoner," I said gently. "Tell me more about it."

Eric turned to meet my eyes.

"All right. We had captured a Viet Cong. This was after a full night and day of being pinned down by a battalion of North Vietnamese. They were holding a hilltop, and they were picking us off one by one. More than a hundred of our guys had been killed or wounded. And all this time, it turned out, the Vietnamese had been moving their personnel out. By the time we finally got in there, there was nothing left. Nothing. We'd had so many losses and we never saw who did it. Our guys were really frustrated.

"We took turns standing two-hour watches. I was asleep—it was about five o'clock in the morning—and someone else was on guard. What happened was the guys had decided to intentionally let the prisoner run so they could kill him." Eric's breathing had become shallow and his voice was barely audible. "I woke up right in the middle of it to hear them shouting. Then the guy right next to me shot him." Eric hunched further forward, his torso eloquent with tension. "I was the senior man in the situation. I keep thinking I should have done something to stop them."

When I asked Eric to sum up his feelings about the incident in a single sentence, he paused for a long moment, then whispered, "I should have done something." Eric rated his guilty feelings about the situation at an intensity of 9 on the 0–10 SUD Scale. When I asked him if there was a positive statement that reflected how he would like to feel about the event, he answered immediately, "I wasn't responsible." This was a good start.

"Fine," I said. "Now picture the scene and keep the words 'I should have done something' in mind." I felt this would activate the aspect of the memory that most needed healing. To stimulate the information-processing system, I started moving my hand, allowing Eric's eyes to track my fingers in short, quick diagonals. Between sets of eye movements, I told him to "blank it out and take a deep breath."

After two sets of eye movements, Eric reported that the picture was unchanged but his feelings had dropped to a 6 or 7. "I hear the sound of the M16 going off two feet from my head, and I realize the effect it's having."

I led him through three more sets. Suddenly Eric gave a short surprised laugh. "The sound is quieter, and my feelings are now a 4. It's more like I didn't have anything to do with it. Yes, somebody's dying, but . . . "

More sets. "It's a 2 now. It's just a scene."

"How do the words 'I wasn't responsible' feel now?" I asked.

Eric took a deep breath. His shoulders dropped a fraction of an inch. "I feel better about it; I wasn't responsible. But it still makes me feel sad. I can sit back and see myself in the scenario, but someone's still dying, and I'm afraid the bad feelings will come back."

Two more sets. "Someone's died. I'm not feeling responsible; I'm less threatened. This gives me some confidence in the mechanism [EMDR]," Eric laughed. "Obviously, if you can drive it away, I can."

More sets. He says the feelings are still at a 2.

More sets. No change.

"What would make them a 1?" I asked.

"Nothing," Eric replied. "Someone still died. I was physically present, I could have physically done something, so I have trouble saying I have no responsibility. Simply as a human being, I had a chance to keep someone from dying." A new thought struck him. "I didn't have the mental presence; I was just waking up, and I didn't see enough to realize what they were shooting at. I saw them shooting at one guy, but there could have been five more behind him."

Eric fell silent for several moments, then shook his head. I waited. "There really wasn't much I could do," he burst out. "I never thought about that part before. I did the right thing."

The spontaneous insight Eric was having was identical to those I had witnessed in an earlier study. I could only hope that the insight was evidence of the same type of changes I had seen in the participants of my study. It was clear that new positive beliefs had to be emotionally held: Intellectual understanding was not enough.

As I watched Eric associate his way through the minefield of his Vietnam memories, it seemed to me that the knowledge that he had indeed acted appropriately by not stopping the shooting had always been available in his mind. After all, it was not new information, and it was objectively true. But somehow Eric had not been able to get at it before. It was as if the method opened a physiological block in the information-processing system, enabling Eric to have access to that information and so resolve his trauma. If this were true, then what Eric had tapped into must be that innate self-healing system I had thought I caught a glimpse of during my study.

It made sense. Our bodies are physiologically geared for survival; we adapt to our physical surroundings in order to live. Why would our minds be any different? They, too, must be geared to make adaptive responses that would increase the odds of our survival. Surely, Eric's feeling sad about the guerrilla's death was more adaptive than feeling (mistakenly) that he was responsible for the death. But until Eric's memory of the shooting, which was stored neurologically, had been opened up by dint of EMDR, Eric couldn't access the more adaptive, more appropriate knowledge, which was also stored neurologically.

Forty minutes of our first EMDR session had passed. "Let's work on the village scene," I said. Eric nodded. His mouth was pressed to a thin line. This one was harder.

"Well, I was out on ambush, and the company was being mortared. I moved into an area and found the Viet Cong doing the mortaring. I called in artillery. The problem I have with it is I had no experience calling in artillery and I wasn't very accurate at it and I was calling it in real close to a village. That's what's so hard." Eric's eyes filled with tears and he turned his face away from my steady gaze. "The children . . . " His words caught in his throat. "I don't know if I landed the shells in the village and killed all the people or not."

Eric summed up the negative lesson he learned from the shelling in the statement, "Anything I do is wrong." He said the intensity of his fear was an 8 out of 10 on the SUD Scale: fear of doing what's wrong, fear of dying, and fear of doing something he isn't qualified to do. I started the sets using horizontal eye movements. After the first set, Eric said, "I'm having trouble bringing it up."

Another set. No change. I switched to diagonal movements and we did two more sets. When I checked in with Eric this time, he said, "I'm put in a situation where I've got to call in artillery, and I have no idea how to do it. Those guys gave me instructions over the radio, but . . . it's at night. The first thing they do when they think they've got your position is they'll send an illumination round. It goes off at about five hundred feet, but it sounds like it's going off right next to you. I tell the guy on the radio and he says, 'Okay, a live one's coming.'"

"Keep that picture and the feeling of danger in mind," I said. Three more diagonal sets. Things were moving much more slowly than before. Eric reported the intensity of his fear was now at a 4.

More sets. "There's a change. In the first sets, I was in 'Nam. I can see now where I am [in the office]. I'm safe, I'm okay."

Another set. Eric's fear had dropped to a 2. "I realize where I am, but it still frightens me. I'm completely here emotionally, but it still frightens me."

Two more sets. The fear was now at 1.5.

"What happens when you see the scene and feel it?" I asked.

"This one's harder to say 'it's over.'"

Another set. Now the fear was back up to a 2 or a 3. "For some reason, when I say, 'it's over,' it bothers me," Eric admitted. "It's not over. I'm still scared."

Another set. Eric's fear held steady at a 2. Two more sets.

I asked, "What about the words, 'I did the best I could'?"

"They bother me. I did the best I could, but it wasn't too good. I did the best I could, but I don't know the results." Eric paused, cocked his head to one side, and frowned slightly. "But the mortaring stopped. So I did do something. I don't know how many people were killed. I don't have enough information to know if I did the right thing. I do know I did the best I could." Eric's brow lifted, and his face seemed to open up and relax. "It's very possible I did do the right thing. The mortaring stopped. I must have got it dead center. The people in the mortaring company were killed, and less people died in our company." He dropped his chin and shook his head.

"What is it?"

Eric was now crying. His fear had shifted to sadness. "People died, people I knew." He drew himself up to sit straight. His elbows dug into the arms of his chair; his hands were tightly clasped. He sobbed. He wouldn't reach for a Kleenex. After a while, I started another set. Eric followed my hand with his reddened eyes. It was a much longer set than any we'd done so far.

"And now?" I asked softly.

There was a long silence. "It's less, but . . . I kept coming back to the sadness."

"Okay. The same thing." I led another set.

"It's a 6."

More sets.

"It's a 5."

"And what do you get now?"

"People still died. It's more as if I'm seeing it on the news. This last time I wasn't personally involved. They weren't people I knew."

Another set. The sadness is down to 4.

Another set. A 3.

Another set. A 3. Now a new fear arises. Eric said, "A bad feeling comes from the thought that it still bothers me twenty years later. That scares me. It makes me feel like I'm never going to get away from this feeling."

More sets. A 2.

Another set. A 2.

"What's the feeling now?"

"An inner sadness about the whole situation, that it happened. Sadness at the deaths. Sadness for all the people who died or were wounded. We were just people there doing our job. I think about the families . . . " Eric broke off. His face was streaked with tears, but he held himself upright in his chair.

"What about yourself? How do you fit into the picture?"

"I had the position I had . . . " More tears. Eric stared at the floor. "I have mixed feelings. I'm glad that I'm still alive and could save some guys from getting killed." Still the tears came. "But I'm feeling scared that it was just the luck of the draw who was there that night. It wasn't that bad people died and good people made it. It was just where you were. I wasn't where the mortars were falling, so I got to live that night." Eric dropped his head and sobbed aloud.

"It's all mixed up with whether or not I should have . . . How do you decide who goes out and who doesn't?"

"Did you?" I asked

"Did I what?"

"Did you decide?"

Eric was still crying. "I could have chosen not to call in the artillery, not fired them, but just a different set of people would have died. I didn't have a choice whether or not people died. I am part of the decision of who. I guess it wasn't a hard decision because I knew the men in my company, and I didn't know the VC, the people in the village. In some ways it was an easy decision to make. But just to be part of it was hard to deal with. Like *Sophie's Choice*."

Another set. Eric continued to cry, his fingers tightly interlaced.

"Now it's a little less."

Another set.

"A bit less."

Another set. Eric had stopped crying and was staring out the window to his left.

"How strong is it?" I asked.

"Four," he replied.

"And what's the feeling?"

"It's still sadness people died. The feeling is less strong because I can be a little more rational about it and realize that I had no choice. I didn't make the choice whether or not people died. Given the situation, I really didn't have a choice of choosing which . . . "

Tears caught in Eric's throat. He shook his head again and again. "I knew the people on one side and not the other. I didn't really give it much thought. It seemed obvious at the time. It still seems obvious to me. We were being mortared, we were being attacked. The obvious thing to do is fight back."

Eric paused and nodded. Then he looked at me sheepishly and gave a rueful laugh. "I did the best I could."

"You sure did. And the mortaring stopped."

"Yes, the mortaring stopped. But it's not over. It's not over for me."

I bent toward him. "Is it possible to separate out this sensitivity, the love you have for all life, to hold that and at the same time allow yourself to feel that under impossible circumstances you did the best you could, you did do well, you helped to save the lives of the people around you?"

Eric shook his head. "I have trouble separating them out. This situation was brought about because I was trying to stop death. Still the results were death." A long pause. "For some reason, I hang on to the fact that the result was still death. I have trouble hanging on to the idea that there was probably less death than there would have been."

"Can you bring up the picture of being involved in it and the words 'there was less death'?"

"Yes."

Another set. "It's better. It's hard to hold on to it, but it's better."

Another set. Eric takes a deep breath. "About the same."

Another set. "It's better. The feeling comes from 'I did do a good job; I found them. I did put an end to it.'"

In this memory, the intensity of Eric's fear started at an 8 (on the 0–10 SUD scale), slowly declined to 1.5, then apparently shot back up to a 6. When I checked with him, I learned that the emotion that he was feeling, and that we were measuring, had changed. Fear had shifted to sadness, and the rise in intensity was about the new emotion. As we worked on it, Eric's sadness decreased, too. In moving from fear and guilt ("anything I do is wrong") to sadness ("people died"), Eric was evolving toward a healthy, adaptive resolution of his trauma.

When he returned a week later, Eric reported that he had not had nightmares since our first session. This was the first time in twenty years that he had slept soundly for seven nights in a row.

At the start of our second session, Eric and I went through his list of five disturbing memories from Vietnam and got new SUD ratings on each one. We found that some of the memories we had not yet worked on had already decreased in intensity. This was the same kind of generalization effect I had seen in my study. It made me feel as if I'd had a glimpse into the fabric of the mind. The memories and emotions not only arose associatively during the EMDR session, but somehow resolving the emotional pain of one traumatic incident was having a ripple effect, defusing similar feelings about other incidents.

We then turned our attention to problems at work that Eric was frustrated and worried about. Toward the end of this second session, we shifted our focus to Eric's intense feelings about the bone-shattering grenade wound that had nearly crippled him for life. After several sets of eye movements, Eric began to cry. He couldn't remember what had happened, and he felt too blocked to continue. We could not get any further with it.

At the beginning of our third session, I asked Eric how intense his feelings were now about having had to call in an artillery attack so near a village. He told me they were a 6 out of 10 and that the feelings were anxiety and fear.

"I don't really know what went on that night, who died or who didn't," Eric said. "I can only guess. I still can't recall much of it. If I could have a video of it, maybe I'd find out something I don't want to know."

"What about the statement 'It's my fault'?" I asked. "Does it feel true?"

"Emotionally it does, but intellectually I know I did what I had to do. I made the right decision with the information I had."

We moved from there to targeting the frightening and painful aftermath of Eric's grenade wound: his lying in a helicopter next to dead and dying men, his shock at seeing what was left of his legs, his feeling of impotence and fear at being confined indefinitely to a wheelchair. Even the treatment itself (six months in the hospital and nearly a decade of outpatient physical therapy) had brought Eric despair; it seemed like it would never end.

This time, although he still couldn't remember the explosion, Eric was able to envision the scene of the blast and feel the fear. At one point between sets, Eric told me he had almost decided to have the more severely wounded leg amputated so he could get on with his life. After several more sets, he said, "I'm glad I didn't give up on it." Another set. "Now I know the result." Another set. "It feels better yet." After one more set, Eric felt at peace with it. "Now I can say it's history."

At the end of the third session, I asked Eric for the second time that day about the artillery incident.

"I feel better. I made the right choice. I can see that more clearly. It's a 1 or a 2."

"How true does the statement 'I did the best I could' feel on a [VOC] scale of 1 to 7?"

"About a 4. The problem is that people did die. There is no good choice. There's no good feeling. There's only a feeling of 'I did what I had to do at that time.' But I can't imagine it ever being a good feeling. Death was the name of the game. I did do the best I could do, but what I couldn't do was keep people from dying." He thought a moment.

"It probably could be a 6 or a 7. I really did do the best I could."[8]

In Sessions 4 and 5, Eric and I used EMDR on other memories from the war, then on situations in the present that were triggering his intrusive and obsessive thoughts at work. These were clearly connected, in that Eric's feelings of having no control over the past events in Vietnam made him hypersensitive to parallel experiences in the present. Therefore, when Eric found himself in situations in the present in which he had no control over events, it triggered his old feelings from Vietnam. It's a vicious circle, but often it is physiologically driven by the need to survive. Either we learn to respond to danger, or we die.

⌢

The past affects the present even without our being aware of it. This knowledge is probably Freud's greatest gift to psychology, and thanks to the extremely rapid effects of EMDR, it is something I have witnessed again and again in working with people. The past does not inevitably cause dysfunction, but it teaches us things we incorporate into our present-day emotional reactions and decision making. Often those teachings are about what constitutes danger or what we perceive as danger, and they trigger a fight-or-flight response.

For example, one of the things that caused Eric a great deal of distress in the present was his intense anger when he felt a situation was out of his control. Anyone who has worked in a high-pressure situation, as existed in the company where Eric was employed, knows that a certain amount of anger and frustration is inevitable. But Eric's anger flared up with an intensity he did not understand. When we targeted a recent incident at work, Eric suddenly stopped me and said, "I just realized that this is the anger that let me get through Vietnam. This is what let me kill."

During the fourth session, we worked through the rage and he came to the positive cognition, "I am now in control." It meant that he not only had choices in the present situations but also no longer had to fear his own anger. He said, "I found when I stayed with it, it didn't overwhelm me. I can handle it." Eric told me later that he was experiencing a new sense of ease at work. He felt free to react naturally to his coworkers and found that both his enjoyment and his productivity increased. It was only by processing the remnants of the Vietnam experience that he could take his place firmly in the present.

One month after our fifth and final session, I called Eric to see whether the effects of the EMDR treatment had lasted. Eric said he had not had any nightmares or obsessive thoughts and that his depression had vanished. I checked again a year later: same story. And a year later: still fine.

Now, eight years after his five EMDR sessions, Eric Smith finds himself a thoroughly happy man. Liberated from the ties of the past, he can be fully and joyfully here in the present. He has started his own software consulting business, has remarried, and is raising another daughter. Life is indeed good. "I have found the light at the end of the tunnel, and it's very bright," he says with a smile.

What had EMDR done that Eric's previous therapy had not? Eric had done a lot of therapy with some very talented people before using EMDR. Previous therapy had helped him get off drugs and alcohol and had given him an intellectual understanding that he was not responsible for all those deaths in Vietnam. It just wasn't enough.

Eric still doesn't know whether the women and children in that village were killed. He thinks they probably were. After all, an artillery shell doesn't know who it should kill and who it should spare. In a mission review after the air strike, Eric's superiors had told him he'd done a very good job. But his heart did not, and never would, agree.

"I didn't realize what being in the Army would mean until I got to Vietnam, and then it was too late," Eric told me. "You just don't know the stakes until you see them. I never felt good about being there, being involved in it. I had to do things I didn't believe in. Even my grandmother said, 'It was war, so it's okay.' But it's not okay. War means nothing to me. The military means nothing to me. We were all people."

Eight years after EMDR therapy, when Eric talked about Vietnam, his eyes filled with tears. But they were no longer tears of shame, fear, and guilt. They were tears of compassion for the nineteen-year-old boy who spent twenty years lost in the violent jungles of Vietnam.

4

The Fabric of Treatment: Uncovering the Hidden Depths of Pain

> What lies behind us and what lies before us are tiny matters
> compared to what lies within us.
>
> —RALPH WALDO EMERSON

ENTERING THE WORLD of trauma is like looking into a fractured looking glass: The familiar appears disjointed and disturbing. A strange new world unfolds, revealing astonishing layers of pain carried around by the people you would least suspect to be suffering. I remember how clearly this was brought home to me by one of my first clients, a "proper" sixty-two-year-old woman from a "nice family" who was active in the community. Looking at her gave no clue that she had struggled her whole life with panic and fear as a result of childhood sexual abuse by her father. Her description of wandering aimlessly around her house after the rape, awaiting her mother's arrival and not knowing what to do, was haunting, as was her sadness at all the years she had wasted wrestling fruitlessly with her pain. Another woman, a sixty-eight-year-old retired professional, lived with flashbacks and intrusive images of a rape committed the year before. Poignantly, she explained that even the sight of the attack dog she had purchased brought back the images and the terror. As we processed the memory, she realized that never in her life had she allowed herself to feel at peace and that this could be a chance to embrace that state once and for all.

These stories and others taught me how important it is to look below the surface of appearances. Disturbing events are an inevitable part of life, but even a person's obvious symptoms may give no clue to the far-ranging consequences of the trauma. Both the women I mentioned responded rapidly to EMDR, and the severity of their symptoms decreased dramatically. However, the additional associations that emerged during their processing made it clear that EMDR was needed for much more than merely getting rid of their nightmares and flashbacks. I began to see more clearly how trauma takes place within the context of a life and larger social system and that a comprehensive treatment mode is needed. I decided that the goal for EMDR therapy should be to help the client generate the most profound and the longest lasting effects possible, while feeling safe, balanced, and in control.

With this aim in mind, I formulated what is now known as EMDR therapy's eight-phase approach,[1] which integrates important aspects of many other types of therapy, such as psychodynamic, cognitive, behavioral, and interactional. The eight phases include client history and treatment planning, preparation, assessment, desensitization, installation, body scan, closure, and reevaluation. For the most part, the cases presented in this book employ all eight phases, although some of the phases have been omitted to save space. Trained EMDR clinicians use all of the phases for comprehensive treatment.

In the first phase of EMDR treatment, the therapist takes a thorough history of the client and develops a *treatment plan*. This phase is vital because EMDR can bring up high levels of emotion, and there are some people for whom EMDR is not physically appropriate. For instance, approximately 10 to 15 percent of people treated with EMDR intensely re-experience their trauma. For this reason, although the period of discomfort is relatively brief, people with cardiac or respiratory problems and pregnant women must consult with their physicians before doing EMDR therapy, to determine if their condition is too fragile.[2]

Once EMDR treatment is deemed appropriate for a client, the therapist asks him specific questions about his personal history, characteristics, and patterns of reaction. This phase includes a discussion of the specific problem that has brought him into therapy, his behaviors stemming from that problem, and his symptoms. With this information, the therapist develops a treatment plan that defines the specific targets on which to use EMDR processing. These targets include the event or events from the past that created the problem, the present situations that cause distress, and the key skills or behaviors the client needs to learn for his future well-being. For instance, a client may indicate that every time his mother calls him, he becomes very anxious. What makes a twenty-, thirty-, or forty-year-old man feel like a little boy? If there is nothing in the present to make this an appropriate response, the reason lies in his history. What earlier events are locked in his nervous system that cause him to feel intimidated? What skills might he need to learn to begin setting appropriate boundaries?

To understand clients more thoroughly, I often ask them to give me a list of the ten most disturbing events from their childhood. For instance, while most people remember a time when they were humiliated in grade school, it affects them to a greater or lesser degree depending on their life experience. I ask clients to hold these disturbing events in mind and rate them on the 0–10 SUD Scale. Even though they happened years ago, many of these memories may still be very upsetting. If so, the memory may shed light on current problems with authority, learning, or other situations. I also try to determine how clients interpret these events to themselves. When a client concentrates on a specific memory, I may ask her what words automatically come to mind that describe her feelings about herself or her behavior in the situation. If her cognitions are negative and she says, "I was a failure, I'm worthless, I'm not likable, I can't stand it," I know that the memory needs to be addressed in treatment. If her cognitions are positive and she says, "I can succeed, I am worthwhile, I am likable, I now have choices that I didn't have then," I assume that the memory has been processed and has taken its proper place in the past. Any event, from any time in life, can have a detrimental effect. Depending on the client's responses, I develop a comprehensive treatment plan that takes into account the far-reaching effects of the lifetime of experiences.

One of the unusual features of EMDR is that people seeking treatment do not have to discuss any of their disturbing memories in detail. Whereas some people are comfortable and even prefer giving specifics, other people present more of a general picture or outline. When the therapist asks, for example, "What event do you remember that made you feel worthless and useless?" the person may say, "It was something my brother did to me." That is all the information the therapist needs to identify and target the event with EMDR.

The second phase of EMDR treatment is *preparation*; I cannot overemphasize its importance. One of the primary goals of the preparation phase is to establish a relationship of trust between the client and the therapist. Clients do not have to go into great detail about their disturbing memories; however, if the client does not trust his clinician, he may not accurately report what he feels and what changes he is or is not experiencing during the session. If he wants to please the clinician and says he feels better but really feels the same, no therapy in the world will resolve his trauma. In any form of therapy, it is best to look at the clinician as a facilitator, or guide, who needs to hear of any hurt, need, or disappointments in order to help achieve the goal. EMDR therapy encompasses a great deal more than eye movements, and the clinician needs to know when to employ variations to keep the processing going.

During the preparation phase, the clinician explains the theory of EMDR, how it is done, and what the person can expect during and after treatment. Finally, the clinician teaches clients a variety of relaxation techniques for calming themselves in the face of any emotional disturbance that may arise during or after a session. Learning these tools is an important aid for anyone. The happiest people on the planet have ways of relaxing themselves and decompressing from life's inevitable and often unsuspected stresses. One goal of EMDR therapy is to make sure that clients can take care of themselves.

Because EMDR is a treatment that centers on the needs of clients, the clinician offers ways to make sure that clients maintain a balanced sense of control. Although it is understandable that people may start off wanting to avoid the disturbing material that EMDR brings up, it is this avoidance that keeps their problem alive. To counter the avoidance without generating new distress, the therapist teaches clients how to maintain a dual awareness of, first, the distressing material from the past that is triggered during the eye movements and, second, the fact that they are safe in the present. Ideally, the person doing EMDR will feel as though she is on a train and the upsetting targeted events are merely the passing scenery.

Assessment is the third phase of EMDR treatment, during which the clinician identifies the aspects of the target to be processed. The first step is for the person to select a specific picture or scene from the target event (which was identified during Phase 1) that best represents the memory. Then the client chooses a statement that expresses a negative self-belief associated with the event. Even if he intellectually knows that the statement is false, it is important that he focus on it. These negative beliefs are verbalizations of the disturbing emotions that still exist. Common negative cognitions include statements such as "I am helpless," "I am worthless," "I am un-lovable," "I am shameful," and "I am bad." The client then picks a positive self-statement that he would rather believe. This statement should incorporate an internal sense of control, such as "I am worthwhile" (or lovable, a good person, in control) or "I can succeed." When the primary emotion is fear, such as in the aftermath of a natural disaster, the negative cognition can be "I am in danger" and the positive cognition can be "I am safe now." "I am in danger" can be considered a negative cognition because the fear is inappropriate; it is locked in the nervous system even though the danger is in the past. The positive cognition reflects the reality of the present.

At this point, the therapist asks the person to estimate how true she feels her positive belief is by using the 1–7 Validity of Cognition (VOC) Scale. Also during the assessment phase, the person identifies the negative emotions (fear, anger) and physical sensations (tightness in the stomach, cold hands) she associates with the target. The client also rates the disturbance by using the 0–10 SUD Scale.

Phases 1 through 3 lay the groundwork for the comprehensive treatment and reprocessing of the specific targeted events. Although the eye movements are used during the following three phases, they are only one component of this complex therapy. The use of the step-by-step eight-phase approach allows the trained, experienced EMDR clinician to maximize the treatment effects for the client in a logical and standardized fashion. It also allows both the client and the clinician to monitor the progress during every treatment session.

Phase 4 is called *desensitization* because it focuses on the client's disturbing emotions and sensations as they are measured by the SUD rating. This phase encompasses all of the person's responses (including memories, insights, and associations that may arise during the sessions) as the targeted event changes and its disturbing elements are resolved. This automatic associative process offers the opportunity to identify and resolve similar events that may have occurred and are linked with the target. That way, a client can surpass her initial goals and heal beyond her expectations. During desensitization, the therapist leads the person in sets of eye movements (with appropriate variations and changes of focus) until her SUD levels are reduced to 0 or, if appropriate, 1 or 2.

For instance, Eric, the Vietnam War veteran discussed in Chapter 3, reported a level of sadness of 2 that would not decrease. When I asked him what prevented it from going lower, he said, "Someone died." Once again, we see that appropriate emotions and beliefs do not change with EMDR. We are not machines, and we shouldn't expect people, even those treated with EMDR, to have no reaction at all to a tragedy they have experienced. However, it is important to make sure the reaction is healthy and useful. Unfortunately, people often assume that the grief, shame, guilt, or anger they are feeling is appropriate, merely because they experience it. As I will demonstrate throughout this book, the negative beliefs we have about ourselves are often the inappropriate residue of the trauma itself. The question we should ask ourselves is, "Am I happy?" If the answer is *no*, we should consider a therapeutic alternative and the possibility of change.

The fifth phase of EMDR treatment is called *installation* because the goal is to "install" (fully incorporate) and increase the strength of the positive belief that the person has identified to replace his original negative belief. For example, the client might begin with a mental image of being beaten up by his father and a negative belief of "I am powerless." During the desensitization phase, he reprocesses the terror of that childhood event and fully realizes that as an adult he now has strength and choices he didn't have when he was young. During the fifth phase of treatment, his positive cognition "I am now in control" is strengthened and installed. How deeply the person believes his positive cognition is then measured using the VOC Scale. The goal is for the person to accept the full truth of his positive self-statement at a level of 7 (completely true). Fortunately, just as EMDR cannot make anyone shed appropriate negative feelings, it cannot make people believe anything positive that is not appropriate. If the person is aware that he needs to learn some new skill, such as self-defense training, in order to be truly in control of the situation, the validity of his positive belief will rise only to the corresponding level on the VOC Scale, such as a 5 or 6.

Body scan is the sixth phase of EMDR. After the positive cognition has been strengthened and installed, the therapist asks the person to bring the original target event to mind and see if she notices any residual tension in her body. If so, these physical sensations are targeted for reprocessing.

Evaluations of thousands of EMDR sessions have indicated that there is a physical resonance to unresolved thoughts. This finding has been supported by independent studies of memory indicating that when a person is negatively affected by trauma, information about the traumatic event is stored in episodic memory, rather than narrative (semantic) memory, and the person retains the negative emotions and physical sensations of the original event.[3] When that information is processed, however, it can move to narrative (or verbalizable) memory, and the body sensations and negative feelings associated with it disappear. Therefore, an EMDR treatment session is not considered complete until the client can bring up the original target image without feeling any body tension. Positive self-beliefs are important, but they have to be believed on more than an intellectual level.

The seventh phase of EMDR treatment is called *closure*. It ensures that clients leave at the end of each session in better shape than they were in at the beginning. If the processing of the traumatic target event is not complete in a single session, the therapist assists the person in using a variety of self-calming techniques to regain a sense of equilibrium. Throughout the EMDR session, the client has been in control (for instance, he is instructed that it is okay to raise his hand in the "stop" gesture at any time), and it is important that this control continue outside the therapist's office. Clients also are briefed on what to expect between sessions (for instance, some processing may continue, some new material may arise), how to use a journal to record these experiences, and which techniques they might use on their own to help them feel calmer.

The final phase of EMDR treatment, called *reevaluation*, takes place at the beginning of each therapy session after the first. The therapist checks to make sure that the positive results achieved (low SUD, high VOC, no body tension) have been maintained, identifies any new areas that need treatment, and continues facilitating processing of the additional targets. The reevaluation phase guides the clinician through the various EMDR protocols (written for different client problems) and the full treatment plan. As in any therapy, the reevaluation phase is vital to determine the success of the treatment over time. Although clients may feel relief almost immediately with EMDR therapy, it is as important to complete the eight phases of treatment as it is to complete an entire course of treatment with antibiotics.

Although EMDR may produce results more rapidly than other forms of therapy, speed is not the primary goal, and it is important to remember that every client has different needs. For instance, one client may take weeks to establish sufficient feelings of trust to begin processing (Phase 2), whereas another may proceed quickly through the first six phases of treatment only to discover, at that point, that something even more important needs treatment. The following story provides an example of just such a case. Through the eyes of a carefully trained clinician, patterns and reactions can be identified that become the doorway to alternatives the client did not know were possible.

ຄ

Jocelyne Shiromoto was one of the first people trained in EMDR therapy. A licensed clinical social worker from San Diego, Jocelyne had heard about EMDR from a psychiatrist with whom she was sharing a case. At that point in her career, Jocelyne was willing to consider anything that might legitimately help her clients. She was tired of taking their money without being able to guarantee that therapy would give them results; she was tired of the circles that talk therapy seemed to go around in; and she was nearly burned out at seeing so much pain and being able to do so little about it.

As Jocelyne started using EMDR in her private practice, she worked it into her existing methods: an eclectic mixture of psychodynamic, cognitive, and behavioral therapies. She used EMDR with some clients and avoided it with others. One of the cases in which it turned out to be extremely useful was that of Emily Zazaroff.

Emily's mother, Mary Beth Ritter, had been seeing Jocelyne for quite a while, trying to sort out her conflicting feelings about her marriage and her husband of more than thirty years. Mary Beth had made some progress but was still in a lot of confusion and pain when her married daughter Emily told her she wanted to meet with Jocelyne on her own. Emily had watched her mother trying to come to grips with her life, and she knew that deep soul searching alone would not give her mother the answers to her questions about her marriage. Her mother needed facts, facts that only Emily could provide.

At their first session together, Emily, who was then thirty, told Jocelyne that her father used to come to her room at night and fondle her when she was seven and eight. At the time, part of her knew what her father was doing to her was bad, but another part yearned for his attention. Bill Ritter was a withdrawn, inattentive, critical, and occasionally violent father. When he began fondling her, Emily experienced the only tenderness she had ever known from him. It made her feel important, and that made her feel guilty.

During her twenties, Emily told Jocelyne, she had found ways to resolve that guilt. She had gone to group therapy and talked a lot about her father. She had realized that she was not responsible for the abuse. She had confronted her anger about the past and taken some long hard looks at her tendency to get involved with violent men in the present. Now Emily felt it was time to break the silence about the incest. She believed it would help her mother in therapy and help the whole family begin to heal. She planned to ask her father to get counseling. She loved him, and she didn't want the abuse to damage another generation in her family: Both of her younger sisters and her brother had young children.

Jocelyne and Emily met with both parents the following week. When Emily revealed the incest, her mother was shocked and grieved, but her father took full responsibility for what he had done. He agreed to get counseling. It looked as if Emily's hope for a united and healed family might come to pass.

Ironically, Emily and her husband, Tom, were having painful problems trying to start a family of their own. Their physician had explained to them that on the average, 90 percent of healthy American couples conceive within one year of trying, but Emily and Tom had been trying to have children for four of their six married years. This was bitter medicine for Emily, who had gotten pregnant twice in her late teens, defying all odds by conceiving once when she was on the Pill and once when she was wearing an IUD. Both pregnancies had ended in miscarriage: the first when Emily was struck by a car, and the second when the IUD was taken out.

A battery of doctors and medical tests had confirmed that there was nothing wrong with Emily's reproductive system; there was no physiological reason she could not conceive. An emergency-room nurse herself, Emily was a savvy consumer of medical care and had gotten expert advice on her condition. She had also taken the fertility drug Clomid for more than two years to stimulate ovulation. The doctors had evaluated her husband, too; they found that Tom had a low-to-normal sperm count, which was not an alarming finding, and they didn't think it was the cause of the infertility. Finally, Emily and Tom had decided to try artificial insemination. Their first attempt was scheduled in two months, at the beginning of August, and Tom would be getting a shot of testosterone in late June to boost the odds when he donated sperm for the artificial insemination. They were told that the usual success rate for intrauterine insemination is 10 percent.

Four years of trying to conceive had brought Emily a lot of grief. She had examined her life for anything she might have done to cause her infertility. Had her two early miscarriages had an effect the doctors couldn't measure? Had God forsaken her? Was she really a bad person who didn't deserve to have kids? At work, Emily searched the faces of the pregnant women who passed her office door on their way to the obstetrics-gynecology department next door. Why did these women get to have babies and she didn't? There was only one reason left that she could think of, and it made her blood run cold. It meant the infertility really was her fault, and she didn't want even to think about it, let alone talk to a therapist about it. She never had.

Over the next three months, Emily saw Jocelyne privately to work on issues concerning her father's abuse and other painful events in her life. During some of these sessions, Jocelyne and Emily used EMDR to work through old feelings and to ensure that Emily really had resolved the sexual abuse. In one of those sessions, Emily told Jocelyne that when she was twenty she had been beaten and raped by a coworker in a utility room at the New York hospital where she had her first job. Although the incident no longer disturbed her, the treatment she had received at the hands of her employers did. Emily had not reported the rape until several days later, and when she did tell the hospital security personnel, they didn't believe her. They called her to the office several times, demanding that she repeat her story of the rape, sometimes interrupting her during her shift or calling her late at night at home. They remained skeptical.

Paradoxically, the hospital management took Emily's story seriously—and caused even more damage. They ordered Emily to see one of their staff psychiatrists for counseling. She refused—it felt like an invasion of privacy—but management pressured her, and Emily finally gave in. She reluctantly attended a few sessions with a female psychiatrist, then quit seeing her. When Jocelyne asked Emily for details about the rape and the hospital's failure to investigate it, Emily spoke about these issues willingly. On the subject of the psychiatric treatment, she was uncharacteristically vague.

One day, Emily told Jocelyne about her frustration at not being able to have a baby. As Emily revealed the details of her four-year struggle to conceive, Jocelyne evaluated whether the incest or the rape could be a hidden psychological factor blocking Emily's path to motherhood. It would be an easy conclusion to jump to, but Jocelyne didn't think that was the case. Neither of these traumas seemed to bother Emily anymore. At least, she certainly appeared to have resolved them and accepted them as part of her history.

At their next session, Emily was more keyed up than usual. Her hands were clenched atop the arms of her chair, driving the points of her nails into her palm. Scenes from yesterday's family gathering played in her mind like trailers for a G-rated movie: her nieces and nephews running circles around and around the house, yelping, chasing, laughing, shouting, bickering, crying; herself sprawled on the living room floor playing with her nephew Matthew and his toy trucks; the four babies with their sticky, bright faces, all born in the last twelve months.

"You know, it's weird," she said. "As much as I love the kids, sometimes it's hard for me to be around them."

"In what way?" Jocelyne asked.

"Well, I feel sort of tense. Anxious. Actually, I've always felt that way around kids. And there's this photo of me and my youngest nephew that I have on our refrigerator door—it's from last Christmas. He was four months old then, and he's got on a red sleeper. I'm holding him with one hand under his butt and my other hand on his back to keep his head up. My sister Jennifer took it and sent it to me. But, I don't know why, it's a beautiful photo, but I feel really terrible when I look at it. Lately, it's been worse and worse. Finally last weekend I ripped it off the fridge and tore it up. I was in tears about it."

"What do you think that feeling is about?"

Emily fixed her gaze on the painting behind Jocelyne's desk.

"Maybe I'm afraid I'm going to molest him."

"What makes you think that?"

"That's what the psychiatrist told me, the one they made me see when I was raped."

⁀

The psychiatrist's name was Dr. Virginia Loder (not her real name), and Emily remembers having only two, maybe three sessions with her. Emily knew her reluctance to see Dr. Loder was right when the psychiatrist asked her to tell her about her childhood and her family. "What has that got to do with anything?" she asked. "It has nothing to do with the rape."

Dr. Loder pressed. Emily still refused. The psychiatrist pressed again. Emily lost her temper.

"Stop pushing me! I feel like I've been abused all my life, and I'm a nice person and I don't deserve this!"

"What do you mean you've been abused all your life?"

At which point, Emily told Dr. Loder about her father and his fondling.

"Then what happened?" asked Jocelyne.

Emily's right hand flew to her left upper arm and squeezed hard, a nervous habit Jocelyne had noticed before.

"Well, she got real quiet and just sat there and stared at me for a few minutes, it seemed like an hour. Then she leaned forward and looked straight at me and she said, 'I want you to know that it is a medical fact that if you were sexually abused, you will sexually abuse your own children, if you ever have any.'"

"What was your reaction?"

"I threw up. Really. On her office floor. Then I cried, I pleaded with her to tell me that wasn't true. She was really cold about it. She just said it was a medical fact. She said, 'I suggest you never have children.'"

Jocelyne Shiromoto took a deep breath. Before her sat a healthy young woman with no physiological reason to prevent her from having children but an overwhelming emotional reason not to.

"Emily, do you still believe that?"

"No, not in my head. Even right after I left her office, I went home and cried and cried and prayed, and then I got mad. I decided this woman didn't know what she was talking about, I decided they were all out to get me, and I just refused to see her anymore."

"So you didn't believe that what she said was true?"

"No! But it still bothered me." Emily's hand was now squeezing her upper arm almost rhythmically. "In the years after that, I tried to find where this so-called medical fact was written, and the only thing I found were a few short articles in *Redbook* or *McCall's* and I thought, you know, some idiot probably came up with some tiny little study . . . and I decided not to believe it. But what's really dangerous is when someone makes a statement like that, even though I know that I don't have it within myself to do that to a child . . . it was still there, what she said, and the silent fear. It was still there inside me."

"Can you put that fear into words?"

Emily ducked her head. Her long blonde bangs brushed the bridge of her nose. "I guess it's that since I have been a victim of incest, the consequences are that I will molest my own children." Emily seemed to be holding her breath as she spoke. "I have to face it that I have a terminal disease. I'm trapped; it's like a life sentence. And I live it even though I don't believe it."

Tears streamed down her flushed cheeks. "So maybe the infertility is my fault. Maybe deep down I know I would molest a child, and not getting pregnant is my body's way of preventing it."

When Emily confessed that she was afraid of molesting her own children, Jocelyne saw an ideal opportunity for using EMDR. The fear stemmed from a clearly defined single incident that might be blocking the client from full health. In Emily's case, full health could include being able to conceive, if her problem were indeed psychogenic. Although infertility seems to be a biological problem, we all have heard of cases in which women, after years of unsuccessful attempts to conceive, have finally given up and adopted a child, only to get pregnant a year or two later. What appears to be happening in these cases is that the psychological pressure or stress the woman feels about having a child (even if the pressure is only self-imposed) blocks her from becoming pregnant. In these days of the exploration of the relationship between mind and body, it is not hard to understand how such stress could cause a formerly fertile woman to produce, for example, an acidic environment in her body that would prevent insemination. One hundred years ago, Freud suggested that certain types of paralysis were hysterical reactions to psychological conflicts. Clearly, something that assaults the body, such as a natural disaster, car accident, or physical assault, can affect the mind. Conversely, many heart attacks occur when some terrible piece of information has "assaulted" the mind.

Another interesting aspect of Emily's case is that her traumatic stress reaction appears to have been caused by an incident that, on the surface, does not seem as damaging as either the incest or the rape she suffered. But the mark of a good psychotherapist is her ability to look at the big picture and identify what negative beliefs are driving the person's behavior or state of mind. Jocelyne was able to look past the obvious, not insisting that either the molestation or the rape caused Emily's infertility.[4]

Emily's present-day feelings of shame and guilt about her long-ago meeting with the psychiatrist were extreme, and they pointed to a block that needed to be cleared—a memory that needed to be processed. The incident was still having a negative effect on her: She felt humiliated and frightened at the thought of it. She was also having physical sensations connected with the experience. The question is, what deeper effect might the incident be having on her body? Even if EMDR had no effect on Emily's infertility, it would be important to clear out her guilt. A therapist must be responsive to each client, tailoring EMDR to the needs of the individual, and in Emily's case, a "secondary trauma" was as damaging as the original one. Good therapy is a dynamic interaction between clinician, client, and method. It is poignant when people say, "It's no use. I've tried therapy and it doesn't work!" What they've tried is one or more particular therapists. They may not have tried the right one.

Even though Emily had recovered from the trauma of the molestation and rape, she was still tormented by guilt and fear resulting from a cruel accusation made by an authority figure in a moment when Emily was extremely vulnerable and emotionally aroused. Emily literally threw up when Dr. Loder made her damning pronouncement—that was how deeply it affected her. The way a rape victim is treated, or maltreated, by hospital personnel, police, friends, and family can do more damage than the sexual assault itself.

⌒

Jocelyne asked Emily if she'd like to try EMDR on the incident with the psychiatrist. Jocelyne said she couldn't promise that it would affect Emily's infertility—indeed, it is against the law in many states to tell a client that any psychological treatment is guaranteed to work for anything—but she told her that it looked like there might be a link.

Seven days later, Emily walked back into Jocelyne's office. During their previous visit, Jocelyne had prepared Emily for the processing session and they were ready to go. Emily had already formulated a negative statement that summarized her fears: "I will molest my children because I am a victim of molestation." When Jocelyne had asked her how intense that fear felt on the 0–10 SUD Scale, Emily had rated her fear at a 9. In a final preparatory step, Jocelyne had asked Emily to come up with a positive statement that expressed what she would like to believe instead. Emily had thought it over and stated, "I would never molest my children. I do have choices." When asked to rate how true that statement felt at the moment on the 1–7 VOC Scale, Emily had said it felt only like a 2 or 3.

"So let's start with the scene back in the psychiatrist's office," Jocelyne said. "Just keep that picture in your mind, along with the negative belief, and notice the feelings that come up as we go along. Okay? Now follow my fingers."

As Jocelyne led Emily in the eye movements, Emily began to relive the moment when the hospital psychiatrist told her she would molest her own children. Emily's stomach clenched and a sour taste filled her mouth. "I feel sick," she told Jocelyne after the first set of eye movements. As the sets continued, Emily balled up her hands into tight fists, moaned, and cried, but she kept her eyes moving. During a pause, she reported a shift from the intense fear she had started with to a feeling of total, utter loss of hope. "It's like someone took my dreams and hopes and pulled them right out from under me. I wasn't the same after that," Emily said. Tears rolled down her cheeks, her head dropped, and her hands fell open, revealing tiny crescent-shaped cuts in her palms where her fingernails had broken the skin.

Jocelyne and Emily took time to talk about how damaging it was for someone in authority to make such an inaccurate statement. Then they started another set of eye movements.

The next thing Emily noticed was a flood of white-hot anger. "She abused me!" Emily shouted, a flush rising to her face. "How could anyone say something like that to me? If she were in this room right now, I'd scratch her eyes out!" Jocelyne directed Emily to "stay with that" and initiated another set of eye movements. Emily grasped her upper arm for comfort and focused on Jocelyne's moving fingers. Now she felt a fresh flood of anger at her employers, who had forced her into seeing the psychiatrist: "The rape itself wasn't as bad as the horrible way they treated me. I got raped twice!" Finally, after several more sets, Emily said she felt angry with herself. "How could I have believed her?"

At one point, Emily's memory of being in the psychiatrist's office shifted, and she recalled another incident when she had felt shame and fear concerning molesting a child. When she was eleven, Emily worked in her church's day care center. One Sunday morning she was cleaning up a baby with a very messy diaper.

"I had washed her off and was taking a look to make sure I'd gotten her clean. (At the time, I had a baby sister and brother and my mother would always yell, 'Make sure you get it clean or she'll get an infection!') Just as I'm inspecting the baby, her mother walked in. She came up to me and took over the diapering. I have always felt so guilty about that, so ashamed, as if I had done something wrong and she had caught me," Emily said. "Now I see what that mother did was normal. She was the mom, so she took over."

As they continued speaking, Emily's intense emotions subsided. Her hand released its death grip on her upper arm and her stomach relaxed. Toward the end of the session, Emily gave her head a shake, then quietly and firmly announced, "It's just not in me." Emily now knew in her heart—not just in her head—that she would never sexually abuse a child. Finally she looked into Jocelyne's eyes and said, "I have spent all these years fearing that I would molest a child. It is so sad, such a waste."

As Jocelyne worked with Emily using EMDR to treat her negative beliefs, she was not trying to contradict, argue with, or restructure the way that Emily thought about that day in the psychiatrist's office. Intellectual insight was not going to work. The trauma went much deeper, and healing had to occur on a physiological and emotional level. She trusted that EMDR would jump-start Emily's natural healing process.

When their processing session was over, Jocelyne asked, "Emily, how do you feel about your statement, 'I would never molest my children. I do have choices'? On a scale of 1 to 7, how true does that statement feel?"

Emily wiped a hand over her damp face, grinned, and said, "Seven. Absolutely."

That was the only processing session Emily Zazaroff and Jocelyne Shiromoto did on the issue of Emily's infertility. The next week—by now it was late June—Emily came back and the two talked over what EMDR had revealed. Emily was still angry at the psychiatrist, appropriately so, Jocelyne thought, but she was calm and clear about what happened all those years ago.

"It's like I had one part of my brain that said, 'Absolutely, no way is this true,' while another tiny little part of my brain was still screaming, 'Oh no! Wha? . . .' That scary part's not there anymore."

Two and a half weeks after the EMDR session, on Independence Day weekend, Emily conceived.

⌘

Did EMDR enable Emily Zazaroff to get pregnant? Or was it the testosterone shot her husband was given in late June? We'll never know for sure. But the fact that Emily and Tom conceived a second child without any medical help makes the cause seem reasonably clear. Emily and Tom certainly believe their daughter was a gift from EMDR. "It was the first time in my life that I actually felt like I was ready," Emily says now. "There was nothing prohibiting me in my mind. Before, I always felt there was something preventing me, but I didn't know what it was."

Emily also says that without EMDR she never would have been able to bond with her baby. "Before, when I would play with my nieces and nephews, I always kind of held back a little, so I never really connected with any of them. When I had my daughter, I felt a freedom that I had never ever felt before. To really be with her, kiss her, touch her. There was an innocence there that I'd never ever had my whole life. With EMDR I think I probably did thirty years of therapy in one year."

By the way, her first baby's name is Elizabeth, and she has a mop of red curls.

5

The Many Faces of Fear: Phobias and Panic Attacks

Once you've been bitten by a snake,
you are very cautious even of a coiled rope.

—THE DALAI LAMA

SOME OF THE STORIES psychotherapists hear from trauma survivors are so extreme, they might be hard for ordinary people to relate to. In the course of this book, for example, you will meet an engineer whose nineteen-ton train ran over a six-year-old boy. You will also hear from a woman who was raped while her young daughter lay next to her on the bed. Even though most of us will never experience ordeals so appalling, we all have certain physiological and psychological reactions in common, and in the face of potential disaster, our general reactions are the same. Fear is one of the common denominators of our shared humanity.

Although each of us is a unique individual, we share adherence to a number of common principles that define and shape the way we develop. One principle that guides the practice of EMDR therapy, outlined in the Adaptive Information Processing model, is that pathologies, or "flaws" of character development, are based on early life experiences. Unless the cause of the problem is organic, or biochemical, everything we feel or do, every action we take, is guided by previous life experiences, because all of them are linked together in an associative memory network.

We are not creatures who respond at random; rather, we react to an internal, associative reality. To allow us to make sense of our experiences, the perceptions of present events automatically link up to the past in the memory network, and the stored negative emotions can flood through the person. In EMDR therapy, the clinician tries to identify the negative experience that set the problem in motion. Sometimes it's obvious. In the case of posttraumatic stress disorder, the experiences are horrendous ones that impact a person with a sense of horror and fear of death. For others, it can be everyday experiences that leave the person permanently marred. For instance, someone may be laughed at during a camp play and, from that time on, feel bad about himself in similar situations. The response can be an everyday, low-key reaction of feeling unsure of himself when he is asked to speak, a confusing and pervasive unhappiness in groups, or a full-blown anxiety reaction in which the person shakes, turns red, and wants to run away whenever he is asked to perform in public. In some way, the experiences are associatively related, such as in the reaction of a woman who developed an inability to leave her house after becoming sick in public when she found out that her husband had had an affair.

Although earlier life experiences are generally at the root of a pathological response in the present, they are given different clinical labels depending on the symptoms they cause. Posttraumatic stress disorder, panic attack, panic disorder, and phobia are subsets of a category known as anxiety disorders. If the person has a life-threatening experience and subsequently has intrusive thoughts of the event and avoidance behaviors, we call it posttraumatic stress disorder. But life-threatening events, or even everyday ones, can contribute to other disorders. If the person has discrete periods of intense anxiety and fear, we call the events panic attacks. If recurrent attacks include at least a month of persistent worry about having another panic, we call the condition a panic disorder. If specific feared objects or situations cause intense anxiety and avoidance, we call it a phobia. In any case, while biological factors may predispose some people to anxiety or panic reactions, the ultimate culprit is generally an earlier life experience or experiences that set the problem in motion and that remain locked in the person's nervous system.

EMDR therapy treats different anxiety disorders with various protocols explicitly geared to the problems. To maximize the treatment effects, EMDR processes not only the distant memories but also more recent events and situations the client can imagine being involved in in the future. We do this because the associative memory network is complex, and we want to reach as many of the problem areas as we can. Because past and present are connected in our associative memory network on many levels, the positive treatment effects spread throughout the system, and the person can begin to respond in a positive way to similar situations.

Although EMDR therapy seems to enter into the memory networks and uses them to special advantage, the reason the earlier experiences can cause such a disturbing response may be found in a complicated chain of stimuli and responses. For most anxiety disorder symptoms, a disturbing experience is the initial cause, and the anxiety that was generated may have become linked to any number of things (such as sounds or objects) that were present at the time. Those things may cause the anxiety to come up automatically at a later date, and the response may then link to everything present during that time. The web of anxiety responses can become more and more complex and all-encompassing. Fortunately, the solution can be straightforward, and the concepts that underlie the treatment all go back to a genius by the name of Ivan Pavlov.

Although different psychological modalities offer varying explanations, one way to look at fear disorders is through the Pavlovian lens of stimulus-response, with the upsetting event as the stimulus and the fear-driven behavior as the response.[1] Nearly a century ago, Pavlov discovered, almost by accident, that he could train dogs to salivate in response to the sound of a bell that was rung shortly before they were fed. Hundreds of subsequent studies with humans have shown that these kinds of automatic responses are elicited by similar pairings in a wide variety of conditions.[2]

In the world of psychology, this stimulus-response phenomenon is called classical conditioning. It explains why a mother's touch can make a hungry child stop crying. The baby has learned to associate mother with food and comfort. The concept of conditioning is the cornerstone of behavioral psychology, and its use has become so commonplace in our culture that we don't even notice it. For example, a variant known as operant conditioning occurs whenever someone makes an association between an action and a consequence. A child who runs into the street is punished in the hope that he will learn to associate that action with the punishment—and stop the behavior. Bonuses are offered to personnel based on the same theory, but with the opposite intention. Although stimulus-response is only one of many mental processes, it is certainly one of the most basic and elemental. Physiological and mental processes are inextricably intertwined.

One of the mechanisms that rapidly enables EMDR therapy to resolve disorders based on fear and anxiety may relate to classical conditioning. Just as fear becomes associated with certain stimuli, causing phobias and panic disorders, there is evidence that EMDR may rapidly decondition the sufferer with a powerful relaxation response. In a study by David Wilson and colleagues,[3] people with a disturbing memory were asked to think about the event during the EMDR procedures, while either doing eye movements or keeping their eyes closed. In both cases, the subjects were hooked up to biofeedback equipment. After treatment, an independent polygraph reader evaluated their heart rate, respiration, blood pressure, and galvanic skin response (the electrical resistance in the skin associated with emotional arousal).

The results showed that the subjects who did eye movements while thinking about their disturbing memory seemed to have an automatic physical relaxation response. The other subjects did not have the same response. This finding appears to indicate that humans have an internal physiological mechanism that activates emotional healing when it is appropriately accessed and directed. The results of this study also underline how powerful the link is between our physiology and our psychology: After a single session of EMDR, the subjects' primary symptoms disappeared.

This interconnectedness of body and mind is most obvious in the study of phobias. Whereas therapists working with phobic clients may disagree on how to treat the phobia, they generally agree that the cause of the problem is that the client has associated a certain stimulus (spiders, for example) with a physiologically based fear response. If the person's fear is so strong that it interferes significantly with his everyday functioning, it is called a phobia. An estimated one out of every ten people in the United States suffers from phobias, which can range from social phobias like fear of public speaking to specific phobias involving fear of a situation like flying or driving (the most common) or fear of animals (the least common).[4]

The usual response of someone with a phobia is to avoid the situation or the object that is causing him fear. Behavioral psychologists maintain that this avoidance simply feeds the phobia. To be cured, they say, people must seek therapy in which they are repeatedly exposed to the object of their fears (either in real life or in their imagination) in such a way that no negative consequences (such as actually being bitten by the spider) occur.

As this happens, the person's fears should gradually diminish until they are no longer a problem. Research has shown excellent results when using behavioral methods on people with phobias. Unfortunately, therapists who work with phobic clients have learned that the remedy for clients with complex phobias is not always as simple as the remedy for heavily screened and selected research subjects. That is why the comprehensive treatment planning used in EMDR is so important.

A randomized controlled study reported that EMDR therapy effectively eliminated phobias in 83 percent of the participants after only three sessions, and numerous other evaluations have reported comparable effects (see Appendix C).[5] The special EMDR protocol we have developed for treating phobias is aimed at the pivotal event that caused the phobia and any extenuating circumstances that may be holding the fear in place. Often the cause of a phobia is more complicated than it first appears. I once had a client who was terrified of flying; ordinarily I would have considered her problem straightforward. On taking this woman's history, however, I discovered that her husband was a traveling salesman. She felt that the only way she could avoid being dragged around the country with him was to be afraid of flying. This wasn't a conscious decision on her part; it was a case of *secondary gain*, a term that refers to the fact that people derive some benefit from their disorders. To treat this woman successfully using EMDR, one would first have to address the couple's relationship using family therapy. The wife would have to learn to stand up for herself and set her own limits so that her phobia didn't have to set those limits for her.

Another important aspect of the EMDR protocol is that it addresses all the contemporary stimuli that might independently trigger the person's fear. For example, if a man is afraid of flying, there are many activities that lead up to being on the plane. To address the full range of the problem, which includes all the anticipatory anxiety, one has the client imagine, scene by scene, a movie of himself going on a plane trip, starting with planning the trip and ending with his safe return. Any of the stimuli surrounding the entire experience of flying (calling the airline, driving to the airport, or walking to the gate) could serve as triggers for him, especially if he has previously gone through the entire experience in a state of fear. Likewise, if a person has claustrophobia, it is important to process all the situations that cause him to be afraid: getting stuck in traffic, being trapped in an elevator, getting on a crowded bus.

Again, the fear response is caused by some earlier life experience, whether it was a personal trauma, seeing someone else get hurt, or being repeatedly warned of danger. Sometimes, however, the pivotal event is buried in the client's earlier history. One person discovered during processing that his fear of flying was based on seeing his mother die and his consequent feelings of inadequacy. After that event was processed, the effects generalized through his associative memory network and made his current problem, his fear of flying, easier to deal with during treatment. Sometimes treating the pivotal event can generate complete healing throughout the entire memory network.

Although many phobias are caused by a single traumatic experience and can be rapidly treated with EMDR, others may be more complicated and the roots may consist of several accumulated events. Layers of distressing incidents can cause some people to lead an existence that is subtly stifled in many ways. Never realizing they can be helped, they spend years in muted pain. Others may be compelled to seek therapy because the tendrils of these long-ago events have wrapped themselves around a perfectly ordinary activity, like driving a car. What seems like an isolated phobia may provide an opportunity for healing on many associated levels.

⏝

Jessica Spenser was twenty-two when she had her first episode of what would become a fourteen-year siege of driving phobia and panic attacks. Jessica was a journalism student living in Los Angeles. She was also a strong athlete who enjoyed demanding sports like windsurfing, sailing, snorkeling, and hiking on the edges of cliffs. Despite all this activity, Jessica felt empty, unstable, and unsettled. She often felt a fear that was difficult to pinpoint but could be boiled down to a terror of losing control.

One night she was driving in the center lane of a Los Angeles freeway at sixty miles per hour. From one moment to the next, she went from taking the sheer act of driving for granted to being stone-cold terrified that she would faint, lose control of her car, and cause a fatal pileup of twisted metal and broken bodies. All Jessica's rational thinking stopped, adrenaline shot into her bloodstream, and her heart and mind started racing. She had fainted in the shower the year before, and as she was driving she had the same feeling of losing control of her body. Terrified that she would black out, Jessica pressed her foot to the brake pedal. She focused on getting to the shoulder where she would be safe, but she had to cross two lanes of traffic to do so. Car and truck lights seemed to come at her from all directions. People were honking and swerving to miss her as her speed dropped.

Jessica made it to the shoulder safely, but the incident didn't end there. Seeds of fear that had been sown long ago had broken through the surface that night. Over the course of the next decade, they would branch out, casting an ever-deepening shadow through her world.

By the time Jessica met psychotherapist Deany Laliotis, a licensed clinical social worker in Washington, D.C., her fear of driving had grown and spawned other fears. Jessica had not driven on an expressway for fourteen years. She only drove on secondary roads, and that only in daylight. Her career was collapsing. She had become a freelance newspaper reporter whose wide-flung assignments required a lot of driving. Sometimes what would have been a twenty-minute freeway ride turned into a two-hour expedition through downtown traffic jams, school zones, and unfamiliar neighborhoods. Gradually, Jessica put less energy into seeking work. She started giving up other activities in which fainting could be life-threatening. She stopped sailing, hiking, snorkeling, and windsurfing. As the years went by, she became more and more socially withdrawn and isolated. The only person she emotionally connected with was her husband.

Jessica had tried to get help for her driving phobia. Over the years, she had had one-on-one counseling, group therapy (which she was still involved in), hypnosis, and biofeedback. Sometimes she got partial relief from her fears, but the relief proved temporary. She came to see Deany because she had heard about EMDR.

Jessica worked with Deany for five months. She began by telling her about the panic attacks and the numerous times in her life, starting from childhood and continuing to the present, when she had fainted and lost control of her body. Jessica was the youngest of three and the only daughter. Her mother worked part-time outside the home, and her father was sometimes left with the responsibility of taking care of his daughter. He resented this and took his animosity out on Jessica. When he came into a room and found her playing there, he got very angry. He raised his voice, threw things around, and changed the TV channel until she left. He forced Jessica to eat food she didn't want and to do chores that she wasn't mature enough to handle. He never hit or molested her physically, but he bullied and terrified her. From the age of six, Jessica was often left at home alone. In this, Deany recognized one source of Jessica's problems.

The picture became more complicated when Deany learned that Jessica had had three operations in her first four years of life, two on her eyes and one on her urethra. She endured most of her hospital stays without company. Occasionally her mother would visit, but her father never would. Jessica was left virtually alone by her family during the frightening ordeal of surgery. By the time the operations were over, Jessica had developed an extreme fear of doctors, needles, and injections. Now thirty-six, she told Deany she hadn't had a physical examination in years.

The childhood abuse and abandonment that Jessica had suffered clearly offered fertile ground for a number of fears and dysfunctions. There was ample opportunity to use EMDR; however, Jessica's primary complaint was her inability to drive freely, and therefore it was decided to target the driving phobia with EMDR. Because Deany and Jessica didn't know the specific cause of the fear, they began by targeting the first (and worst) panic attack (the one on the L.A. freeway) and the intense feelings and beliefs that went with it: "I'm inadequate," "I can't control this," "There's something wrong with me," and "I'm the problem." As Deany and Jessica did set after set of eye movements, the images that came up for Jessica flowed into one another like a movie that goes from the past to the present and back again. The feelings that accompanied the images that Jessica saw in her mind's eye were excruciating: intense fear, guilt, grief, and despair.

In one session, Jessica started out with a frightening image of driving into a tunnel. The image shifted to being trapped with speeding trucks all around her, blocking her, forcing her. Then one of the large trucks turned into her father, creating the same sense of intimidation and domination she had felt as a child. The associations spawned by EMDR opened a flood of emotions, and realizations followed. This was how she'd lived all her life. In fear. She panicked because she was terrified of losing control. She was terrified of losing control because it reminded her of the many times when her father did.

With this realization, Jessica and Deany began to target Jessica's family issues. In one session, she remembered a hot and muggy summer day when her father told her to mow the lawn. Only eleven and small for her age, she pushed the heavy lawn mower out of the garage but could not get it started. Eventually she yanked on the starter cord so hard it broke. Her father was enraged and ordered her to get it fixed. Jessica hung her head and let her tears drop silently onto the grass. She couldn't get the lawn mower fixed; she had no money.

Jessica and Deany did other sessions around her driving phobia: going across bridges, being struck by tractor-trailers, going onto interstates with concrete barriers. In all these situations Jessica felt trapped, unable to control either her own body or what was going on around her. Deany thought that these themes might also have been present during Jessica's childhood surgery, so they targeted that. During the eye movements, Jessica recaptured the specifics of those painful times, even smelling the odor of ammonia that permeated the hospital. With the eye movements, she felt again the grief and fear of being left there alone and unprotected. There were strange people around her doing painful things to her body. Targeting those experiences not only reduced the impact of Jessica's self-denigrating beliefs but also got her over her fear of doctors and injections. She started to trust herself and her body more, trust that it would not let her down by making her faint.

Slowly Jessica began to come out of her shell. Because so many of her issues had taken root in childhood, they pervaded her sense of self; as the upsetting memories were processed, Jessica's personality seemed to change. She became more sociable, more assertive, more secure, and more self-confident. Deany was pleased with this progress; however, she and Jessica had been working together for a couple of months, and Deany felt things weren't moving as quickly as they usually did with EMDR. Ironically, none of these EMDR sessions had yet relieved Jessica's driving fears. Something was holding her back. She would leave a session with Deany feeling encouraged about the prospect of freeway driving, but when she was on her own, she could not make herself go out and do it. She was paralyzed with anxiety about what might happen. Unfortunately, the one time she did try, it was nighttime—an adverse condition they hadn't targeted—and she panicked. It was a major setback. What if she fainted and hit someone? Maybe killed them? Maybe got killed herself? More processing didn't budge the anxiety. Something was feeding the fear that they just weren't getting to.

Finally Deany decided they'd better just get out on the freeway together and see what happened. Whenever Jessica started to feel panicky, they pulled over to the side and immediately did EMDR on whatever had triggered her. They spent four sessions doing this, drawing quizzical stares from passing drivers but making tremendous progress. In addition to offering Jessica the support she had never had from her family, Deany was combining EMDR with the more traditional in vivo ("in real life") exposure technique typically used by behavioral therapists. All of Jessica's fears and the stimuli that caused them were not fully accessed in the office; this procedure allowed EMDR to process them quickly on the road.

Jessica's life changed dramatically after her "highway therapy" resolved the last of her fears. Her self-esteem continued to grow; she started marketing her journalistic skills again; and she drove wherever and whenever she pleased. Jessica even got the necessary shots to accompany her husband on a business trip to the Far East. Her fear of doctors and needles was gone.

It is not unusual for the identified problem targeted by EMDR to lead directly to related incidents. These connections are always logical, although that fact may not be immediately apparent. A client who starts by targeting a traumatic event, such as the day his father abandoned him, may go on to remember similar events, such as abandonments by other people or other situations in which he felt the same overwhelming despair. He may also remember other upsetting experiences he had with his father or other times he believed self-denigrating thoughts such as "I don't deserve love." As I have explained, this is because our previous life experiences are physiologically linked together in a memory network, along with similar events that occur in the present.

EMDR's ability to open memory networks and process old experiences allows people to emerge from treatment healed beyond their original complaint. Jessica left EMDR therapy with far more than a renewed ability to drive a car. Her processing led to a rapid alleviation of problems that had been seeded long before her phobia arose and had affected her self-esteem in many ways. The overt symptoms that finally propelled her to seek help offered her a doorway to far greater changes.

This interaction of past and present was found when a group of EMDR clinicians flew to Florida to treat victims of Hurricane Andrew. They saw each of the clients for a single treatment session that was offered specifically to deal with symptoms caused by the storm. The therapists reported that in the middle of that one session, approximately 30 percent of the clients began processing the memory of a childhood trauma that gave them similar feelings of chaos and lack of control. The hurricane had given them a window of opportunity to clean out the residue of the long-ago events.

The old experiences can exacerbate the negative reactions to new experiences, and the new can exacerbate the reactions to the old. In fact, one of the things that EMDR has shown us repeatedly is that the past is present.

Although we think we have buried it, the past can reach out with a stranglehold of fear when we least expect it.

⟲

In March 1990, Susan Rafferty and her second husband, Sam, were sitting on their sofa listening to the blizzard raging through the Colorado night. In fact, it was Sam who was listening; Susan was trying as hard as she could to block out the howl of the wind and snow against the window-panes. Ever since childhood she had been afraid of storms. This fear wasn't characteristic of her personality: Susan was a confident, articulate, assertive, and even feisty woman in her forties. The mother of two grown sons, she was a woman who could manage a home, hold down a full-time job, and still find time to dress meticulously with never a hair out of place.

Susan's mind had shut the door on the storm but had opened an internal debate on an equally stressful topic: her new job, which she'd had for less than a month. She was handling accounts receivable for a large defense contractor in Colorado Springs, and although she had worked for the firm earlier as a valued secretary, she now felt out of her league. Very large amounts of money were at stake. The result was that she had spent her first weeks on the job in a panic, an unnerving contrast to her usual supercompetent performance in life.

Susan turned to say something to Sam when suddenly one-half of her face went numb. Sam bundled her into the car and rushed through the icy streets to the emergency room. They both were terrified that Susan had had a stroke, but the doctors found nothing wrong with her and sent her home.

What no one knew at the time was that Susan had just had her first of many panic attacks. Although a pounding heart is the physical reaction most people associate with panic, other symptoms include numbness or tingling sensations, shortness of breath, dizziness or lightheadedness, shaking, trembling, chest pain, nausea, abdominal distress, chills, and hot flashes. As we saw in Emily Zazaroff's case (the woman who couldn't conceive), the body is an inseparable part of the psychological process. Often it is the physical symptoms that tell the real tale of the turmoil the client cannot express verbally. This is especially true of the "doers" and caretakers among us. They are so busy making sure that everything is handled for those around them, they leave little time to review their own needs, psychological or otherwise. Often they view their emotions as a weakness they refuse to indulge. Ironically, it can be the strongest people who suppress the most and fare the worst.

The months that followed were stressful for Susan, as the pressure continued at work and escalated at home. Her brother, who had AIDS, and her sister-in-law both had recently been diagnosed with cancer and undergone major surgery. Her youngest son, Ernie, was in the Air Force and expected to be sent to the Persian Gulf soon to join the U.S. war effort there. Sam's oldest son, also in the armed forces, was sure he would have to go too. Susan was also worried about herself. She had more numbness, this time in her hands and feet. She also had difficulty breathing, dizziness, and embarrassing and unexplained bouts of diarrhea. These symptoms seemed to come in waves, as often as four or five times a week. Susan's doctor ordered an MRI to see if she had multiple sclerosis. The results were negative.

One day about six months later, Susan was pushing her shopping cart down the crowded and noisy aisles at Wal-Mart. The public address system was issuing loud announcements, and Susan felt like the merchandise piled high on shelves was looming over her. Suddenly she couldn't breathe. Her chest tightened, her heart raced, her entire body trembled, and her skin turned clammy. I'm going crazy, Susan thought. If I don't get out of here, I'm going to die. She turned and literally ran for the door, bumping past other shoppers and leaving her half-filled cart behind.

Back in her car, Susan gripped the steering wheel for several minutes until her feelings subsided. Then she pulled herself together and got practical. She'd handled a lot of tough things in the past six months and she could handle this situation too. "Okay," she told herself aloud. "Fine. I just won't go to Wal-Mart. I don't like Wal-Mart anyway."

One week after her disastrous morning at Wal-Mart, Susan took her shopping list and drove to Kmart. The same thing happened. In the middle of the bustling store, she suddenly found herself in a blind panic and had to run for the door. Her physical symptoms were the same: chills, trembling, racing heart, and trouble breathing. Sitting in her car afterward, Susan spoke to herself sternly: "This is ridiculous. You can't go all your life without going to Kmart."

Susan went back to her physician. He thought her attacks might be due to low blood sugar and set up a complete glucose tolerance test for her, which involved measuring five blood sugar levels over the course of five hours. Susan had plenty of time between the readings, so she and Sam walked up the block and stopped at a large drugstore. All of a sudden, Susan felt every symptom she'd ever experienced: the diarrhea, the difficulty breathing, the sweats, the panic, the jelly legs. Sam took her arm and hurried her back to her doctor, who called for an immediate blood test. Susan was shaking so hard that the lab technician couldn't take blood from her inner arm. He had to prick her finger instead. But Susan's blood sugar level was normal.

When the doctor came back into the consulting room, he was carrying a book whose cover bore the words "anxiety disease." "Susan, I think you are having panic attacks, and I want you to read this so you'll understand more about them. Also, I am going to put you on some antianxiety medication."

Susan read the book she was given and everything else she could find about anxiety and panic disorder. Everything she'd experienced was described in these books. She wasn't crazy or dying. She had an anxiety disorder, just like the people she was reading about. She thought it ironic that knowing that thousands of other people were suffering from this condition actually made her feel better. The anxiety medication, which Susan took religiously at first, relieved the attacks for a while but had less and less impact on her panic as time went by. The medication also had an unnervingly familiar side effect: Every time she took one of the three-a-day tablets, Susan felt falling-down dizzy for forty-five minutes afterward.

Eventually Susan gave up on the medication, but she refused to give in to the disease. Her reading had told her that panic attacks often escalated into full-blown agoraphobia: Susan vowed she would not become housebound because of her fears. She forced herself to go into grocery stores and Kmart when what she really wanted to do was go home and sit alone in the dark. Despite her efforts to fight the panic, however, Susan continued to have attacks as often as four or five times a week. They seemed to come out of the blue, sometimes at work, sometimes in noisy crowded places, sometimes in the car. The net of stimuli was expanding, but each time Susan fought back. If she was in the car, the minute she felt a lump rising in her throat and constriction in her chest, she'd turn up the radio and sing at the top of her lungs until the panic subsided. She'd breathe deeply and keep driving. Sometimes the numbness and the chest pain felt so much like a heart attack, she would stop trying to tough it out and get herself to the emergency room.

In the hours and days following an attack, Susan found herself overwhelmed with fear, worrying when she would have another attack—and where. This anticipatory fear, combined with the panic attacks, made her a prime candidate for the diagnosis of panic disorder. This condition is more difficult to treat than panic attacks alone because fear about having another panic attack feeds the original fear. For many people, even a hint of the physical sensations can cause a panic attack; there is no need for an external stressor. Being afraid of one's own body's reactions can feel inescapable.

Susan tried many things to calm herself, including biofeedback and a thirty-day intensive stress-reduction program. None of them worked. Finally, she changed her medical insurance and joined a health maintenance organization that ran a clinic with a psychotherapist on staff. George Dunn, a psychological social worker, gave Susan a battery of tests (which showed she had anxiety and depression) and took an in-depth history, which was when Susan told him about the tornado. The one in 1984. The one that had ripped her house from its foundations and hurled its contents across the county. The one that had killed Susan's first husband and abruptly ended their happy twenty-year marriage.

ↅ

Susan had grown up in Missouri and, like all children born and bred in the Tornado Belt, before she learned to talk, she had absorbed a healthy fear of storms and the twisters they were apt to spin off. Susan knew to run straight to the basement when the wind started howling like a squadron of fighter planes. She knew to crouch in the southwest corner, where a tornado usually strikes first, before it has a chance to pick up your stove, your sink, your sofa, and your standing lamps and slam them into you at bone-breaking speeds.

In 1984, Susan and her first husband, Keith, had been living in tiny Barneveld, Wisconsin, where Keith was the athletic director at the local high school. Barneveld, a placid dairy-farming community with a population of six hundred, is set in the emerald hills of southern Wisconsin. Legend had it that Barneveld was tornado-proof thanks to its sheltering hills, known locally as Blue Mounds. When Susan, Keith, and their two sons moved there from Colorado in 1979, they bought a new two-story Cape Cod reassuringly located next door to the fire station and right at the foot of Blue Mounds. The moment the moving van pulled away, Susan went down to the basement and located the southwest corner of the house while Keith, Joel, and Ernie—all native Coloradans who had never seen a tornado—exchanged accommodating grins. Over the years in Barneveld, they would wear those grins repeatedly: Every time a storm blew up, Susan rushed "her men" down to the basement just in case the storm spun off a tornado. They went, but only to humor her.

June 7, 1984, was hot, humid, and windy. Susan came home from work, kissed Keith and called a hello to Ernie, then went upstairs to change. Then the three of them walked uptown to the Village Restaurant for dinner. It was much too hot to cook. When they got back, the wind was still blowing violently, and Susan convinced Keith that they should abandon their air-conditioned bedroom upstairs for the night and sleep downstairs in the guest room, where the constant howling of the wind would be muffled.

At 12:50 a.m., Susan was awakened by a loud clap of thunder and a flash of lightning. It was pouring rain. As she got her bearings, Susan heard a persistent low whistling, like wind blowing in the eaves or a car horn that doesn't have enough power. Just then Ernie ran into the guest room in his undershorts; the whistling had awakened him, too. Maybe it was the tornado alarm from the next town. Susan looked out the window into total darkness. No lights were on in town, not even at the fire station next door. The loud whistling was not a tornado alarm, it was the tornado itself.

"Keith, come on! We're going to the basement," Susan shouted and started running. Ernie followed her. Keith was awake, but he wasn't rushing; over the years in Barneveld, he had adopted a patronizing attitude toward what he thought of as Susan's tornado-alarmist tendencies. He reached for his pants as Susan sprinted through the kitchen and flung open the door to the stairs that led down to the basement, where the pets slept. The cat streaked past, headed for her food bowl. The dog was still down there in the dark, barking wildly. Then Susan heard a loud cracking as the siding on the house started to break up. After that, everything went black.

When Susan came to, she found herself in complete darkness, soaking wet, and buried in three feet of rubble in the southwest corner of her basement. Rain was still beating down, drenching her hair and thin nightgown. The air was acrid with the smell of heating oil, oozing no doubt from a break in the basement oil tank. There were no stairs. There were no rows of shelving stacked high with storage boxes, old luggage, and other junk that had been relegated to the basement. There was no ceiling above her. There was no house above her.

Ernie was beside her. Keith was not, but Susan felt instinctively that her husband was all right; she could feel it with that "sixth sense" she'd come to rely on over the years. Somewhere in the dark, their dog, Samantha, was still wailing.

When the storm let up, Ernie crawled out from under the rubble, climbed precariously out of the sinkhole that used to be their basement, and ran for help. Left alone, Susan hugged Samantha's small wet body to hers and did what she usually did in times of crisis. She got practical. She started making a mental list of the things she would have to do. First was to cancel their credit cards in case someone found them and tried to use them. Next she would get the power turned off and cancel the telephone. Then they'd all have to get new driver's licenses. Susan's mind had switched into automatic pilot, ignoring the emotional devastation and taking refuge in the practical.

Eventually a team of paramedics—every one of whom Susan knew—came with lights and laid down planks into the basement so that Susan, now oil-stained as well as soaked, could climb out. The emergency lighting set up by the rescue teams lit up a scene most notable for what was not in it. The family car was gone, as were the walls of the house, the floors, the roof, the furniture, the plumbing, the appliances, and nearly all their personal possessions. Her neighbors' houses were gone, too. Worst of all, there was still no sign of Keith.

A friend arrived and got Susan out of the rain and into her car. A while later, another friend offered Susan and her dog a bed for the night. Susan accepted, knowing Ernie was off helping the rescue workers and probably wouldn't sleep at all that night. The next morning, he showed up with clothing and shoes he'd borrowed for Susan. Then they went back to Barneveld, or tried to. Their way was blocked by the police.

"I'm sorry, ma'am, we can't let anyone in," said a tired cop. "You'll have to wait here."

"Not likely! I live in this town, and my husband has not been accounted for. I'm going in whether you like it or not."

Susan and Ernie were put in a police cruiser and taken to the command center set up in the middle of the town. On the way, they saw the damage the tornado had done. The devastation was almost impossible to take in. Eleven of the twelve houses in their immediate neighborhood were flattened. Three-hundred-mile-an-hour winds had destroyed three churches, the municipal building, the fire station, the American Legion Hall, the Village Bar and Restaurant, and the Thousand Curls Beauty Shop. At the bank the only thing left standing was the vault. At the Lutheran church, only the bell tower remained. In just twenty seconds, as *Time* magazine would later put it, Barneveld had been "wiped right off the map."[6]

When Susan and Ernie reached the command center, they were taken to see their local policeman. His face was haggard and sad.

"Susan," he said. "Keith's dead." Then he turned to her son. "Ernie, you found him last night. Why didn't you tell her?"

"I d-d-didn't want to believe that was my dad," he said in a shaky voice.

Susan felt her eyes widen with amazement. "You knew?" Maybe that was why Ernie had not come to the friend's house last night.

"Yes, Mom."

Before the reality of the news could hit her, Susan clicked back into automatic pilot. "Okay. Where is Keith? Dodgeville? Well, come on. We're going to Dodgeville." And she marched out of the command center.

During the twenty-mile drive to the hospital in Dodgeville, Susan got more details about the tornado from the friend driving them. Nine people had been killed in Barneveld by the tornado, seven of whom were Susan's immediate neighbors, including her best friend, Jill, Jill's husband, and their eight-year-old daughter. Their infant son had survived but was permanently paralyzed from the waist down. Eighty-eight people in all had been injured.

Once at the hospital, Susan had to talk her way past the authorities to see Keith. They told her it wasn't necessary—he had already been formally identified—and it wouldn't be good for her. (Every bone in Keith's body had been broken.) But Susan would not be swayed.

When she finally pushed open the doors of the morgue, Susan saw nine corpses covered head to toe with white sheeting. On one gurney, the sheet had slipped to the side a bit and she could see a man's elbow. No, not just a man's elbow. Keith's elbow. It was Keith's. Susan's heart tilted, and the energetic and assertive face she had been putting on began to crack. It wasn't until later that Susan realized that the other eight bodies in the room had been her friends and neighbors.

In the days that followed, Susan became more and more depressed. The town had been opened to residents, but she had little desire to see what could be saved. In early July, *People* magazine ran a photo-essay on the resilience of Barneveld's plucky citizens, who were continuing to get married, give birth, meet the weekly payroll, and rebuild their silos in time for the haying season and their school in time for fall.[7] Susan read the article and wept. She wasn't feeling "plucky"; she was going through the motions.

Unfortunately, one of Susan's impediments to her recovery was her own self-sufficiency. She was able to ignore the destruction of her home by focusing on what she had to do. She was able to cope with the loss of Keith the same way. But not taking sufficient time to grieve, partially because she had to take care of her son and pick up the pieces of her life for his sake, left the wounds unhealed. She had decided to stay in the area for another full year, until Ernie graduated from high school. They had found an apartment (with a basement) in Mount Horeb, twelve miles from Barneveld, but they were miles she would rarely travel. Without the support of her friends and neighbors in Barneveld, she was left to find her own way in isolation. Rather than explore her fears and sorrow with others who could understand and sympathize, she walled them off. After she had done what she could to salvage her belongings, Susan focused strictly on the future.

However, the weather didn't cooperate. June, July, and August brought many summer storms, a number of tornado warnings, and another tornado (which touched down a half mile from Susan and Ernie's new place). The two of them spent most nights sleeping on pallets they had rigged up for emergencies in the southwest corner of their cellar, trying to ignore the chillingly reminiscent sound of high winds howling through the eaves. Each storm compounded the feeling of chaos and lack of control. The repeated exposure did not help; instead, the real lack of safety linked to each storm drove the problem deeper and deeper.

Everyone from Barneveld, whether he had suffered losses or was one of the few lucky ones, was encouraged to get psychotherapy. Susan made an appointment with a therapist who was covered by her medical plan. When the therapist asked her how she was doing, Susan told her that she was terrified of storms and that the sound of high winds set her heart racing.

"I think you're doing really well," the therapist said. "I could treat you—we have treatment for people with irrational fears—but your fears aren't irrational."

Susan smiled. To her mind, the psychotherapist had just confirmed that she was handling her losses the right way: taking care of business in the present, doing what she needed to, and not looking back. It would be years before Susan realized that the therapist was probably not trained in working with victims of natural disasters and that "handling it" wasn't the way to handle it at all.

After Ernie graduated from high school and started college, Susan decided to move back to her hometown, where her parents lived and where she and Keith had spent their first fourteen years together. Once she got settled, her life improved. She got a job as secretary to the controller for a defense contractor and began to put her life back together. Several years later, she met and married Sam Rafferty, who came from a big Irish Catholic family.

⁓

Talking over the terrible events with George Dunn helped Susan begin to understand how the aftermath of the tornado that destroyed her life ten years before was creating fresh chaos for her now. The convergence of factors, including the extreme stress in her life and the storm outside, had been sufficient to tip the balance and launch her into that first panic attack. Then the fear had taken on a life of its own. She understood it now, but month after month, she continued to have panic attacks.

One day she heard a news story about a rape victim whose panic and other traumatic symptoms had been successfully treated with EMDR. Susan was interested. If she could just get enough insight or a little relief from her persistent panic attacks, she could make more progress in her regular therapy. It was September 1994, and Susan had been suffering from panic attacks for four and a half years. She located an EMDR clinician and scraped together the cash—Susan's medical insurance wouldn't cover it—to pay for the five or six sessions, ninety minutes each, that the therapist had estimated would be needed.

Susan's EMDR therapist was a licensed professional counselor named Beverly Schoninger, who had been practicing psychotherapy for six years. The first time Susan and Beverly met, Susan spent the session filling Beverly in on her history. When she came to the part about the tornado, her face flushed and she started hyperventilating. Susan was on the verge of having a panic attack right there, but she kept on telling her story in vivid detail. During this narrative, it came out that Susan had once wished their house would blow away so they could get the insurance money and start new lives.

Beverly diagnosed Susan as suffering from panic disorder. As an EMDR therapist, she registered the need not only to change Susan's beliefs about the panic and teach her the appropriate skills to deal with her feelings and physical sensations, but also to address the pivotal event that precipitated her panic response.

Before their first ninety-minute session was over, Beverly had taught Susan how to create a safe place inside, where she could go to calm herself when intense feelings came up. Susan pictured her bed from childhood, which had been her own little corner of the world. Made of fruitwood, the bed was part of a Queen Anne–style bedroom set given to her by her parents when she was ten. Beverly had Susan imagine the bedroom and experience the feelings of safety, and then she used sequential sets of eye movements to help strengthen the positive emotions.[8] Soon Susan was able to bring up the image on her own and have the positive feelings emerge strongly along with it. With this tool, Susan could let go of any feelings of disturbance that came up during the session, and she could use it also if any distress arose outside of Beverly's office.

In their second session, the following day, Beverly asked Susan to fill out a questionnaire specifically about her panic attacks. In answer to the question, "What are the feelings, emotions, and sensations you most often experience?" Susan wrote, "Anxiety, lump in my throat, light-headedness, dizziness, spaciness, disorientation, pain in my chest, neck and shoulders, tingling in my hands and feet. And I'm very tired." In answer to the question, "When are you most likely to lose control of your body?" Susan's written reply was, "When something happens in my body I don't understand, pain that is not explained, or in crowded stores or at the office."

After completing the questionnaire, Beverly guided Susan through the safe place exercise once more. She wanted to be sure Susan could calm herself should she panic during EMDR.

In their third session, two weeks later, Beverly and Susan started delineating the target for reprocessing. Beverly began by asking Susan what "bad" lesson she had learned about herself from the tornado.

"I'm not in control, and I don't know who I am anymore. I'm not the person I thought I was." Susan picked up a pillow and positioned it carefully behind her head for support.

With great gentleness, Beverly asked, "Susan, do you have any feelings of guilt about what happened to Keith?"

"No. No, I don't feel guilty."

"Well, some people might feel guilty about this. You know, when people die, very often their loved ones feel it was their fault in some way, even if it wasn't. Even if it couldn't have been. Check deep inside. Let your gut answer, not your mind. Do you think you might have any feeling that it was your fault?"

"Oh!" Susan's eyes widened. There was a long pause, and then Susan said, "My gut does feel like that, like it was my fault, like I was the cause of Keith's death." Tears spilled down her cheeks.

"Okay," Beverly said, "so 'it was my fault' is the negative lesson you learned from the tornado. What would you like to believe instead?"

After a slight hesitation, Susan said, "Maybe . . . I did the best I could?"

"That's fine."

When Beverly asked Susan how true this statement felt right now on a scale of 1–7, Susan gave it a 3. (Beverly thought it was probably even lower but said nothing.) Susan rated her disturbing image of the event at an intensity of 8 on the SUD Scale of 0–10. She identified the negative feelings as sadness. When Beverly asked where in her body Susan felt this, she said it was in her chest and throat.

Concentrating on the body sensations is often the easiest way into the memory network. The mental image and the negative belief are sufficient to access the dysfunctional information, and attention to the body can allow the processing to occur without getting bogged down in too many verbalizations or self-recriminations. It is also especially important for the client to concentrate on physical sensations when dealing with panic disorders and phobias because the body itself has become such a constant source of fear. Susan could focus on these sensations fairly easily now because of the safe place exercise, but this was only the beginning.

The first target Susan and Beverly decided to work on was the night of the tornado. They would start with the moment Susan woke up and retrace her every step.

As soon as they began the eye movements, Susan started crying. She was reliving it all, moment by moment: being violently awakened by thunder and lightning, hearing the chilling wail of the tornado, trying to rouse Keith, speaking to Ernie, running to the window. When she reached the part when she was standing at the top of the basement stairs, Susan's face crumpled.

"What do you get now?" Beverly asked.

"I just realized that my sixth sense was wrong that night. It told me Keith was okay, but deep down I knew he wasn't. Deep down, I knew he was dead. I just couldn't stand the knowledge," Susan cried.

"Okay, see if you can stay with that."

Through set after set, Susan's emotions went down and up like a roller coaster, sometimes plunging into chest-tightening guilt, other times rising to an exhausted acceptance. "I didn't want him to die," she moaned, choking on her tears. Then, "I caused his death." With this came chest pain. A bit later, "I feel better." Breathing more easily. And back to, "Why didn't I die too?"

Susan was frustrated and angry with herself. She thought she should have been able to protect Keith because she was the one who knew about tornadoes; she'd grown up with them. A little later, Susan came upon a fresh wave of guilt welling up in her throat because the tornado had broken every bone in Keith's body, whereas she had walked away without a scratch.

Guilt at having survived is a common response to the death of a loved one, especially during tragedies such as these. We also see it in combat veterans and emergency personnel who wanted to help but had no power to save the victim. Knowing intellectually that there was nothing to be done is not sufficient. Our emotions just don't follow logic, as we wish they would, and it's our emotions that ultimately lead the way.

After their final set that day, Susan told Beverly, "There's a piece inside about my being a no-good person." She shook her head. "It doesn't make sense to me. I don't know where I got this stuff that I was bad." Working through her guilt with the eye movements, Susan had arrived at its toxic core: shame, the feeling that we have not only done something bad but that we *are* something bad.

By the end of the session, the intensity of Susan's guilt had dropped considerably, from an 8 to a 5; however, because of the shame she felt, her desired positive belief that she had done the best she could had diminished from 3 to 2. Most of the time using EMDR, a person's positive belief increases as her negative feelings decrease. Not this time. This was the first time Susan consciously realized that her abiding belief that she had done the best she could for Keith was a facade and that it always had been. EMDR made her see that behind that facade, Susan had always felt guilty about Keith's death. In addition, other aspects of how she might have failed him were coming to the surface. Therefore, the level of truth in the positive belief Susan stated at the beginning of the session ("I did the best I could") had, in fact, dropped.

This is an example of the fact that EMDR will not make someone believe anything that is not true. Part of the natural healing process is for people to take the appropriate level of responsibility for what happened and work it through. In Susan's case, more processing was needed, but all the work could not be done in one session. However, once the processing begins, people often continue to make spontaneous changes.

Beverly scheduled another session with Susan for two days later. She didn't want her sitting with a significant level of distress (a 5 on "it's all my fault") or a low level of self-esteem for too long. But when Susan arrived for her next session, she was a lot calmer, and she reported having no panic attacks since doing EMDR the last time.

"Do you remember the negative belief we ended with last time?" Beverly asked her.

"Yes. It was, 'I believe the tornado was my fault.' You know, in my conscious mind, I had no idea that feeling was in me. I'm way too smart to believe something that irrational. But there it is."

"Check your gut feelings now about that. How intense are they? From 0 to 10?"

Susan closed her eyes for a moment, then replied, "It's a 2. I've been thinking about it a lot, and I feel much better, as if I've been processing this stuff ever since."

Susan was quiet for a moment, then she said in a sad voice, "But I should have been able to make Keith understand the seriousness of the situation." A long pause. "Someday he would have learned to listen to me."

"So that's sadness."

As if in reply, tears streamed down Susan's cheeks.

"Let's do some eye movements on that statement, 'I should have been able to make Keith understand.'"

As they did so, the intensity of Susan's grief increased from 8 to 9 to 10. Her positive cognition still hovered at 2. She told Beverly she was feeling sadness and frustration—"Why did he leave me alone?" she cried—and that she felt it in her chest and her throat.

After several more sets, Susan became calmer.

"It was a choice he made," she said. "It had nothing to do with me. Our soul chooses."

"Stay with that and follow my fingers."

After that set, Susan said, "I can take care of myself," and started crying again. "But it was his choice to live or die, and he was ready to go."

Another set.

"I'm feeling sorry for myself."

Another set.

"I'm rationalizing now; I'm feeling abandoned by my family. They've pretty much dismissed what happened to me."

Susan's distress had now dropped to 2 or 3. Then she said, "I feel guilty about the money. I benefited: We had homeowners' insurance."

Another set.

"I do feel he did the best he could. He was a dreamer, you know, 'Don't think about it and it will just go away.' I was the practical one."

After another set, Susan asked, "What is there about me that I can still trust?"

"What do you mean?"

"I'm not the person I thought I was. I'm not the totally competent person who handles things and gets things done. That was the basic me. Now . . . who am I, anyway?" It was a profound question. She had to come to grips with the fact that, ultimately, we cannot control it all.

The last set. After this one, Susan rated her distress at 0, and said that her positive cognition ("I did the best I could") now felt like a 7, completely true.

Three days later, Beverly and Susan had their final session, a half-hour follow-up. Susan seemed almost to float into Beverly's office. She said she was feeling great, even though she had had one minor panic attack, "in a store, of course," she added. But processing had continued after the experience and it was now clear to her that the attacks had occurred in busy stores because of the fear response to the stimulus of several environmental cues that she associated with being in the tornado: the high shelves overhead stocked with goods (like those that had lined her basement walls), the din (like the chaotic noise of the house being ripped away by the twister's three-hundred-mile-an-hour winds), and the turmoil of so many things happening at once on all sides. But another trip to a store showed her that the power to devastate her was now gone.

"The things that were happening in my body don't happen anymore," Susan told Beverly. "Even at work, where I'm now doing the job of two people, I can let things roll off my back."

A broad smile broke across her face. "I still don't like those big mega-stores, but I think I'm allowed to not like them. I don't have to have a panic attack over it."

6

When Terror Stalks the Night: Sleep Disorders and Childhood Trauma

You can't turn off the darkness, but you can turn on the light.

—OLD SAYING

MY ORIGINAL THEORY connecting EMDR to REM sleep seemed even more reasonable when I discovered that disrupted REM sleep is considered a marker of PTSD.[1] Victims wake up in the middle of nightmares, often sweating or screaming in the middle of their traumatic experiences. We do not yet know whether these dreamers are awakened by their physiological reactions to the nightmares (racing heart rate) or by an overload of the sleep mechanism that might normally enable them to master their upsetting experiences. Either way, the dreamer is stuck. Perhaps doing the rapid eye movements in a conscious state allows people to progress further in their recovery than they can during sleep.

Researchers have investigated the physiological phenomena of sleep since the middle of the last century.[2] One tool they have used is the electro-encephalogram (EEG), a device that records the electrical activity of the brain. The EEG has shown that there are several different stages of sleep. Stages 1 through 4 are called non-REM sleep, or NREM. The REM state, which alternates with non-REM sleep, is characterized by a rapid back-and-forth movement of the eyes. Eugene Aserinsky and Nathaniel Kleitman,[3] who first identified this phenomenon in 1953, did pioneering research in this, discovering that if they woke people during REM sleep, 80 percent reported vivid dreaming. The same types of vivid descriptions were not given during non-REM states. In fact, if subjects were awakened during other stages, they usually reported no memories of dreaming. A minority reported some experiences but without the vivid or storylike imagery. Later research suggested that there may be more dreamlike activity in non-REM states than originally thought, but non-REM states do not provide the rich, personally referenced stories we normally associate with dreaming. For all intents and purposes, what occurs during Stages 1 through 4 is not dreaming as we know it.

EEG readings indicate that brain waves during REM sleep are very much like those of the normal waking state. However, REM sleep is also called *paradoxical sleep* because, although the brain appears activated and alert, the muscles of the dreamer are flaccid and relaxed. These two findings seem interesting in light of observations during EMDR treatment. Clearly, the client is alert and aware during EMDR sessions, but perhaps part of the successful processing entails linking into physiological parasympathetic systems that cause muscles to be relaxed. Research has indicated that the saccadic eye movements generated by the midbrain and the muscle relaxation caused by the reticular formation occur simultaneously during REM. It may be that the pairing of the two is responsible for a deconditioning effect.[4] Perhaps the same two associated mechanisms are stimulated by the externally induced, rhythmic eye movements of EMDR and are the cause of the "compelled relaxation response" identified by David Wilson and others using biofeedback equipments.[5]

In light of work with EMDR, it is interesting to see that research has established a link between REM sleep and a variety of psychological complaints.[6] Although REM sleep and the four stages of non-REM sleep continue in ninety-minute cycles throughout the night, the amount of time proportionately devoted to REM sleep appears to lengthen as the night progresses. Depriving people of REM sleep can cause a variety of reactions including irritability, increased anxiety, and disorientation. The dream state appears so necessary that when dreaming is disrupted, according to sleep deprivation studies, the sleeper shows a "rebound effect," or an increase in dream time on subsequent nights. It is possible that trauma victims who wake in the middle of REM sleep are caught in a vicious cycle, in which the sleep deprivation itself makes them more anxious.

The purpose of dreaming has been debated for decades. Freud theorized that dreams were unconscious wishes that emerged during sleep, when they could not be repressed.[7] He believed that the psyche soft-pedaled the violent and erotic nature of these wishes by disguising them with symbols so that the dream would not be too disturbing. On the other end of the spectrum are those who believe that dreams are merely random brain activity.[8] These researchers initially suggested that the disjointed images that arose in dreams were caused by the random activation of various parts of the cortex and that the dreamer's brain simply attempted to synthesize or make sense out of these random phenomena. But this theory was revised[9] because it did not stand up for long against common sense: It did not explain repetitive dreams and the fact that many of our dreams include the easily explainable content of our daily experiences.

The sleep theorist whose work is most compatible with EMDR's Adaptive Information Processing model is Jonathan Winson,[10] who believes that mammals process survival information during the REM state. Much of Winson's research is based on animal studies that show that a specific brain activity (a theta rhythm in the hippocampus) is generated when the animal has experiences related to its well-being or survival (foraging, scanning the environment for danger) and during REM sleep. Winson suggested that during REM sleep, what the animal has experienced during the day is synthesized and stored in memory to help it survive in the future.

Similar correlations have been reported between emotional memory processing and theta activity during REM sleep, and it is interesting to speculate that the rhythmic eye movements used in EMDR stimulate a process connected with the rhythmic theta waves identified in other mammals.[11] Although the possible connection is highly speculative, there is no doubt that emotional and cognitive processing occur during EMDR. The person integrates the information about the upsetting event ("I am in danger") by processing it and then storing it with a more appropriate emotion ("It's over. I am safe now").

The idea that similar processing of emotional information occurs during REM sleep is supported by a number of studies on both animals and humans. Research has demonstrated that emotional memory benefits from sleep and that this benefit correlates both with the amount of REM sleep and with local theta power during that sleep.[12] Also, studies have shown that depriving subjects of REM sleep after they have learned a specific skill results in loss of that skill or retarded learning. Given that people who dream about the memory show more memory improvement after sleeping,[13] it seems reasonable that dreams generally reflect the adaptive integration of material, whereas nightmares indicate insufficiently processed events. It is clear that trauma negatively affects sleep and can even damage the hippocampus, the part of the brain most closely identified with memory.[14] In turn, perhaps the eye movements in EMDR reopen an apparently crucial window of REM-like activity needed for integration and learning to take place.

Research has also shown that the amount of rapid eye movement is related to the intensity of the negative emotion in dreams.[15] The angrier the person is, or the more disturbed, the more rapid eye movements occur. What all this seems to suggest is that REM sleep enables emotional processing, which is certainly paralleled in EMDR. Clients begin with feelings of shame or guilt and progress to anger, acceptance, or forgiveness. In addition, EMDR clearly processes experiential information, as is the case with REM sleep. That is why dream images seem to make perfect EMDR targets. For instance, one woman complained about a nightmare in which she was being chased by a monster through a cave. We targeted the image, and after a couple of sets, the symbolic overlay peeled off and she said, "Oh, that's my stepfather chasing me through my childhood home." When a recurring nightmare image is targeted with EMDR therapy, people generally uncover the real-life experience involved and process the incident, and the dream does not recur.

Another parallel between EMDR and the REM state is that a vast amount of learning can take place in a very short period of time. Although REM states last only between twenty minutes to an hour at a time, dreamers can feel that they have lived a whole day's experiences. Likewise, processing occurs rapidly with EMDR, and numerous events can unfold with each set. A person targeting a hurricane or car accident generally jumps from one salient element of the experience to another, without having to see the whole event occur. Just as in a dream, the experience is rapid, and it is unique for each individual.

All of this speculation is intriguing, but it is not proof. As the science of neurobiology progresses, we may learn that what happens during the REM state is merely a good analogy to what occurs during EMDR. Because much more than eye movements are involved in EMDR, at the least we can expect that any one theory will not explain all of the treatment effects.

However, one thing we do know is that EMDR can have a profound effect on the sleep disturbances of trauma victims of all ages.

Although the exact function of REM sleep remains open to debate, it has been found that infants spend nearly 50 percent of their sleep time—approximately eight hours a day—in that state. Because adults spend only about two hours per night in REM sleep, many researchers assume that the extra REM time infants spend serves to stimulate the nerve growth they need to develop normally.[16] It is not until they reach about the age of two, when the hippocampus is believed to be mature enough to store distinct memories, that the adult REM pattern emerges. Because the hippocampus is not fully functional in infants, some researchers have conjectured that children do not retain much of their earlier experiences; others speculate that a person's early experiences have no bearing on their later development.

These interpretations, however, do not jibe with clinical findings about early childhood trauma and deprivation.[17] Not only can severe stress inhibit brain development, but traumatic early childhood events can set a dysfunctional pattern that can continue into adulthood. Sometimes these events have to do with the child learning that no one will come to rescue him from his fears. Although few things are more disturbing to most people than the despairing cry of a child at night, sometimes the parent is unwilling or unable to help still the child's pain. The terrors this situation can inflict on a child can have a hazardous effect on the psyche. Neurobiologists such as Joseph LeDoux, who has long studied the substrates of emotional memory, have indicated that although some events may not be stored in visual or verbal memory, they are nonetheless stored on a sensory or feeling level.[18] Early experiences of deprivation or distress may not be visually remembered or verbally expressed, but they can be deeply and devastatingly felt.

In the present and the following chapters, I explore how children react to disturbing experiences and the various ways they can be treated with EMDR therapy. In the first case, a child is stalked at night by fears he cannot describe or define. We see clearly that just because a child cannot verbalize his experiences does not mean he is unaffected. Although many daytime fears can be ignored or brushed aside, the special cry of the infant to attract care and solace at night evokes a powerful automatic pull in every species.[19] The parents also need the balm of sleep; perhaps the disruption to their own rest has lifesaving properties for the infant (and the species) by forcing them to find a solution to the child's problem.

Claire Tibbett sat in the hospital waiting room, tapping her foot on the worn linoleum and trying to feel calm and confident. Her husband, Jack, sat at her side. Down the hall their fourteen-month-old grandson, Davy, whom they were raising as their own, was undergoing cleft palate surgery, the second major operation in his young life. Claire carefully closed the paperback she'd brought and tucked it into her purse. Her mind couldn't stay with the plot. It kept returning to the present: to the operation and to Davy.

Ten months ago, she and Jack had sat in this same room, waiting for their adopted son to emerge from his first plastic surgery, an operation to repair his cleft lip. When four-month-old Davy was finally brought out to them, he had splints on both arms (to keep him from touching his stitches); he wore a U-shaped metal mouth guard; and blood caked his lips. Tears filled Claire's eyes at the memory. Sometimes people asked her and Jack why they were taking on another child—and one with birth defects to boot—now that their three were finally grown. The answer was simple, though hard to explain. Although Davy came into this world with several strikes against him, he was full of love. Even at four months old, he would cuddle up and bury his face in her neck when she cooed at him. Claire liked the way Jack always expressed it. "Davy gives far, far more than he takes." What a joy he'd become in her life, and what a surprise!

"Mr. and Mrs. Tibbett?" A nurse's tense voice interrupted Claire's memories.

"Yes?" Claire leaped to her feet, knocking her purse on its side. Jack rose slowly and curved an arm around her waist.

"Please come with me to the recovery room. We need your help with Davy."

Davy's anesthetic had worn off and he was awake and crying, very scared and very shaky. He'd kicked the IV out of his leg. The nursing staff could not get him to calm down. Claire went to her son, picked him up, and held him gently, patting him repeatedly on the back. Davy clamped his arms around her neck and hung on for dear life. He refused to be put down. When Claire's arms got tired, Jack took over. Davy had been given a large dose of a sedative so he would sleep, but the moment he drifted off and his parents tried to lay him down, he woke up screaming. Even with Jack and Claire there, the nurses could not get Davy onto the gurney to wheel him back to his room. Eventually Claire carried him herself, Davy gripping her more tightly than ever.

Davy couldn't tell his "mom" and "pop" what was the matter, but something was clearly wrong. The child was utterly terrified. Jack and Claire stayed at the hospital and held Davy in their arms for seventy-two hours straight while the little boy slept off the effects of the surgery. At least he's getting the rest, Claire thought. And when we get home, things will be better.

His first night home, Davy had to be patted to sleep. About thirty minutes later, he woke up screaming. Claire and Jack went to him, held him, soothed him, but Davy kept on screaming. He didn't seem to hear them or recognize them, and he had no words for what was happening inside, just wild shrieks of terror. Eventually, after nearly an hour, Davy quieted down and let himself be patted back to sleep. Though Claire and Jack didn't know it at the time, this was to become a heartbreakingly familiar routine in the months to come.

Davy was having night terrors. Night terrors are similar to sleepwalking in that the sufferer may appear to be awake but is not. Davy would sit up in bed, eyes open, and scream. Jack and Claire thought he was awake and were confused and upset that he did not calm down when they tried to comfort him. They didn't realize that, according to some writers who experienced night terrors as children,[20] attempts to restrain and comfort the child can be frightening because the parents are entering the child's horrifying dream-world. In an irony of evolutionary process gone wrong, instead of having his pain dispelled by dream sleep or finding comfort in his parents' touch, Davy was being traumatized over and over again.

ᖇ

Night terrors are more intense than nightmares. Unlike dreams, they do not take place during REM sleep, and the child does not remember them in the morning. It has been suggested that it is a disorder in which the cognitive content that should be dealt with in REM sleep overflows to the wrong sleep state.[21] In fact, the treatment effects of EMDR have offered researchers a possible explanation for the horrific emotions experienced by the victim.[22] Perhaps the terror is so intense because the possible deconditioning properties of the rapid eye movements (linked to the muscle atonia) found in the REM state are not available during the night terror to help process the information.

Experts writing in the popular press disagree on the causes of night terrors,[23] but because there is no known cure, parents are generally advised just to wait until the child "grows out of it," usually sometime between ages five and twelve. Unlike most children's night terrors, however, which last from ten to thirty minutes, Davy's went on for nearly an hour. Sometimes when Jack and Claire tried to touch and reassure Davy, he would lash out at them, his little arms and legs flailing, seeing not his parents but the monsters in his mind. These were not the occasional bouts that the magazines said were normal in children, and Claire felt the situation merited immediate attention. She took Davy to a pediatrician to see if her son's nightly screaming was caused by physical pain. But the doctor could find no physical cause for Davy's outbreaks.

As the weeks passed, Claire noticed other problems. Besides being afraid to go to sleep (he had to be patted to sleep at nap time, too), Davy was scared to be alone. Before the second surgery, Claire was able to put Davy in his playpen in the living room and go into the kitchen to clean up or start a meal. Davy would be fine as long as he could hear Claire moving around. Now, if Claire so much as stepped out of sight, he screamed and burst into tears. In addition, if Davy woke up during a nap or during the night, he would be so frantic to find his parents that he would literally lean over the edge of his baby bed until he fell onto the floor. It was the only way he knew to get out. Eventually, Jack built Davy a bed at floor level so he could get up without hurting himself.

Davy had also developed a fear of the dark and of strangers, neither of which had particularly upset him before the cleft palate surgery. Even more distressing, he had started banging his head against the wall. In fact, Davy seemed so different in so many ways, some indefinable, that about three weeks after the operation, Claire found herself telling one of the surgeons, "It is almost as if I've got a different boy. What's next? It's nothing, but it's everything. He's just different. He's afraid of the dark. He's afraid to go to sleep all of a sudden." The surgeon said that perhaps the boy came to a little bit during the operation, but that, whatever it was, Davy would probably outgrow it.

This was the first of a legion of unhelpful opinions Claire got from the medical professionals she talked to about Davy in the coming months. Other responses included, "It's your imagination," "you're overprotective," "they [Davy's symptoms] are not real," "you're exaggerating," and even "you're making the situation worse by harping on it." The ordeal left her feeling confused, helpless, and very afraid for her little boy.

Over the next year, Davy's night terrors came less frequently, two or three times a week instead of every night, but his other symptoms remained, and new ones developed. One day Claire had driven him to a mall to have his photo taken, and he'd started screaming the minute the photographer's floodlights came on. She also found out he was terrified of being wrapped tightly in clothing. About a year after Davy's fears began, the Tibbett family moved from Georgia to Colorado. It was January when they arrived, and Davy had never seen snow before; like any child, he was entranced. But the moment Claire bundled him into his first snowsuit, he started screaming. The move to Colorado and being in unfamiliar territory had turned up the heat on Davy's night terrors, too. Now they were coming once or twice every night.

In hindsight, Claire can see how all these symptoms pointed directly to what had happened during Davy's cleft palate surgery, but at the time no one could see the forest for the trees. All along, Claire had been asking Davy what was wrong, but he wouldn't, or couldn't, say. (In fact, for a period of time after the operation, Davy lost his ability to talk, a reaction not unusual in very young children who have had surgery.) Claire and the medical professionals she consulted could not figure out what was happening. Davy, now two and a half, had a lot of different symptoms that had to be accounted for.

For example, he would sometimes bang his head and stare into space, causing one doctor to note in Davy's file that he had autistic tendencies. A psychologist tested Davy and found he was developmentally delayed—a full year behind other children his age in acquiring language and other skills. Another noticed Davy was hyperactive, made poor eye contact, and had an extreme attention deficit. She inquired as to whether Davy's birth mother had used alcohol or drugs during pregnancy. Claire said *yes*, her teenage daughter had drunk while carrying Davy, but she didn't know how much. Taking this fact together with the existence of Davy's birth defects—the cleft lip and cleft palate—a neurologist at Children's Hospital in Denver diagnosed Davy as having fetal alcohol effect, a milder version of fetal alcohol syndrome. This diagnosis, an accurate one, explained a lot of Davy's behavioral and developmental problems, but it did not explain his night terrors, extreme fears, and head banging.

Claire had not forgotten what the surgeon back in Georgia had said, however, and she moved heaven and earth to get copies of the operating-room reports from the hospital where Davy had been treated. When she finally obtained them, a former surgical nurse she knew explained them to her. The nurse skimmed the transcript from the operation and carefully unrolled the readouts from all the various monitors Davy had been hooked to.

"There's something here."

"What?" Claire asked urgently.

"He came to."

"He what?"

"Davy regained consciousness during the surgery. It's not that unusual with kids, especially hyperactive kids. Children metabolize anesthesia differently than adults do, and they try not to sedate a child that age too much because it's hard for them to come out of it." She unrolled another foot of the chart and pointed. "Yes, and here is where they sedated him again."

To Claire, this explained the pain and confusion of the past sixteen months. Of course, Davy was afraid of strangers and bright lights. Of course, he was afraid of being wrapped up in tight clothes, going to strange new places, or being left alone. Of course, he was afraid of being put to sleep. Now that they knew what was wrong, Claire felt sure they could help Davy outgrow his fears.

By this time the family was settled into their new home in Colorado. Davy's night terrors were still a serious problem, but Claire felt they were getting a grip on the situation. She was wrong. Jack was about to be assigned to an eight-week training stint in Alabama, and from the moment he left home, things got much, much worse. With Jack gone, Davy's night terrors escalated again. They were now coming two or three times a night. He would shake and babble and thrash around in the bed, screaming at the top of his lungs, "No! Don't! Stop! Get away from me!" The neighbors across the street called the police and reported Claire for child abuse.

A few nights later, Claire nearly went over the edge. She had been trying to hold Davy down during one of his night terrors so he would not hurt himself—ostensibly an easy task, because at less than forty pounds Davy was underweight for his age—when one of the child's wildly flailing fists hit her smack in the face. She ended up with a black eye and a despairing heart. Nothing she did seemed to be helping her little boy.

Besides being physically and emotionally bruised, Claire was exhausted. Each of Davy's night terrors lasted about forty-five minutes, and it took her another thirty to forty-five minutes to get him back to sleep afterward. With two or three episodes a night, every night, and without Jack to spell her,

Claire couldn't take much more. When it got so bad that she'd gone several days without any sleep at all, she finally cried out for help. "I was ready for a padded cell," she recalled. "I broke down in the doctor's office and told them everything."

The result was a referral to a psychiatrist, who, with Claire's information about what had happened during Davy's operation, recognized the child's myriad symptoms as PTSD, brought on by coming awake in the middle of surgery.

～

One of the saddest things about Davy's case is how long he suffered— eighteen months—before anyone was able to diagnose the cause of his numerous symptoms. Sad, but not surprising. The sheer range of Davy's fears, plus those behaviors stemming from fetal alcohol effect, must have been confusing to the people who tried to help him. How did his fear of the dark connect with his fear of bright lights? And what did snowsuits, nap time, and strangers, all terrifying to Davy, have to do with one another?

The breadth of Davy's fears is another example of stimulus generalization, in which a person develops extreme fear not only of the main event, so to speak, but also of all of the different stimuli that were present at the time of the trauma. In Davy's case, stimulus generalization caused him to develop fears not only of having surgery (a situation that didn't arise but that surely would have terrified him) but also of oversize bright lights, the absence of his mother and father, the presence of strangers, the feeling of having fabric wrapped tightly around him (like the sheets that secured him to the hospital gurney), and so on.

We see the effects of stimulus generalization in many PTSD cases. That's why a woman who has been raped jumps with fright when her husband comes up behind her unexpectedly when she's washing dishes. To an outsider, this reaction may seem extreme, but in the context of the stimulus generalization encoded into the woman's nervous system, her actions make perfect sense.

The good news about stimulus generalization is that there is a central trauma from which the client's constellation of symptoms stems, making the treatment relatively straightforward. Treat the core event with all of its sensory cues, and a diverse, generalized range of symptoms will often disappear. If some don't, one can easily target the remaining triggers in subsequent sessions. We see this pattern again and again in using EMDR therapy with trauma victims: Just because the symptoms appear pervasive does not mean the case has to be complicated.

Diagnosing Davy's problem was not the same as solving it, however. Just as Susan reacted automatically and physiologically to triggers associated with the tornado, Davy was doing the same to triggers associated with his surgery. But Davy couldn't reason with himself; he couldn't choose to avoid the triggers; and he couldn't communicate his problem. He couldn't express his panic and terror in any way other than screaming, crying, and clinging. He was a classic example of a child who had been traumatized, complete with sleep difficulties and separation fears. Even his head banging can be explained by his condition. Research studies have shown that this type of self-destructive behavior can be associated with fear and isolation.[24] Therapy sometimes helps, but Davy was too young to be treated using play therapy, especially because he was developmentally and verbally much younger than his thirty-three months of age. The psychiatrist tried prescribing nighttime sedatives, but they only served to delay the onset of Davy's night terrors; they did not reduce their frequency. He could see something had to be done quickly to help this family. The child's adoptive mother was exhausted and could not go on much longer without sleep. In a last-ditch effort, the psychiatrist referred Davy to a child psychologist he had met who was trained in EMDR therapy. Maybe, just maybe, it would work with Davy.

࿔

By the time the psychologist Dr. Robert Tinker met Davy and Claire Tibbett in August 1993, Davy had accumulated a battery of weighty diagnoses: PTSD, fetal alcohol effect, attention deficit hyperactivity disorder (ADHD), and developmental language disorder. Bob had been working with children since the early seventies and had been using EMDR with his young clients for nearly three years.

Bob grinned broadly at his first sight of Davy. With those wide-set eyes, upturned nose, shaggy dark bangs, and long thick eyelashes, Davy was adorable. Claire explained Davy's history, and Bob tried to talk with the boy. No luck. Davy did not reply. Next, Bob tried to get Davy simply to look at him, to engage in eye contact. No luck. Davy was not sullen, stubborn, or uncooperative, but his attention jumped from one part of the room to another, with frequent stops at his mother's face.

Bob's heart went out to the boy. Davy's speech problems, his hyperactivity, and his short attention span would make it impossible to use EMDR with him. How could Davy follow Bob's moving fingers if he could not keep his attention focused? How could Bob know if the child was thinking about the traumatic moment if Davy didn't speak? Later that day, Bob called the referring psychiatrist. "I've just seen Davy and Claire Tibbett," Bob said. "But there's not much I can do to help Davy right now. It'll probably be about a year before I can treat him using EMDR. He's got to be able to make eye contact and have a longer attention span for EMDR to work."

"Too bad. If this doesn't let up, I'm going to have to consider hospitalizing Davy for a time so Claire can get some sleep. She's right on the edge. She can't take much more."

By this time in its history, EMDR had already been shown, through numerous clinical reports, to be highly successful with children, even with toddlers as young as two years. Of course, the procedures had been adapted to take into account the fact that children don't have the verbal skills or the attention span of adults. EMDR clinicians had gotten children to do the eye movements by holding their attention with finger puppets or toys moved back and forth in a left-right-left pattern. In Davy's case, Bob Tinker had to invent his own variation, one that could grab, and keep, the attention of a developmentally delayed, hyperactive, and attention-deficit-disordered little boy.

Bob's mind raced. He remembered something in the EMDR training about working with kids, something about using hand taps or audio tones with people who couldn't do the eye movements. He set up another appointment for Davy to give this alternative approach a try. When he explained to Claire what he wanted to do, she talked it over with Jack. They thought it sounded a little odd, "but at that point," Jack recalls, "we were willing to try anything."

⁀

Bob's reaction was the same as that of some creative EMDR therapists who devised alternatives to the eye movements for clients with special needs. The first of these was Robbie Dunton, who wanted to use EMDR with learning disabled students who could not track the hand movement with their eyes and with shy or uncooperative children who wouldn't look up. Other clinicians, such as Priscilla Marquis, independently developed the same procedures for use with blind clients. Both found that the variations that worked best were doing hand taps that alternated from one of the client's upturned palms to the other and delivering audio tones in alternating ears.[25]

Bob Tinker had never tried either of these methods, but he knew from the EMDR training that the research on how the brain processes information was beginning to shed light on why the alternatives worked.[26] In one study, neuropsychologist Gregory Nicosia had examined a number of EMDR clients by using a technique called *quantitative electroencephalography* (QEEG), or color brain mapping. This procedure plots the electrical activity of the brain and allows the therapist to see the type of brain waves that are generated when a person thinks of a disturbing event. Nicosia reported that after EMDR, the brain waves of the right and left hemispheres go into greater alignment. He had suggested that the hormone norepinephrine, which is released during trauma, suppresses the REM state and causes the two hemispheres to go out of synchronization. He then conjectured that it was this misalignment of the hemispheres that prevented the brain from processing the traumatic event. What happened with EMDR, he argued, was that the rhythmic, repetitive eye movements resynchronized the right and left hemispheres by mimicking the "pacemaker" mechanisms in the cortex that exist for that purpose.

Although too few subjects had been studied to be sure of the resynchronization theory, it opened up an interesting area of investigation. It also called into notice an independent line of research that had begun ten years earlier and seemed to give the theory some support. In EMDR training, Bob had learned about the researchers in the United States and the Netherlands who had done controlled studies on the functions of the two hemispheres by examining the effects of gaze manipulation.[27] They found that when a person gazes at an object (such as a color photo of a nature scene) to the right, his response is more positive than when he gazes at the same object to the left. These studies were testing the hypothesis that the dominant hemisphere, which is activated when the normal right-handed person looks to the right, processes positive information and that the non-dominant hemisphere, which is activated when the same person looks to the left, processes negative information. Practical applications of this research might indicate that if you want to impress someone, you should sit to his right. The research also suggested that by alternating the client's gaze from left to right in EMDR, both hemispheres get activated.[28]

The researchers found that auditory and physical manipulation have the same effect. For instance, when an argument is piped into a right head-phone, the subject reacts positively. When the same argument is piped into a left headphone, the subject reacts negatively. It appears that the type of stim-ulation used is not as important as the act of shifting the person's awareness from one side to the other. With this research in mind, Bob Tinker began EMDR with Davy. He used a well-known childhood game and his own clin-ical intuition.

᷒

Davy was three months shy of his third birthday when he had his first EMDR session; he had been having violent night terrors for more than half of his short life.

Bob and Davy sat cross-legged on the floor of Bob's office. They were encircled by piles of toys: cars and castles and houses and airplanes strewn in a bright array of yellow, blue, and orange. Davy sat in sheer wonderment, his body half turned away from Bob, silently taking in the unimaginable abundance before his eyes.

Bob held up a piece of hard candy about twelve inches from Davy's face. "Watch this," he said brightly. "What is it? Look at it." Davy looked at the candy in Bob's hand for less than a second, then turned away. His big brown eyes were dark and wide and dreamy. His mouth was slightly open.

"Davy, watch this," Bob coaxed. "What is it?" Again, Davy glanced briefly at the candy before his gaze wandered off. "Good!" Bob said warmly.

Then he tried moving the candy from side to side in front of the child's face. "Davy, look at me. Watch this. Where does it go? Watch!" This earned him a third brief glance from Davy. "Good!" Bob cheered, giving Davy the candy. But not good enough, he thought.

Bob laid his hands lightly on Davy's shoulders. He had to get Davy to face him if this was going to work. "Look at me, Davy. Turn around this way a little bit. Yes, this way." Davy let his small body be turned toward the man in the metal-rimmed glasses. Now the two were squarely facing each other. Bob gently picked up Davy's left hand, turned it palm down, and used it to slap his own upturned palm.

"Look, Davy! Do that."

Davy looked down at the toys on the floor. Somehow he had managed to turn his body away from Bob again. Bob took one of Davy's small hands in each of his and turned them palm up. "Now hold out your hand, like this. Play a game," he urged, slapping Davy's left palm lightly with his.

"Okay, you do that to me." Davy gave an awkward slap that half missed Bob's outstretched palm. "That's good!"

Davy grinned widely and looked up with delight at his mom, who was sitting off to the side. Then he looked back at the floor. The EMDR session was two minutes old.

In fits and starts, Bob lured Davy into playing a simplified version of patty-cake, in which Bob held his own hands still while Davy slapped first one, then the other. It took a minute or so for Davy to get the hang of it. After every slap, Bob cried, "Good! Now this one!" and nodded toward his opposite hand. "Good! Now this one!" "Good! Now this one!" Gradually, Davy got absorbed in the game, smiling from ear to ear as he slapped Bob's hands left then right then left, the slaps coming louder and louder. Davy was delighted by the noise the slaps made, but no sound—not words or laughter—came out of his mouth.

After eight or nine successive slaps, Davy's attention started to wander, and he turned away. Bob carefully pulled Davy back to face him, took his hands, and started the game again. This time when Davy's attention wandered, Bob invented a variation: After each slap, he grabbed Davy's hand and cried, "Gotcha!"

Davy's whole face lit up, and he laughed out loud. Now this was a game he really liked! "Good!" Bob cried. "Faster!" "Faster!" Davy was going great guns now, slapping with his whole arm and laughing so hard he was falling all over himself, rocking back and forth after each slap as he tried to pull his hand back quickly so Bob couldn't catch hold of it. "Faster! Gotcha! Faster! Gotcha! Good, good! Gotcha!"

Five minutes from the time they sat down together, the EMDR session was over. Davy had learned the patty-cake game and, for brief stretches of time, had managed to alternate his attention from his left hand to his right and back again. "Great! Good job!" Bob said as he rubbed Davy's back in encouragement. "Okay, now you can go play!"

∽

In this first EMDR session with Davy, Bob was not even trying to get him to think about the targeted event. He focused on teaching Davy the muscle movements necessary to play the patty-cake game and on giving him a positive experience of both the game and of Bob himself. This preparation was especially important in Davy's case. Because he was developmentally delayed, he needed extra time to learn the left-right game, and Bob didn't want to risk opening up the blocked trauma (by speaking of the operation) until Davy had the skills needed to process it.

EMDR usually works with children more quickly than with adults. It appears that whereas adults may need ninety-minute sessions, a child can tap into and process a frightening memory in ten to thirty minutes. That's probably because children haven't had as many different experiences in their lives that have reinforced the original fear and their reactions to it. Even in situations in which there have been multiple assaults, a child's symptoms can often be relieved by focusing on one of the events. I once worked with a five-year-old who had been physically abused on several occasions. We concentrated on the most recent incident and the words "don't tell," which had been repeatedly said to her as a warning. She was soon laughing and calling EMDR her "magic." More important, one can generally tell if EMDR therapy has been effective with children because their symptoms disappear rapidly. Nightmares and bed-wetting, for example, may go away after one EMDR treatment.

In Davy's case, the left-right alternation of attention is a good example of how the information processing model works in treatment. By deliberately targeting a disturbing event, the processing taps into, and resolves, whatever feelings were dominant at the time of the original trauma. If the agitation Davy showed in this first session was a result of the trauma (rather than a symptom of attention deficit hyperactivity disorder), then Bob's patty-cake game would have connected, through that agitation, directly to the other aspects of the traumatic event. If that were true, we would expect to see some immediate improvement in Davy's night terrors and other fears.

⤳

Ten days later, Bob and Davy met for their second, and what turned out to be their final, EMDR session. This time they sat on chairs in Bob's office, far away from the distracting toys. Claire had told Bob that Davy's night terrors were a little less frequent since his first EMDR treatment and that he seemed different somehow, maybe quieter. Bob noticed the difference, too. Davy was still lively and still had a mischievous glint in his eyes, but he was calmer. He perched quietly on the edge of the grown-up-size chair, back straight, head up, and short legs dangling.

Bob got Davy to play the patty-cake game with little difficulty, shouting, "This one! This one! Harder! Harder! That's it!" as Davy slapped one of Bob's palms and then the other. Davy smiled quietly and turned to look over at his mom, but he kept on slapping. "That's it, Davy! Look at it," Bob called to get his attention back.

Davy had an expression of bemusement on his face, almost as if he knew something was going on but couldn't quite figure out what. After a couple of minutes, Davy's attention wandered again, and he stopped the game by asking Bob a question about something he saw on the bookcase behind him. Bob answered briefly, then started the patty-cake game again. This time Davy really got absorbed in what he was doing. His arms were moving methodically, and his mouth was pressed into a thin line of concentration. His eyes, unfocused but intent, were staring straight ahead at Bob's chest. Davy had gone into his own world.

When they were two minutes into the session, Bob stopped the game briefly and held on to Davy's hands. "Can you say . . . Davy, look at me." The boy's gaze had strayed to his mom. "Look at me. Can you say *bright light*?"

"Bright light," Davy echoed in a tiny but willing voice.

"Okay. Hit my hand!" An awkward slap. "That's it! Say it again."

"Big light," Davy said a little louder. Slap. Bob was astonished. He had asked the child to say "bright light," and he had responded with "big light." Somewhere inside that little head, it appeared Davy already had made the connection between what was happening in this room and his terrible experience in surgery.

"Say *bright light*," Bob repeated.

Davy complied. "Bright light." Slap.

"Say *big light*."

"Big light." Slap.

"Okay, hit my hand." Slap. "Big light."

"Big light," Davy said again. Slap. And again. Slap. And again. Slap. His face took on a serious, almost determined look. Bob kept Davy at it through seven or eight more repetitions of "big light" before the child's attention wandered and he stopped repeating the words. Now they were three and a half minutes into the session.

"Davy, can you say *hurt*?"

Davy grinned. "Hurt."

"Hit my hand." Slap. "Hit my hand." Slap. "That's it." Slap. "That's it." Slap. "That's it."

Davy's expression was thoughtful. He pumped his arms up and down rhythmically, his effort and concentration visible.

"Okay. Say *lip hurt.*"

"My lip hurt," Davy said promptly, and he slapped Bob's hand.

"That's it. Say it again."

Davy smiles. "My lip hurt." Slap.

"That's it. Now say *mouth hurt.*"

"My mouth hurt." Slap.

"That's it." Slap. "That's it." Slap. "That's it." Slap. "Good." Slap. "Good." Slap. "Good." Slap. "Harder!" Slap. "Harder!" Slap. "Harder!" Slap. "Harder!" Slap. "That's it!" Slap!

But Davy was starting to slow down. He looked over at his mom, his face blank.

"Now can you say *doctor*?" Bob persisted. Davy continued to stare wide-eyed in his mom's direction. "Look at me." No response. "Look at me." No response.

Finally Bob turned Davy's face gently toward him. Then he held up a hand with two fingers raised. "Watch my fingers," Bob said as he moved his hand horizontally at Davy's eye level.

Davy looked briefly at the funny movement Bob was making, then turned his head away again, this time in the other direction. It took Bob several tries to get Davy's attention again. When he had it, he held up both his hands at once and alternately raised and lowered his left and right index fingers. "Look at this," he coaxed. Davy looked and laughed at the new game, but now he was kicking his legs alternately against the chair and rocking his torso. Then his eyes wandered away. He had had enough.

Bob decided to end the session. Eight minutes had gone by. He thought Davy had begun to process his long-blocked surgery trauma, but he couldn't be sure. Bob hadn't used EMDR before with hand taps, and Davy wasn't verbal enough to tell the psychologist how he was feeling. Certainly, Davy showed some positive signs—saying "my lip hurt" and "my mouth hurt," for example—but was that enough? Bob didn't know. He asked Claire Tibbett to watch for any change and told her they would consider scheduling another EMDR session once they saw how Davy was doing.

A few days later, Claire called Bob Tinker. In an astonished voice, she told him that Davy's night terrors were gone.

Davy received a total of thirteen minutes of EMDR treatment, during which no one could be sure what was happening in the child's mind. Looking back at the treatment, Jack Tibbett says he is still "totally dumbfounded by the change that it made in the amount of time it took."

Bob Tinker agrees. "What happened in the sessions was not all that significant. What happened that was significant was the change in behavior that occurred afterward."

"I'll never forget that first night," Claire recalls shaking her head. "I woke up the next morning and panicked. I literally jumped out of bed! 'What's wrong?' Jack asked. And then he realized. 'Davy! Davy didn't cry!' We both went flying into his room to make sure he was all right. It was that scary: Davy slept all night; we slept all night; something must be wrong! But he was sound asleep. It was such a relief."

Claire and Jack had survived nearly two years of sleep deprivation and the agonizing heartache of not being able to help their terrified child. As for Davy, he had, at long last, survived the horror of coming to during the middle of surgery to find his body bound to the table, his eyes blinded by the operating-room lights, his mouth in excruciating pain, and his parents nowhere in sight.

Since his EMDR treatment, Davy has weathered further surgery and his father has gone away for another long stint of training, but the night terrors have not returned. Davy is able to go to sleep at night after a story and a kiss and he stays asleep until morning. He is no longer afraid of being alone. He's still not crazy about being bundled up in a snowsuit, but no more so than other little kids. As is usual with children, the positive effect of the EMDR treatment had generalized from the main target—the operation—to most of the associated fears Davy developed as a result of stimulus generalization.

Davy now sees other professionals to work on the developmental delays that stem from fetal alcohol effect. He also attends speech therapy sessions and goes to a developmental preschool. All of this work is helping Davy curb his hyperactivity, while his mom and pop get counseling on how to raise a hyperactive child. "He's much more like the little boy we knew before all this happened," Claire says with delight. The family is returning to normal.

Being treated by EMDR did not erase the terrible experience for Davy. Now five years old, he has started talking about what happened that day in surgery. He repeats the phrases Bob Tinker had him say during their session (like "bright light"), and he tells his mom that he lay on a bed and his mouth hurt. When one of Davy's counselors gave him a toy operating room, he assembled it perfectly, lay the doll in its hospital gown on the tiny operating table, and announced that *he* was the patient.

Recently Davy and Claire were snuggled side by side on the couch watching a TV program, when a scene in an emergency room came on. Claire tensed slightly, wondering what her son's reaction would be. Davy turned his velvet brown eyes on her, tugged her sleeve, and asked calmly, "Does his mouth hurt?"

Davy's sleep hasn't been disrupted since the EMDR session, and neither has his parents'. In their dreams, they are processing the everyday disturbances of childhood and parenting just fine.

7

The Ties That Bind:
Disorders of Attachment

We cannot live only for ourselves. A thousand fibers connect us
with our fellow men; and among those fibers, as sympathetic threads,
our actions run as causes, and they come back to us as effects.

—HERMAN MELVILLE

EMDR HAS OPENED a new window on the age-old debate of the relative
significance of nature and nurture. A person's physical and psychological
development is dependent on two factors—genes and environment—and
the interplay of these two factors has fascinated scientists for years.[1] For instance, there is a great deal of evidence that intelligence is initially based on
heredity, but no one denies that environmental factors also have an important impact. An innately bright child raised in a family that denigrates learning and education will generally show less ability than a child of average
intelligence who is raised in a more supportive family. Genes may determine
the potential levels of achievement, but a person's actual behavior seems to
depend on environmental experiences.

Because EMDR processes early life experiences, it can potentially allow
greater insight concerning the issue of which psychological problems are
based on heredity, or organic factors, and which are based on the environment. In this way, it may help to liberate people from prisons that were
thought to be genetic. For instance, early studies indicated that schizophrenia
is hereditary,[2] whereas later studies have clearly indicated that environment,

stress, and coping skills play an important role.[3] There is evidence that the children of schizophrenic parents can be prevented from succumbing to the disease if they are parented in a warm, positive, and stable environment and that they often become dysfunctional if they are not;[4] it will be important to see if EMDR can be used to reverse the negative effects of dysfunctional experiences with this population. Although EMDR cannot be expected to reverse the effects of heredity (such as a biological predisposition), it may be possible to process the environmental stresses that cause the manifestation of the disorder. A recent pilot study of EMDR therapy with psychotic participants reporting the elimination of hallucinations after trauma processing has indicated that this may well be true.[5] Heredity is not necessarily destiny!

Of course, EMDR will not be able to give definitive answers to every aspect of the nature versus nurture question. It's hard to determine the cause of specific traits, impairments, or behaviors, because people's experiences begin at the time of conception. Studies have shown that infants who repeatedly hear their mother's voice in utero, when tested after birth are able to distinguish that voice from other female voices.[6] Fetal environment also plays an important part in the child's physical development. (In Chapter 6, it was explained that Davy's nervous system was impaired by his mother's use of alcohol.)[7]

Biochemical conditions, whether caused by an experience in the womb or by genes, can play a part in children's capacities. An example is a child with ADHD (like Davy), whose difficulty concentrating is apparent very early in life. He may always have the biochemical tendency to be easily distracted; however, with medication (if it is found to be useful) and, more importantly, the proper education and support, the child can learn to cope with his disorder and lead a successful and productive life. On the other hand, if a child with ADHD is left too long without help, he will have a number of experiences that can reinforce his shortcomings and damage his self-image. The trauma and anxiety of failure lead to more difficulty concentrating, and the problem becomes compounded. The "failure experiences" perpetuate a cycle of lowering expectations and diminished success. The good news is that the negative effects of environment and experience can often be remedied with EMDR, and the sooner it is done, the better.

In Davy's case, only two EMDR sessions were necessary to turn things around. But Davy had had only one major trauma along with a happy family life and two parents who were devoted to him. Once his trauma was healed, he could start learning all the things he needed to know about having good relationships and succeeding in the world. But when early trauma is left untreated, its effects not only interfere with the person's life but also can undermine the next generation. Parents suffering from trauma can explode in violent fits of temper if unresolved feelings are triggered by present-day events, or they can emotionally shut down, becoming withdrawn and unavailable. No parent does this intentionally, but the consequences to a child can be devastating.

The next story illustrates how integrally (and unconsciously) parent and child are linked and that for EMDR to be effective, it must be woven into the entire clinical picture. Because the symptoms in this case presented a confusing spectrum of behaviors, the therapist needed to work as a detective to identify the right targets to focus on. The case also shows how strong the interaction is between nature and nurture; experiences that go directly against the survival mechanisms we are encoded with genetically can be directly responsible for the most chaotic, debilitating psychological effects. Bonding of mother and child is one of the first laws of nature, and it is clearly designed for the survival of the species. What happens when nature's law is broken and that mutual attachment doesn't take place?

∽

Dr. Joan Lovett took a deep breath, let it out gradually, and began to assimilate the confusion of symptoms she'd just heard about into a coherent picture of a little girl. What a tragic tangle. The exhausted woman sitting across from her might not be the most desperate mother she'd met in her twenty years as a pediatrician, but she was close.

Joan shut her notebook, lifted her head, and found herself looking straight into a pair of very frightened eyes. Okay, she told herself, here's what we've got. The child's name is Ashley. She is cute, blonde, and five years old. She's in kindergarten. Her mom thinks she will grow up to be a drug addict. Her grandmother thinks she ought to be put in a foster home. Her little brother thinks she's trying to kill him, and he's probably right.

The term *sibling rivalry* didn't begin to describe what Ashley felt toward her younger brother, Charlie, who was born a scant eleven months after her. Ashley hated Charlie with astonishing ferocity. She hit him frequently, leaving dark mottled bruises on his arms and chest, and she poked him in the eyes with her fingers. Recently, she had shoved Charlie clean off the top of their bunk bed, quite a fall for a four-year-old. Every day Ashley told her little brother that she hated him. When Charlie was wheeled off to the hospital with a severe asthma attack, Ashley told him she hoped he would die.

Ashley hated her mother, too. She wouldn't let her mom cuddle her, wouldn't make eye contact with her, wouldn't do even the simplest things, like put on her pajamas for bedtime, without a scene. Ashley had temper tantrums worthy of a tin-pot dictator, during which she threw things, screamed, cried, and vomited for half an hour at a time. She had recurring nightmares of animals biting off her hands, of threatening strangers, and of terrible accidents. Recently she'd stolen a bracelet from her baby-sitter's house and lied about it. She often bit her lips until they were swollen. One day she dug a razor blade out of the trash can and used it to cut herself. She was phobic to the point of terror about dogs and about doors closing; when Ashley's mother so much as opened the door to get the mail, the child started screaming.

The incident that pushed Ashley's mother over the edge and into psychotherapy had occurred six weeks earlier during the Thanksgiving feast at Ashley's kindergarten. All the parents had been invited for a holiday lunch served by their children. Ashley had picked up a plate piled with turkey and dressing, then walked swiftly over to her mother and pitched it at her. "I don't want you here!" she screamed. "I hate you!"

Joan Lovett felt real compassion for the woman sitting in her office. Maura Sullivan looked frightened, overwhelmed, and exhausted, but determined. At thirty-three, she was a single mother earnestly trying to get her life together while raising two young children on very little money. She was a recovering alcoholic and drug addict, and she blamed herself (and her use of heroin during early pregnancy) for Ashley's violent behavior. Maura's ex-husband, Charles, was an actor who had often been out of work during their marriage and more often strung out on drugs. He was also physically abusive. The night Ashley was born, Charles was picked up by the police, and Maura had to go through labor alone. When her newborn daughter was brought to her bed, Maura was too exhausted, too woozy, and too overwhelmed to spend much time with her. Looking back, she felt she had missed her chance to bond with Ashley after her birth and now it was too late.

Eleven months after Ashley's troubled arrival, Maura gave birth to a son. Ever the optimist, she named him Charlie, after his father. But by the time

Charlie was one and Ashley was two, their emotionally abusive, on-again, off-again father had abandoned the family for good. One scene from those days stood out in Maura's mind: Ashley balancing precariously on her pudgy legs, silently holding up her arms toward Daddy in the universal toddler gesture for "pick me up!"; her father turning and walking out, the door banging closed behind him.

"Those years were so hard," Maura explained to Joan. "I was close to an emotional breakdown. What with my husband's problems and me coming down from a two- to three-year run on speed [methamphetamine], I just wasn't there for Ashley. I mean, I know I took care of her physical needs—feeding her, changing her diapers, things like that—but emotionally I wasn't there for her. My God, I needed somebody, so I'm sure she did, too! She really didn't have her mom."

Maura shifted restlessly in her chair. "Dr. Lovett, I'm scared to death, and I don't know how to help Ashley. She can get so out of control. Then she'll be crying and Charlie will be crying and suddenly I'm crying, too; sometimes they are both so impossible I have to lock myself in my bedroom to give myself time out." Maura's sentences were tumbling out of her mouth in her passionate yearning to explain. "I'm trying to be a good mother. I love my children. I see they eat healthy meals; I keep them clean and get them all their shots; and I always treat them fairly. But it's not enough. It's not working. I don't know what else to do."

"What does treating them fairly mean?" Joan asked.

"Well, if one of them is hungry, I give them both a snack. If one of them is tired, I put them both down for a nap." Joan noted that a slightly didactic tone had crept into Maura's voice. "When one of them needs shoes, they have to wait until I have money to buy them both shoes. And when one of them has a birthday, I give them both presents. I never let one of them have something the other can't have. It wouldn't be fair. I think that's really important," Maura concluded almost aggressively.

"So it sounds like 'being fair' means that you treat the two children exactly the same."

"That's right. You have to treat all the children exactly the same." Maura paused and waited for Joan's response. Joan looked at her encouragingly but said nothing.

After an uncomfortably long silence, Maura went on. "If my parents had treated all of us fairly, we wouldn't have had a lot of the problems we had."

Joan quietly stood up, walked to a shelf on the far side of the room, and picked up a purple velvet pouch. She returned to her chair and offered the bag to Maura.

"Would you like to use the 'sticks and stones' game to show me more about your family? Inside this pouch are lots of colored stones. First you pick a stone for each member of your family of origin. Then you arrange the stones on this piece of paper, trace each one, and draw lines to show the bonds between the different family members."

Maura slid her hand in the pouch and fingered the smooth, highly polished stones. One by one, she dug out six stones and placed them just so on the paper. Mother, father. Both alcoholics. Herself, the oldest. Sara, three years younger. Stephanie, three years younger still. Finally, an adopted brother, Bill, ten years younger. Maura drew heavy lines showing strong relationships, wiggly lines for more tenuous connections. Joan watched with interest but said nothing. Maura seemed to be finished, but she had picked up the pouch again and was working it restlessly in her fingers.

"You know, I had a brother, another adopted brother. Before Bill." A long pause. "But he's gone." There was no emotion in her voice. Slowly the story emerged. When Maura was eight, her parents decided to adopt a six-month-old baby boy. They named him Shannon, and Maura fell head over heels in love with him, as only an eight-year-old girl can. Shannon was *her* baby. He had great big blue eyes and corn-silk hair. He smiled all the time. Maura thought he was the most beautiful baby in the world. She cooed over him, bottle-fed him, diapered him, and carried him everywhere.

One evening when Shannon had been with the family for about two weeks, they were all in the kitchen cleaning up after dinner. Maura's dad was putting away a cast-iron frying pan when it slipped from his hands and fell to the floor with a loud clang. In a flash, all eyes were riveted on the baby, ready to calm and comfort him. But Shannon didn't flinch. Maura's father picked up the frying pan and, watching the baby closely, banged it noisily against a pot. Still no reaction. Shannon just sat and stared. Maura's mother began to cry.

The next day Shannon was taken to Children's Hospital for testing. The doctor who examined the child found he was deaf and recommended further tests. Over the course of the next few weeks, Shannon was also diagnosed with cerebral palsy and digestive problems so severe he would have to be tube-fed. He would need extensive care. He wasn't expected to live beyond age three or four. Maura's parents decided to keep the bad news to themselves.

One day about two weeks after the incident in the kitchen, Maura came home from school and found that Shannon was gone. "My parents had given him back to the adoption agency," Maura told Joan without emotion. "They said Shannon would have to live in a home for the rest of his life and we couldn't afford that. They said the agency would find a family who could afford it. I never saw him again."

"How was that for you?" asked Joan.

"I'm sure my parents thought they were doing the right thing. You know what's strange?" Maura said, shaking her head. "I haven't thought about that since the day it happened."

"Tell me a little more, like how you feel about it."

"I don't feel anything," Maura declared. A moment later, she broke down and sobbed. The wall that had been holding back her pain for twenty-five years had finally been breached. Now it was crumbling.

⁓

One can only imagine the pain felt by an eight-year-old girl who has had "her" baby taken away from her and the terrible grief that drove her to close off her heart. Apparently, losing Shannon shattered Maura's ability to bond with the significant people in her life, including her own daughter many years later. Deprived of her mother's attachment, Ashley behaved accordingly; she showed no positive feelings nor made any loving gestures to anyone around her.

But it was not the loss of Shannon alone that set in motion this complex intergenerational pattern. The pattern was rooted in Maura's family background: her alcoholic parents, her unpredictable and uncontrollable home environment, and the erratic ways in which parental love was given and withheld. In this emotionally chaotic setting, Maura had found one stable object for her love—her adopted brother Shannon—only to have it wrested from her. Maura's reaction cascaded into the next generation. The impact could be seen in Ashley's angry behavior. Children tend to blame themselves for their parents' shortcomings. Not only do they feel unwanted, they feel that they deserve the treatment they get. When their innate need to bond is not fulfilled, children begin to feel that no one can be trusted and that nothing can be done to change the situation.

The complex interactions of nature and nurture radiate through the entire clinical picture. Some clinicians would note that Ashley's parents and grandparents were alcoholic, so that some of her characteristics were inherited.[8] Other clinicians would say her characteristics were biologically determined by her mother's prenatal alcohol and heroin use. Either analysis would paint a bleak picture of Ashley's chances for emotional health. Fortunately, EMDR clinicians like Joan emphasize the role of environment. For instance, Maura's ability to dissociate from emotional pain, which she had learned when Shannon was taken away, meant that Ashley had a particular kind of upbringing that is likely to spawn psychological problems.[9] The impact of having an emotionally unavailable mother is so great, according to a number of studies, that babies in this terrible situation have been shown to be at increased risk of death.[10]

Children who are traumatized in this way can become either passive or reactive. They may fill their emptiness with fear or anger, or both. The result can be a cycle of violent and inappropriate behavior that alienates the people around them. The more they act out, the more isolated they become, which reinforces their view of themselves as unloved and unlovable. Also, Ashley's tendency to hurt herself (biting her lips, cutting herself) is often seen in people who dissociate, some of whom use pain as a way to feel *something*, to remind themselves they are alive.[11] Self-injury may also be a much-needed distraction: The new pain takes the person's attention away from the old or existing pain or produces feelings of well-being through the release of endorphins.

Ashley's rage at her brother, Charlie, was probably based on several factors. First, Ashley had to share with Charlie what little caretaking their mother had been able to do. Second, she could have been acting out her pain at her father's desertion. Third, Maura unconsciously may have been using Charlie as a substitute for her beloved Shannon, whom she had lost so many years before. She might have been favoring and identifying with her son, thus causing Ashley even more pain.

Although all the problems in this family cannot be traced solely to Maura's loss of her brother, that event, in combination with Maura's general upbringing, certainly laid the groundwork for the patterns of parenting and emotional deprivation that prevented Ashley from forging bonds of attachment with those family members closest to her.

Maura had to process her memory of losing Shannon, going through the full range of attendant emotions (from grief to guilt to anger), before she could reconnect with her own capacity to love. This progression of feelings mirrors the natural healing process that was derailed at the time Maura's traumatic loss took place.

∽

While Maura cried, Joan thought about the devastating impact that losing her baby brother must have had on this woman. A full quarter of a century later, this early loss was affecting Maura's ability to parent her children. Joan knew that they would have to address Maura's residual pain before starting therapy with Ashley. Although Joan had been trained as a pediatrician specializing in children's behavioral problems, she believed in treating the parent as well as the child. She had seen too many parents whose own unresolved problems were reflected in the behavior of their children.

When Maura's sobs quieted, Joan told her about EMDR therapy and asked her whether she would like to use it in their next session to say good-bye to Shannon. Maura, who had been shocked at the intensity of her own reaction to the telling of Shannon's story, agreed.

When Maura returned to Joan's office for their first EMDR session, she brought with her a long typed poem she had written to Shannon as a way of finally saying good-bye. She told Joan that the day after their first session, she had taken a bike ride and thought about Shannon with tears running down her cheeks. "It felt good," she said with astonishment. "And if you hadn't taken out your pouch and asked me to pick a rock for each member of my family, I wouldn't have realized how I felt about Shannon. I wasn't going to mention him." But simply talking about Shannon and the relief she had felt was not enough. It did not change the underlying feelings that were poisoning Maura's relationship with her daughter.

Joan began the EMDR session by asking Maura to put into words the painful lesson she'd learned when she lost Shannon. Maura answered promptly, "I don't want to be close to anyone again." She rated the disturbing feeling that went along with it as having an intensity of 9 on a scale of 0–10. Next, Joan asked her to choose a positive statement that described how she would like to feel instead. Maura closed her eyes for a moment, then said tentatively, almost as if she were asking a question, "I loved him as well as anyone can love a brother, and now I'm free to love again." When Joan asked Maura to rate how true that statement was on a scale of 1 to 7, Maura shook her head and said it was only a 2.

"Let's start with the scene in the kitchen," Joan said. "See if you can bring that scene to mind as you follow my fingers with your eyes. Ready?"

Maura nodded gravely. Almost as soon as Joan started moving her hand back and forth, Maura's eyes filled with tears. All of a sudden she was eight again. She could hear the clang of the frying pan hitting the floor, feel the anxiety building in the room, see her mother's face crumple with misery. At the end of the set, Maura said through her tears, "My parents didn't feel they could take care of Shannon."

"Stay with that," Joan said softly, and she led Maura in a second set of eye movements.

"It was so lonely when he left. They were also relieved. My mom was crying, and lonely, and sad, but no one else even talked about it. Like when I came home and heard my grandfather had died. I thought, why isn't anyone crying for Grandpa? Our family didn't know how to grieve."

Another set.

"I wasn't going to allow myself to get involved again." Maura's sobs shook her whole upper body, but her tightly clasped hands remained almost maidenly on her lap. "And I didn't. Not till much later, way after we got Bill. He was hyperactive. I remember Mom asking Dad to give Bill his bottle and Dad punching her. Dad was drinking. I slept on the couch with Mom." Tears still streaming down her face, Maura shook her head back and forth, back and forth, her long black hair following a fraction of a second behind the swing of her head. "It was my fault about Shannon," she said miserably. "If I'd been home from school, if I'd been there, they couldn't have done it. I could have stopped them."

At this point in the EMDR treatment, Maura's information-processing system needed another jump-start. It is not unusual for people to get stuck in an undue sense of responsibility. To help Maura along, Joan combined the eye movements with a question designed to elicit a positive assessment. In EMDR, this is one variation of a procedure called a *cognitive interweave*. Its goal is to weave together the new, positive statement with the previously stored negative (or dysfunctional) information in the client's brain, so that it can be processed. When the therapist asks an appropriate question, the memory network containing the positive information is stimulated and it can connect to the target network. As we have seen (particularly with Eric when he realized he was not to blame for the Viet Cong prisoner's death), the positive and more adaptive information already exists internally. It simply may not be automatically accessible to the client in pain.

Joan started another set. While Maura was flicking her eyes back and forth, Joan asked, "Whose decision was it to send Shannon back?"

"My parents', but I could have stopped them."

Another set.

"Can an eight-year-old really make the decision to keep a baby?"

"No."

Another set. As the realistic information connected with the target being processed, Maura's false sense of responsibility, and her guilt, dissolved.

Now Maura was angry. She balled her hands into white-knuckled fists, one planted on each thigh, and set her jaw, her eyes still following Joan's fingers. "My parents weren't fair to Shannon! They would never have given away one of their own kids; why did they give him away? They should have treated him the same as us! It wasn't fair!"

Another set. Maura's anger had cooled, and she was imagining holding Shannon on her lap and talking to him in the way she wished she had been able to. She was telling him some of the things she'd written in her poem— and finally saying good-bye. "I'll always remember your smiling face. You'll always have a special place in my heart. When I look at the stars, I'll name one after you."

Another set. Maura stopped crying; she was breathing deeply and regularly. She told Joan she felt calm but at the same time keenly aware of all her senses: the feel of the nubby fabric covering the arm of her chair, the sound of cars rolling by outside. With eyes closed she said, "I loved him as well as anyone can love a brother. Now I'm free to love again."

"Stay with that." Another set.

Maura remained calm. "Maura," Joan prompted, "how upsetting does it feel now when you remember the scene in the kitchen? From 0 to 10?"

"Zero," Maura replied. She looked slightly puzzled with her answer.

"And how true does that statement feel, 'I loved Shannon as well as anyone could love a brother, and I'm free to love again'? On a scale of 1 to 7?"

"Seven," Maura said with a smile. "Definitely."

"Now you're also free to be fair by giving each of your children what they need. You're free to parent from a sense of protection and meeting your children's needs, not from a sense of guilt. Guilt brought you here, but you don't need guilt anymore to get yourself to be an effective parent."

Sixty minutes had gone by when Joan and Maura ended the only EMDR session they would ever do about Shannon. Joan could see the shift in Maura, hear the change in her voice when she spoke of the brother she'd lost. Maura was already a little bit brighter, a little bit happier. But the real winner from this session, Joan knew, was going to be Ashley, the desperately angry and lonely little girl whose mother had finally taken her heart out of deep freeze.

The following week—it was late January—Joan met Ashley for the first time. What she saw was a fair-haired little girl who was very pretty and very unhappy. When the two were alone together, Joan introduced herself and invited Ashley to sit on the floor with her. Ashley plopped herself down and looked around as if taking inventory. The playroom was crowded with bright plastic toys, paints, clay, stuffed animals, wooden blocks, and dolls.

For Joan, this first meeting with Ashley was to prove memorable. "It was a nightmare of an hour," Joan recalls. "Ashley went through everything in the playroom. Everything. She'd take the clay and break it up and say, 'That's no good.' She'd say, 'I want water.' We'd get water. She'd say, 'I don't want water.' She'd pick up a doll. Dress it. Undress it. Say, 'This is no good.' Start a game. Say, 'This game is boring.' Wanted her mother. Then didn't want her mother. Started a painting. Threw it out. Started another one. Tore it up. There was no real play; it was just messing around with one set of stuff and moving on to the next. She went through everything we have. I didn't really know what was going on, but what I did begin to learn in that first hour was what it felt like to be Ashley. Her experience of the world was that nothing was satisfying. Everything was disappointing. It was as if she were saying, 'I'm a disappointment. I can't do this, I can't do that, I can't do anything. Nothing has meaning.' That's what it felt like to be Ashley. It was terrible." It was no wonder that everyone had difficulty being around her.

Because of Ashley's inability to bond with or trust anyone, Joan knew she would need to spend considerable time developing a relationship with her in which the child could feel safe. This feeling of safety is critical to EMDR treatment, as it is in any type of therapy. Unless Ashley felt safe, she would not be able to learn from Joan the skills she so sadly lacked: how to bond, how to care, and how to care take. This was not going to be quick and easy EMDR therapy. Ashley was not the victim of a single trauma, as Davy was. She also was not an adult who had had a variety of experiences that Joan could use to represent positive alternatives. Ashley had to be weaned from a pattern of actions and relationships that had gone on for her whole life. She had to be given examples that showed her there was a cause-and-effect universe, that she was a unique and important individual, that she could express herself in ways that would lead to happy relationships, and that she could safely love and be loved. Until she had a sense of a positive alternative, her negative and dysfunctional attitudes would have a firm hold; there was no positive or adaptive information to connect up with.

During their second session, Ashley began painting picture after picture, only getting as far on each one as making a single circle for the head before declaring, "That's no good," and throwing it away.

At their third session, Ashley wanted to make believe that the dolls were babies crying, and she asked Joan to make wailing sounds, which she did. Ashley really liked having the babies cry. Then she asked Joan to be the mother comforting the babies. This was the closest Ashley had come so far to actually playing, but it was not yet real play, in which a child makes up stories about the characters and scenes she invents. At this point, Ashley was still dissociated—removed from any nurturing emotions. Though she may have heard stories or watched TV programs about happy families, they didn't relate to her. She had to ask Joan to make the babies' wailing sounds and act as their loving mother. In this session, as in earlier ones, Ashley was the observer; she neither comforted the babies nor received comfort herself.

In late February, Joan gave Ashley some magazines and told her she could cut them up and make a collage. Ashley cut out a picture of a mother holding a baby. Then she cut off the mother, snipped her into little pieces, and said, "I hate mommies. The baby's glad it's alone to do what it wants."

In March, Ashley wanted to play babies again and asked Joan to be the baby crying. Joan said, "Waaaaaah!" Ashley looked straight at Joan and let her cry. Then Ashley announced that she had to go to a meeting. Joan responded by acting angry and upset that her mother hadn't come to her. Ashley watched with interest.

This was the first step in Joan's campaign to introduce Ashley to relationships that were far different from the dissociated or abusive example set by her parents' marriage. Joan had begun by showing Ashley that it's okay to get angry and express feelings. In later sessions, she offered Ashley new ways to express her fear, sadness, or guilt, and she did so in a way that allowed Ashley to experience those emotions in someone else for the first time. Maura had been taught never to let her children see her "bad" feelings. Only through games and playacting in the comfort of a safe relationship would Ashley gradually be able to connect with and express her feelings of pain without lashing out.

The next week, Ashley started playing a little. She and Joan took turns creating a drawing, each one making marks with a different colored crayon. As they did this, Ashley asked, "What will happen to me if my mom isn't waiting for me?" Instead of answering, Joan responded by asking, "What?" Ashley replied, "I will die." Joan felt that this response summed up Ashley's experience of feeling abandoned as an infant and of having no bond with her mother. On a very elementary and evolutionary level, the feeling was completely valid. Any infant (of any mammalian species) needs the care and protection of a loving parent or it will die.

In April, Ashley started to play. She showed an interest in learning to play a board game by the rules. This gave Joan a spark of hope: Ashley wanted to "do it right." Next, Ashley got Joan to make big mommy stars and little baby stars out of pink Play-Doh. When they were done, Ashley announced that she loved babies and hated mommies, and she smashed the mommy stars. Joan waited until the mommy stars and baby stars came up again in Ashley's play, signaling that they were important symbols to her. Using the stars as a focal point, Joan decided that it was time to start EMDR processing.

By now, Joan had devoted about three months to establishing a relationship with Ashley that was strong enough for them to do EMDR together. EMDR can work beautifully with children, producing rapid effects, but it must be used within the context of a nurturing and comforting therapeutic relationship. Because EMDR can stimulate intense feelings, the client, whether she is four years old or forty, must work with someone who provides a safe "home base," a trustworthy, stable, and loving place from which she can risk forays into the powerful territory of her feelings and to which she can always return. Although this safety was easy for Davy to experience, it was painstakingly difficult for Ashley to achieve. The goal was to build a positive and adaptive relationship for Ashley to connect with before the EMDR processing started.

In early May, Ashley asked Joan to make mommy stars and baby stars again. After doing so, Joan picked up a mommy star and, saying nothing, simply began moving the star back and forth, from left to right, about twelve inches in front of Ashley's face. Ashley watched the star closely for a while, then grabbed it and smashed it. Joan repeated this "game" until all the mommy stars were squashed. In the sessions that followed, Ashley spent a lot of time teaching herself how to draw stars. She made whole universes of them and was quite proud of her new skill.

As Ashley's therapy continued, Joan began interspersing EMDR sessions with regular play therapy; she used various figures, toy pieces, or clay shapes to represent the significant problems in Ashley's life. On various levels, Ashley learned to associate these different objects with specific situations like her troubled relationships with her mother and her brother, her own deprived childhood, and other experiences of being lonely or shut away. Once the association was made, Joan could use the objects to stimulate the stored experiences that were causing Ashley's disturbance.

By using these different toys and symbols as focal points during EMDR, Joan created a link between Ashley's consciousness and the place where the pertinent information regarding the important people and situations was stored in her brain. For example, when Joan held up a symbol, like the large star that represented Ashley's mother, and led the child into eye movements, theoretically it had the curative effect of linking an area of dysfunction (the relationship with her mother) with Ashley's innate information-processing system.

Over time, as Joan created a safe relationship between herself and Ashley, and then between the symbol and the problem so that the EMDR processing could be done, Ashley became calmer and more receptive. Her receptivity allowed the important links to be made, so that one by one the primary areas that caused Ashley so much pain could be addressed.

In mid-May, Ashley asked Joan to make mother ducks and baby ducks out of Play-Doh. When Joan had accomplished this, Ashley looked intently at the results, but she did not smash the mother ducks. Ashley had now been in therapy with Joan for three and a half months and had had one modified EMDR processing session.

In a parent conference shortly afterward, Maura reported that Ashley was doing a little better at home and had started asking, "Can I help you, Mom?" "She seems at times to *like* me almost," Maura added with embarrassed surprise.

In July, Ashley surprised Joan by asking her to make a dog out of Play-Doh. Joan, remembering how terrified the child was of dogs, set to work immediately. Joan formed the head and body and got Ashley to make the legs. As soon as all the bits were assembled into a complete dog, Ashley smashed it flat with her fist. They made another dog. Ashley smashed it, too. They made a third dog, and Joan held it at eye level in front of Ashley's face. Then, timing her words to her movements, Joan made the dog jump from left to right and back again, while chanting, "It's . . . safe . . . to . . . decide . . . whether . . . to . . . play . . . with . . . the . . . dog . . . it's . . . safe . . . to . . . decide . . . whether . . . to . . . play . . . with . . . the . . . dog." Ashley watched wide-eyed, her attention riveted on the clay figure moving back and forth before her eyes.[12] When Joan stopped, Ashley smashed the dog. Later in the session, Ashley wrote on the board, "I love Mommy. Mommy, No, No, No."

Offering a specific positive statement (usually before a set of eye movements) is another form of the cognitive interweave. As we will see, this interweave did not cause any profound change in Ashley immediately. What it did do, theoretically, was open the memory network in which Ashley's fear of dogs was held, resulting in long-lasting changes in her behavior that took place after the session.

A few weeks later, Ashley came into Joan's playroom and discovered a board game called Cabbage Patch Kids. It had a brightly colored board showing various destinations: an abandoned mine, a hospital, and so on. The game pieces were little disks showing the faces of various Cabbage Patch babies: some sad, some happy, and some very angry. The game was played by twirling a spinner and seeing which character the arrow stopped on. One character, for instance, would scoop up the babies and take them to the abandoned mine. Another character would rescue them and rush them to the hospital. If you landed on a stork, you got to adopt another baby.

As Ashley started playing, Joan talked for the Cabbage Patch babies. "Oh no! Why did we get abandoned in this cold dark mine? Are we bad? Or ugly? Or mad? Don't they love us?" By the end of the game, Ashley had "adopted" six babies, five angry ones and a happy one.

"Can you hold the babies?" Joan asked, as she picked up Ashley's disks. Ashley nodded. "Okay, put out your hands. Good. Now let's put one angry baby here," Joan said as she pressed a grubby and well-worn disk into Ashley's left palm. "And let's put another angry baby here in your other hand. Okay? Good. Now, see, I have the happy baby right here, in my hand." Ashley was following this operation avidly. Then Joan used her happy baby to tap first Ashley's left hand and then her right, saying in rhythm to the movements, "You're . . . safe . . . now . . . and . . . you're . . . okay . . . you . . . can . . . have . . . your . . . sad . . . and . . . mad . . . feelings . . . and . . . you're . . . okay . . . you're . . . safe . . . now . . . and . . . you're . . . okay." This was the positive cognition Joan had been planning to use with Ashley, and the game was a natural for it.

On August 30, Joan was standing at her office door chatting briefly with Maura when she saw Ashley push over her little brother. When Charlie struggled back to his feet, Ashley pushed him over again. A few minutes later, when their session had started, Ashley picked up a boy doll and shoved it into Joan's hands. Then she picked up a girl doll and crowed, "She hates the little boy!" Next, she picked up an old telephone Joan kept as a toy and used the handset to beat the boy doll. Then she took the boy doll, crunched him between the folding halves of a Scrabble board and pitched the whole thing across the room. Joan had often seen Ashley angry, but this was something different; today the child wanted to kill.

Eventually Ashley's rage subsided, and she picked up another doll. She told Joan it was the daddy doll. He had come home, and everything was okay. Once again we see the interaction of nature and nurture. It doesn't matter how unavailable or abusive a father like the one who abandoned her might be. The need and the desire for Daddy's love overrides all. Charlie, her brother, would be a scapegoat until Ashley's pain was healed.

Joan asked Ashley to hold the girl doll in one hand and the boy doll in her other. Ashley did so. Then Joan picked up the daddy doll—which was sure to rivet Ashley's attention—and started a version of the EMDR tapping game they had played with the Cabbage Patch babies. "This . . . daddy . . . doll . . . wants . . . to . . . teach . . . you . . . something . . . I'm . . . okay . . . when . . . I . . . share . . . I'm . . . okay . . . when . . . I . . . share . . . I . . . can . . . have . . . my . . . feelings . . . and . . . I . . . can . . . share." The tapping game went on for less than a minute, perhaps the length of five or six repetitions of the positive cognition Joan had selected. Ashley said nothing, but later in that session she had the girl doll and the boy doll get married.

As the months went on, Joan continued painstakingly to defuse the earlier experiences and weave new threads into Ashley's developmental tapestry: that it was all right to trust others, express emotions, and reach out without hurting or being hurt. All the while, Joan offered Ashley loving acceptance and continued associating positive beliefs and emotions with play objects during the EMDR processing.

In mid-September, Ashley went back to kindergarten. Joan and Maura had decided that Ashley should repeat the grade because she had a wonderful teacher and she had missed so much skill development the previous year owing to her angry, erratic behavior.

By early November, when Joan had been seeing Ashley for about ten months, she started noticing a definite change in the child's behavior. At one session, Ashley was calm and controlled for the entire hour. She played games with Joan by the rules and "called" Joan on the phone after each move to tell her it was her turn. She expected Joan to "call" her, too.

In the following weeks, Joan and Ashley started playing a version of peekaboo in which Ashley would hide in the bottom shelf of the bookcase and Joan would bob back and forth, in and out of Ashley's line of vision, asking aloud, "Where's Ashley? Where's Ashley?" Joan did not incorporate any positive statements into the game, as in conventional EMDR, but simply used the child's alternating attention to affirm to her that she existed.

During the same period, Joan started talking with Ashley about the fact that even before a baby is born, even before anyone can see her, she's there, inside her mommy. Ashley loved this information and asked to hear it over and over. "I wanted to give her the message, 'You were meant to be,'" recalled Joan. "There was a sense of emptiness about Ashley, a sense of never having been wanted or liked, perhaps even a sense that she wasn't supposed to have been. In the peekaboo game, the implicit meaning in asking 'where's Ashley?' and then finding her is, 'I see you. You're here. You exist.'"

In December, Ashley had to have her adenoids removed, and Joan arranged to have a talk with Maura beforehand. "You know how you told me you weren't really there for Ashley when she was born?" Joan asked. "Well, this is your chance. I want you to really baby her before and after the surgery. Be with her until they put her to sleep and be there when she wakes up. When children come out of surgery, they temporarily regress to a baby state, so this is the perfect way to redo Ashley's lonely birth experience." Maura's eyes lit with excitement. Joan continued, "This will be your chance to tell her everything you wanted to say that you never got to say when she was born."

The next time Joan saw Maura, she was grinning from ear to ear. "I did it!" she laughed. "Ashley loved it. And it was so much fun! I even offended the surgeon by dashing off in the middle of his advice when I heard a nurse say they were about to wheel Ashley in."

At her first session after the operation, Ashley wanted to make crowns, one for herself and one for her mom. When Ashley put on her crown and dubbed herself "Princess Shannon," Joan looked at her curiously. To the best of her knowledge, Ashley had never been told the story of her mother's baby brother.

One day Maura called to read Joan a comment from Ashley's report card: "Ashley's having a great second year. I love watching her bloom."

When Ashley wanted to play with magic wands, she and Joan made some. Joan used the wand to talk with Ashley about wishing and wanting and about how she deserved to have wishes and wants, even if she didn't get everything she asked for. At first, Ashley didn't even know how to make a wish, but she was a quick learner.

"I wish for a diamond ring!" Ashley declared.

"You mean when you grow up?"

"No, I mean now."

So Joan made her a "diamond ring" out of paper, and occasionally in later sessions they used the magic wand to do EMDR processing on thoughts and feelings that came up during their wishing-and-wanting games.

Progress reports from Maura told Joan that things were continuing to improve at home. Ashley was now protective of Charlie and wasn't as afraid of being abandoned by her mom anymore. However, she was still terrified of seeing doors closed. Maura had learned not to close herself in her bedroom when the children were out of control, but Ashley still had to reprocess her feelings from those experiences as well as her grief at having the door closed on her relationship with her father. Then, one day, Ashley walked into the playroom, paused at the door, and flipped the sign from "Out" to "In." Joan watched this, thinking perhaps they might try some EMDR today on Ashley's phobia about doors closing. There was a children's song that would provide a good framework.

"Ashley, do you know the song 'Open, Shut Them'?"

"No."

"It goes like this." Joan sang softly, "Open, shut them. Open, shut them. Give a little clap! Open, shut them. Open, shut them. Put them in your lap!" Joan's voice rose and fell with the four notes that composed the singsong melody as it wound its way through several more verses. Ashley followed along, then chimed in when she got the hang of it.

"That's great, Ashley. Now let's try this. Remember the time you hid in the little nook under the sand tray?" Ashley nodded. "Want to try it now?"

Before Joan could finish her question, Ashley was scrambling into the opening beneath the rolling table that held a miniature sandbox. Ashley wiggled around until she faced Joan. Being in this hidey-hole was one of her favorite things to do.

"Okay. Now let's play a game." Joan picked up a big pillow covered with bright flowers and started to sing. "Open . . . shut them . . . open . . . shut them . . . " As Joan chanted the words, she slid the pillow back and forth to cover and uncover the opening to the "cave" where Ashley was hiding, matching her actions to the words in the song. Ashley moved her eyes back and forth, following the pillow. Then she added some words of her own.

"Open . . . shut them . . . open . . . shut them . . . you are . . . safe inside . . . open . . . shut them . . . open . . . shut them . . . you are . . . safe inside." It was another version of their peekaboo game and one that, Joan hoped, would open up the block that kept Ashley afraid of closing doors. Joan hypothesized that this fear originally stemmed from Ashley's being abandoned by her father. But Joan couldn't know for certain.

As it turned out, it didn't matter. Ashley and Joan played "Open, Shut Them" with great delight for a little while, then went on to other things. Maura later reported that Ashley was having no more problems with doors closing.

In May, Ashley's kindergarten teacher told Joan during a phone consultation that Ashley had much more self-confidence, good skills, and plenty of friends. "She's more argumentative with her friends," the teacher added, "but I think that's because she feels safe enough to disagree. She seems very happy."

On June 14, 1994, Ashley made a book. She dictated the text while Joan wrote it down: "I like making forts with Joan, and I like playing school with Joan, and I like playing Barbies with Joan, and I like coloring with Joan, and I like going swimming with Joan, and I like going to the zoo with Joan, and I like going to Disneyland with Joan." Joan earnestly recorded Ashley's words. She was touched and delighted: Ashley was now able both to feel and to express love, and judging by the fact that some of Ashley's story was pure fiction, she'd definitely mastered the art of wishing and wanting. Joan noticed that she always looked forward to playing with Ashley, too.

At home, Maura, who had also been seeing a counselor, reported that Ashley was now willing to make eye contact with her. She allowed her mom to touch her now, too. When Maura read a story, Ashley would come sit in her lap. She liked to be cuddled and asked for hugs and kisses. There was still sibling rivalry with Charlie, the normal kind, but Ashley was not pushing him off beds and giving him bruises. Her phobia about closing doors was gone, and her frantic fear about dogs had shifted to simple cautiousness. In fact, Ashley had recently spent the night at her aunt's house and had allowed their Great Dane, Reckless, to sleep by her bed.

Maura Sullivan looks back in wonder at the changes in Ashley and in herself. "I am so grateful that I was able to find the help. It's taken a totally desperate, sad, and lonely situation and turned it into a situation that is now full of love. We are a happy family.

"The EMDR didn't take away my feelings of missing Shannon," Maura adds, "but it helped me get them out of the way of raising Ashley. I had been afraid of really loving her because I was afraid of losing her the way I lost Shannon. I hadn't realized that I was cutting myself off from my daughter. But Ashley felt it, and that's probably the biggest reason why she had such a hard time loving me, because I hadn't allowed myself to really love her."

The most critical factor in Ashley's recovery may well have been Joan's decision to work first with the child's mother. Had Joan not attended to Maura's problems, any progress by Ashley would have been futile. The child would not have been able to connect with her mother, and she would not have had a safe and loving home environment in which to change her behavior.

"After the EMDR, so much of me opened up," Maura recalls. "There was an inner peace as well as a lot of grieving. I felt I wanted to be with Ashley, even if she didn't want to be with me. I didn't force myself on her, but I would always open up and ask, 'Ashley, do you want to come and sit by me? Do you want me to read a story? Do you want me to help you with this?' At first she wasn't open to the change, but gradually it has really worked. Now I can't get her away from me; she has a lot of time to make up for! She has opened up so much now that she knows that I love her."

In December of 1994, a little more than two years from the miserable day when four-year-old Ashley heaved a plate of Thanksgiving turkey at her mother in front of the whole kindergarten, Ashley's first-grade class put on a Christmas buffet and invited the parents. Maura arrived and, a bit nervously, started helping the other mothers set out the steaming dishes. She looked up in alarm when she heard the sound of stomping feet headed her way. Ashley was coming at her quickly, shouting, "Come on, Mom! Let's get in line. I'm hungry!" Maura felt that she was indeed blessed and had something to be truly thankful for.

☙

As EMDR was used more extensively with both children and adults, it was clinically reported that it could help clients and therapists fill in the deficits that were caused by failure to receive the proper care and attention dictated by nature and the evolutionary-survival process. It is important to remember that the Adaptive Information Processing EMDR offers really means accelerated learning. It can help to mitigate the consequences of abuse and incorporate new skills and adaptive behaviors in the nurturing environment of the clinical relationship. However, it is also clear that not every case of attachment disorder is caused by a lifelong history of deprivation or disruption, and the treatment does not have to take as long as Ashley's did.

For instance, Todd Long was a fourteen-year-old boy with a classic attachment disorder who wouldn't make eye contact, hated to be touched or held, and was socially withdrawn and avoidant. When EMDR processing was used to target Todd's anger at his parents, the boy remembered an incident when he was three or four years old. He had had an utterly miserable time after having been left at a day care center. Following that, he had stopped trying to connect with other people for the next ten years. He also remembered that he had chosen to be dropped off at day care instead of accompanying his parents to another destination. At the time, however, Todd became terrified that his parents were not going to come back and pick him up. Possibly, his fear was triggered by thinking that because he had "abandoned" his parents, they would abandon him in return.

Processing this memory appeared to change Todd's attitude and behavior completely. His parents reported, "He can't seem to get enough of us. He's making eye contact now. He sits next to us, touches us, and wants to be hugged. We can't believe this change."

Of course, many attachment disorders have to do with losing a parent, being in multiple foster homes, or experiencing bad parenting. Sometimes, however, something one might not imagine would be disturbing turns out to be a serious trauma to a child. Millions of children go to day care every day with no problem. For Todd, however, it was a trauma and one he did not recover from until he had processed his locked-up fear of abandonment and remembered that he had chosen to be at the center. Sometimes, it is just as simple as that.

Whether EMDR treatment takes three sessions for a child who has had an otherwise solid foundation or three years for a child who needs a new sense of reality built bit by bit, or any amount of time in between, it doesn't matter. What is important is that the healing is done. The sooner it starts, the sooner the child's life can begin.

8

Healing the Ravages of Rape

> In the midst of winter, I finally learned that
> there was in me an invincible summer.
>
> —ALBERT CAMUS

OVER THE YEARS that I have worked with EMDR, I have seen it prove widely successful in the treatment of rape victims who have PTSD. Like combat veterans, rape victims can develop a "domino effect" of symptoms ranging from negative emotions, thoughts, and behaviors to recurring physical sensations. The fact that EMDR therapy deals comprehensively with all four types of aftereffects is what makes it so effective in helping rape victims recover from their traumatic experiences.

In these enlightened times, the effects of sexual assault are acknowledged to be devastating. Before the 1970s, however, the psychological community largely ignored rape victims in favor of investigating the rapist. Except for emergency-room care, treatment of rape victims was nonexistent. The prevailing social attitude was that the rape victim was in some manner to blame for the attack, and any of her problems following the rape were based on her preexisting personality issues.[1]

It was not until the advent of the feminist movement in the early 1970s that the psychology community began to pay attention to the emotional repercussions of rape and how to treat them. Interviews with rape victims and the details that emerged began to inspire more interest in the psychological process. The patterned response was labeled the *rape trauma syndrome*, and serious investigations began to examine the specific effects.[2]

As previously noted, the influx of suffering Vietnam combat veterans had caused an increased awareness of the response to trauma. Clinicians began to describe rape symptoms in much the same way that they described the symptoms of combat-related PTSD. Finally, in 1980, rape was officially recognized as a potential cause of PTSD in the third edition of the therapist's "bible," the *Diagnostic and Statistical Manual of Mental Disorders*.[3] Despite this apparent progress in the recognition of rape as a serious cause of psychological problems, the first controlled studies of how to treat rape victims successfully did not appear until over a decade later.[4]

Today, sexual abuse survivors constitute the largest number of PTSD victims. Although there are estimates that only one-fifth to one-half of all rape victims file police reports, it has been noted that the number of assaults appears to be growing. In the 1980s, estimates of the prevalence of rape in the United States ranged from 5 to 22 percent of the female population.[5] Ten years later, a study indicated that between 24 and 53 percent of a community sample of women reported a sexual assault.[6] Regardless of the prevalence, the effects can be devastating. A U.S. survey indicated that about 620,000 women eighteen years and older were raped in 2010 alone.[7] And those are only the ones who reported the crime. A just-completed survey of nine colleges reported that approximately 25 percent of female students had been sexually assaulted, although most had never reported it.[8]

Although verbal, emotional, and physical assaults certainly leave their mark on the victim, it is difficult for many women to imagine anything more violating than a sexual attack. Establishing some sense of safety and boundaries in relation to others generally involves a sense of physical distance. We get uncomfortable when a stranger stands too close to us in line or at a counter. Our own skin is a boundary that marks our sense of physical self. Therefore, it should not be surprising that to have another person forcefully enter one's own *body* goes beyond the breaking point for practically anyone.

Once a woman suffers such a horrendous event as rape, the physiological state she experienced at that time can become locked in place. She may have endlessly cycling obsessive thoughts about the assault along with feelings of disgust and terror. Like combat-related PTSD, rape engenders a fear response that manifests as intrusive symptoms (flashbacks, nightmares, ruminations about the rape, and panic attacks), avoidance of situational and psychological reminders of the attack (through social isolation, emotional numbing, and substance abuse), and hyperarousal (insomnia, hypervigilance, and an exaggerated startle response that does not diminish over time).

Sometimes this event-specific fear response expands to a general fear of being attacked. Women who have been raped by a stranger may fear all unfamiliar men, whereas women who have been date-raped typically start to mistrust all their male friends. Over time, this fear can result in a life spent in nearly total seclusion. One woman who had been raped stayed home behind barred doors with her guard dog, leaving only to go to work. Getting raped in a place a woman considered perfectly safe, like a neighborhood parking lot or the laundry room in her apartment building, can shatter the ability to trust herself and her own perceptions. Sometimes it feels like the only thing left to do is hide.

Now that I have seen the results of using EMDR with rape victims, I know that many others continue to suffer needlessly. Without proper treatment, the aftereffects of rape can last for years. Studies show that between 33 and 63 percent of victims who get no treatment continue to suffer symptoms of PTSD so intense that they disrupt daily functioning.[9] The woman's social life, job performance, and ability to parent all suffer. It is impossible for someone to stay psychologically balanced and focused on the task at hand when she is physiologically conditioned to be continually on guard and to react to minor stressors with fear and anxiety. Even more disturbing is the fact that spontaneous recovery can reverse itself in time.[10] The woman thinks she is free of her symptoms only to be caught again, suddenly, in their choking grip.

Before EMDR, the primary treatment available for rape victims was a type of behavioral therapy called *exposure*. This approach consists of several different techniques (such as one termed *flooding*). It calls for the victim to bring to mind the most painful moment in her rape and stay with it, and the intense feelings it engenders, for as long as forty-five to ninety minutes at a time for 7–15 sessions, and to supplement clinical sessions with daily exposure homework. The goal is simply to tolerate the extreme emotions and physical sensations that arise. If treatment is successful, over time the woman will no longer have such intensely painful feelings about the assault. Many therapists are reluctant to use exposure techniques, however. They are unwilling to urge a terrified rape victim to stay in contact with the worst moments of her assault for a prolonged period.

Fortunately, EMDR uses an associative process, so prolonged, extended focus on the trauma is not an issue, and since homework is not needed, all the treatment is done in the presence of the therapist. Most importantly, research on EMDR therapy with single-trauma rape victims shows that 90 percent no longer had PTSD after only three sessions.[11] An additional advantage of EMDR therapy is that it addresses the person's negative self-beliefs, such as feeling she was to blame or feeling that she is tainted. This is especially important because society at large reinforces these beliefs. We still occasionally hear reports of rape trials in which defense lawyers are allowed to point out what the victim was wearing, where she was walking, or what her previous sexual behavior was. These factors have no bearing on someone not taking *no* for an answer, and such treatment can have a negative impact on the vulnerable and shaken victim.

The picture for the sexual assault victim becomes even more complicated. Not only do the recurrent intrusive pictures, emotions, and physical sensations need to be dealt with, but also it is vital to address at least three basic human beliefs that may have been shattered by the victimization: the belief in personal invulnerability, the belief in the meaningfulness of life, and the belief in one's own self-worth. These beliefs, first enumerated by Dr. Ronnie Janoff-Bulman,[12] can be badly shaken for months or even years after an assault. The victim may be flooded with feelings of worthlessness, an obsession with being dirty, and the conviction that she is a mere object to be controlled and used by others.

In EMDR treatment, some of the negative self-beliefs therapists hear from sexual assault victims are "I am damaged for life," "I am powerless," "I am bad," and "I am worthless." When a woman utters words such as these, she is not partaking in an intellectual exercise. She is verbalizing the emotion she feels when she thinks of the sexual assault or when memories of the attack are triggered. Although she may understand intellectually when friends or family remind her that she is now safe, this reassurance may make no dent in her automatic physiological response. As we observed with combat veterans, although the victim may have been in numerous group therapy sessions and read various self-help books, she is not able emotionally to incorporate the helpful information given to her. The high level of emotional disturbance is locked in her nervous system and chains her to the past event.

Although self-help techniques can show the rape victim how to cope better with her distress, they don't go far enough. The goal of EMDR therapy is for the victim to become entirely free of emotional turmoil. The woman who is plagued with intrusive pictures of her rapist's face, the feeling of his hands on her body, and the heat of his breath on her face needs to process all of this information. When she has completed EMDR, these physical sensations and the negative emotions that go with them will no longer be stored in the memory network about the rape: They may be remembered as facts, but they will no longer be felt. With EMDR, part of the treatment includes facilitating the emotional adoption of positive self-beliefs such as "I'm now in control," "I am fine," "I did the best I could," "I am a worthwhile person," or "I now have choices." Once all of this has happened, the bonds of the past are essentially broken, and the rape survivor can take her proper place in the present.

Because EMDR treatment targets all of the information related to the trauma, often it can help clients to heal more than the rape itself. As we saw in Emily's case in Chapter 4, the aftermath of the rape can be as upsetting as the rape was. How many marriages have faltered because the husband cannot deal with his wife having been assaulted? How many times has the victim been abandoned by friends who have tired of her unremitting suffering? It is not surprising that research with sexual assault survivors shows the recurrent themes of sadness about their losses, discomfort about their vulnerabilities, guilt about "their" responsibility for the assault, and ongoing fears of attack.[13] All of these factors need to be dealt with for complete recovery to be achieved.

Sometimes the effects of the assault can be subtle, and it is clearly true that women are not the only victims. One male client came into therapy because he found it impossible to maintain close and intimate relationships. Although he was a successful executive, he found himself prone to violent fits of anger. During the EMDR session, he was able to see the connection between his present problems and a childhood sexual assault by his priest. The breaking of trust, the violation of his innocence by someone who should have protected him, was the undercurrent that caused him to withdraw when anyone got too close. After processing the memory, he no longer responded that way; he became involved in a serious relationship a few months later.

It is important to remember that what happens in EMDR is that the person's internal information-processing system is stimulated so that the core of health that is within can blossom forth. When a woman is raped, she may go into shock and her body may shake and bleed, but with the proper medical care it can heal in a matter of weeks. We *expect* this to happen. The mind can also go into shock after a rape and can cause the victim to relive the assault over and over. With the proper psychological care, the mind can heal at the same rate as the rest of the body.

People do not have to go through years of therapy for the healing to take place. Naturally, if sexual, emotional, or physical assaults occurred repeatedly over many years the therapy will not be brief. This is particularly true for adult survivors of childhood abuse. However, the EMDR therapy will generally be more rapid than traditional treatments since the underlying mechanisms of recovery are the same. The brain and its information-processing system are part of the body and are governed by the same laws of cause and effect. When a physician taps our knee, it jerks in response. Our minds give similar knee-jerk responses to external pressures and experiences. Some responses are healthy and serve us well. Others do not but can be changed.

In this chapter, we look at a case of rape that involved a convergence of factors that would push the outer limits of anyone's ability to cope. The fact that the victim was able to heal so rapidly with EMDR is a tribute to an inner resilience that is our heritage. It does not make the assault any less reprehensible. It doesn't take away the moral obligation to act responsibly. It doesn't in any way minimize the suffering. But it does show that we are capable of ultimately triumphing over evil and its legacy.

～

If the two men hadn't been so scary, they would have been pathetic. They were skinny. They were dirty. They smelled. They were obviously destitute. One of them wore hand-me-down pants so large they nearly fell down every time he stood up. He had to keep yanking them back up with his left hand. His right hand held the knife.

Dawn Baumgartner, a single mother, was awakened with that kitchen knife at her throat just past midnight on February 10, 1993, in her house at Albrook Air Station in Panama. Dawn was a buck sergeant from the United States who worked fueling aircraft on the six A.M. to three P.M. shift. She had been assigned to nearby Howard Air Force Base for a four-year hitch, half of which she had already served. Not that she was in a hurry to leave Panama; it had been a dream assignment, until tonight.

Dawn loved the tropical climate of Central America and spent as much time as she could out of doors. She was drawn to the ocean and often went horseback riding on the empty palm-fringed beaches. She took expeditions into the jungle and, with the help of some rudimentary Spanish, went off the base and met the locals. Tall, attractive, and outgoing, Dawn had made a lot of Panamanian friends. Times were good. She was content and so were her two young children, Amanda, five, and Tommy, three.

All that changed within the space of twenty minutes, the time it took two local men to climb in Dawn's bathroom window (left open a crack to temper the smell of the cat box); beat, threaten, and tie up her five-year-old daughter and lock her in a closet (in the futile hope of muffling her loud cries); stuff VCR, stereo equipment, jewelry, and other valuables into duffel bags; and rape Dawn. Luckily, little Tommy slept through the whole thing.

Looking back at that dreadful night, Dawn isn't sure which was worse: being sexually violated or being unable to protect her daughter from harm. Dawn did succeed in convincing the men that she could quiet Amanda if they would let the child out of the closet. As Amanda ran sobbing to her mother, a chill went up Dawn's spine at the sight of the livid bruises on the little girl's face and arms. One of the men had clamped his hand over Amanda's mouth with such force that Dawn could see the marks of his fingers bruising her daughter's cheeks. Amanda also had a huge swelling above one ear, where one of the men had slammed her head into the concrete wall of the closet. Her small, delicate hands were roped at the wrists with a pair of Dawn's bootlaces. The laces had cut deep into the child's skin, and her fingers were turning purple.

Dawn, still in bed with a knife at her throat and wearing only a nightshirt and underwear, took Amanda onto her lap, hugged her, rocked her, and hummed "Hush, Little Baby," a song that had always quieted her daughter when she was an infant. "These are bad guys, Honey," Dawn told Amanda, "and we have to do whatever the bad guys say." It was at this point, Dawn remembers, that her emotions totally shut down. She stopped feeling anything. She couldn't even cry. All she could do was focus on Amanda and keep her daughter's head turned away so the child couldn't see that the man holding the knife to her mother's throat had started running his free hand up and down the inside of Dawn's thighs.

Dawn begged the man to cut Amanda's purpling hands free; when he agreed, she had a soul-sickening moment when she saw the point of his knife move toward her daughter. What if he's going to kill her? she shrieked in her head. What if he slits her wrists? But he didn't; he wasn't the angry one.

His partner, clearly the one in charge, was. He had taken two empty duffel bags from Dawn's closet and gone to search the house for valuables.

When he returned, he went over to the bed, flipped Dawn onto her right side, and tied her hands behind her. The other man put a gag in her mouth. Then the angry one raped her.

In that moment, all Dawn could think of was Amanda. She felt no grief or rage or fear for herself, just an icy determination that Amanda must not be allowed to see what was happening to her mother. The child was lying beside her, facing her. Dawn, still propped on her right side, leaned her left shoulder over her daughter until she was sure she had blocked Amanda's line of vision. She held that position with a fierce determination that overruled all other emotions. It seemed like hours. When the rape was over, Dawn realized with shame that she had wet herself, a common physical response in moments of extreme fear. Her body had been deathly afraid, even if her mind had not.

Three days later, the Air Force shipped Dawn and her children home to her mother's house in Colorado Springs, near Peterson Air Force Base. Dawn was out of control. In Panama, she was not able to go back into her own house and was having violent rage and panic attacks. Every Panamanian man she saw, she thought was her attacker. The Air Force mental health authorities had wanted to remove Dawn from the source of her distress and send her someplace where she would feel safe. But Dawn's source of distress was no longer external: The rape was over; the men were three thousand miles away. It was Dawn's inner world, the footprints left on her psyche by her two attackers, that was so painful.

Even back home, Dawn's panic did not subside. She saw a dark-haired deliveryman approach the house and hid in the hall closet, heart racing and frantic with fear, until he was gone. She could not bear to be naked and would not take a shower unless she wore a bathing suit. Her parents were at a loss to help her. She paced the carpet obsessively and rubbed at her thighs until she had sores. She was too afraid to leave the house, even to go to the corner store. She saw danger in every stranger's face.

There was more. Dawn often broke down in uncontrollable fits of sobbing and was afraid to go to sleep at night. She had flashbacks at the sight of a kitchen knife, and she panicked if anyone, even her children, touched her. After one major panic attack, Dawn was taken into the base clinic. A female physician showed Dawn how to use deep breathing to calm herself. Dawn came back the following week: The deep breathing was useless to her; it was like trying to drain a lake with a shot glass. The doctor prescribed a tranquilizer for Dawn's panic attacks. It was to be taken "as needed" (which, in Dawn's case, was every day). The medication slowed down the frequency of Dawn's panic attacks, but it didn't stop them, and it had no effect on any of her other symptoms.

Three weeks after Dawn arrived home, her parents insisted she get some counseling. It was either that, they told her, or check into a mental hospital. Someone at the base chapel referred Dawn to a local agency called the Center for Prevention of Domestic Violence. Peterson Air Force Base had no female counselors, and there was no way Dawn could handle working with a man. Once Dawn started conventional therapy with a woman counselor at the center, things got a little bit better. It helped to have somebody to talk to. Dawn got herself assigned to a desk job and was able to return to work part-time, although her coworkers had to be briefed on her condition: "Don't go near her, don't touch her, don't spook her." They also were told where she kept her anxiety medication; a couple of times, someone had to pull Dawn aside when she went into a panic and make her take her medication. Dawn felt ashamed, as if she were a child who had made a scene. Although her body was locked into the physical nightmare of the assault, there was a part of her mind that judged herself harshly, a characteristic of most victims. After all, the assault was over. Why couldn't she just drop it? Why couldn't it just go away?

Dawn's work schedule dwindled to a quarter of a workday. She was very nervous, fearful, and shaky. She had trouble concentrating and sometimes broke down in tears at her desk. Her coworkers and her supervisor were understanding, but Dawn knew she wasn't performing to military standards. She knew they weren't expecting her to do that yet, but she felt people were looking at her and wondering what her problem was.

Just as Dawn's work was suffering, her home life was suffering, too. She and her kids had moved into a place of their own, but Dawn didn't feel she was being a good parent: she couldn't be there fully for her kids. She let Amanda and Tommy run wild for fear that getting upset with them or yelling at them would trigger one of her panic attacks. She knew that her body couldn't distinguish between strong negative emotions arising for a logical reason in the present and those arising from memories of the rape. She was afraid one would trigger the other, and she was right. With her body physiologically frozen in time, the best she could do was try to keep herself calm. With all her resources aimed at keeping herself steady, things that previously bothered her a little bit became more bothersome. Things that used to bother her a lot would now send her out of control.

Although she tried not to affect her children, it was impossible. The kids felt the lack of boundaries and developed their own sense of being out of control. The safe world that had been bounded by their loving mother's restraints was shattered. Their own emotions started to expand to fill the void.

Amanda developed night terrors and started wetting her bed, but she wouldn't talk to her mom about it. Tommy poured chocolate syrup on the furniture, the carpet, and the dog in the middle of the night. He got a dozen eggs out of the refrigerator and pitched them, with surprising strength for his age, onto the ceiling.

The more Dawn pushed herself to get better, the worse she seemed to get. She had heard about, and tried her hand at, exposure therapy: forcing herself to confront the things she was terrified of. She was still afraid of going to the store (because of the strangers she might see there), but she tried making herself go. On these outings, she had to have someone with her all the time in case she went into a major panic attack, which often happened. Of course, each panic attack compounded the problem by making her feel more and more powerless. She always had to carry her anxiety medication with her, which she hated to do because it made her feel she was dependent on the drug.

Six months later, despite psychotherapy, Dawn was still a physical and emotional wreck. She was slipping further and further into depression. She felt angry, helpless, sad, fearful, lonely, and guilty. She still wasn't sleeping at night. She couldn't date. She had myriad physical problems. She was unable to relax. She still couldn't take a shower without her bathing suit on. Besides panic attacks, she had sudden crying jags and outbursts of temper.

These fits could be triggered by crowds, strangers, being touched, and sometimes just the sight of a man. Sometimes Dawn had no idea what set her off. One day she was horsing around with the kids when Tommy grabbed her hands from behind and pulled. Dawn's body went into panic and she started screaming at the children, frightening both them and herself. It was the last straw. When Dawn calmed down, she thought, this is not fair to my children; they are suffering for what I went through.

Dawn went to her next counseling appointment in a state of desperation. "I need something more. It helps having somebody to talk to about it, but it's not getting at the root of the problem. I'm not getting any better. I can't stand it much longer. Maybe I should get admitted to a mental institution for a couple of weeks." Her therapist suggested that Dawn try EMDR as a last-ditch effort, and two days later, Dawn walked into the office of a woman whom she prayed could help her.

Sandra Wilson was a licensed psychotherapist based in Colorado Springs. When she met Dawn, she was conducting a large study to determine whether people could be healed from the disturbing symptoms of traumatic stress in just three ninety-minute EMDR therapy sessions. Sandra was handling all the initial screening and history-taking interviews with prospective clients herself. Those accepted for the study were assigned at random to one of five therapists who would conduct the three free EMDR treatment sessions.

Haltingly, Dawn told Sandra her personal history and the story of her rape in Panama. Next, she completed several psychological tests designed to identify her symptoms and measure how severe they were. As Sandra listened to the young woman's story, she was struck by how much of Dawn's trauma was showing up in her body: vomiting, back pain, dizziness, constipation, numbness, headaches. As it had during the rape itself, Dawn's body was testifying to the overwhelming feelings she carried.

Sandra accepted Dawn for her study and randomly assigned her case to Laura Knutson, a licensed clinical social worker in Denver who had been trained in EMDR and had volunteered her time to the study. Reviewing Dawn's history before their first session, Laura noted that the formal diagnosis given to Dawn's myriad symptoms was posttraumatic stress disorder.

Laura and Dawn met for their first session on September 23, 1993, seven months and two weeks after the rape. The time for spontaneous remission had passed. These symptoms were not going to go away without effective treatment. Laura had read over the notes from Dawn's initial screening regarding her trauma and her symptoms, but she wanted to hear Dawn tell her the story aloud.

"I was raped while I was stationed in Panama by two men. And my daughter was lying next to me in the bed while this was happening to me. I'm really worried about my kids, especially my daughter."

"Okay," Laura said gently. "And what do you want out of our time together?"

"I want to be calmer. Less anxious. Less frantic about every little thing happening around me. And I want to take a shower without fear."

Then Laura outlined the therapy they would do together and explained to Dawn that they would start by singling out Dawn's worst memory of the rape.

"That's easy. I am in my bedroom. It's dark. I can hear Amanda crying and the two men shouting at her and pushing her around. They had her in my closet."

Dawn's negative cognition that went with this scene was, "I am powerless to protect us." The feelings it brought up were anger and fear, which Dawn said she felt as tightness in her throat. She rated the intensity of these feelings as a 10 on the 0–10 scale. The positive belief Dawn wanted to have instead was, "I'm in control. I'm safe now." She said this felt true at about the level of a 4 on the 1–7 scale.

They started with Dawn focusing on the moment when she had first known something was wrong. As they progressed from set to set, Laura watched as the eye movements took Dawn back to that night and seemed to make her relive it step by step, scream by scream, writhing, legs shaking, cursing at the perpetrators, her own pain compounded by the impotent rage she felt at what they were doing to Amanda. Four sets. Six sets. Eight sets. Ten sets. The rerun continued with the jerking, clutching gestures of Dawn's rigid body telling Laura the story her words could not form. At one point, Dawn was holding her wrists together as if they were still tied; a moment later, her fists flew apart, breaking her bonds. But she said nothing about it. Dawn's rape had been mostly silent, and so was her EMDR-stimulated experience.

Dawn knew how to signal Laura to pause by raising her hand in the "stop" command; although she used this signal frequently during that session, she seemed determined to get through the worst part of the memory. It took eleven very long sets. Dawn had said little in their ninety minutes together, just an occasional exclamation or remark: "It's like I'm there," "I can see them," "I can smell how bad they smelled," "Amanda is shaking," "oh, my God, my daughter," and "the bastards."

After the last set, Dawn told Laura, "It was so scary, so close to what really happened. Like I was reliving it but even worse. When the rape was going on, it was like I was outside of my body watching this movie. It wasn't me that it was happening to, it was a movie. That was my best way of coping with it.

"But this time, it was me. It was terrible, but it's like I had no choice but to deal with it."

The experience Dawn reported, feeling like she was outside of her body watching a movie, is called *dissociation*. It is a common reaction during sexual assault, and it helps insulate the victim from the overwhelming pain of the moment. Unfortunately, this natural survival mechanism does not protect the victim from the symptoms that follow the trauma. In fact, one theory is that because the experience is dissociated, it is not stored in memory as a whole but as separate fragments of images, thoughts, and feelings, which makes healing more difficult.[14]

During EMDR, all the aspects of the trauma reconnect, thus allowing the person to process the experience fully. Being able to go in and out of the disturbing memory during each set of eye movements, plus having a hand signal to tell the clinician to stop if necessary, allows the rape victim to control how much of a "dose" of memory she exposes herself to. If she finds her feelings too painful during processing, she can stop for a while and rest or turn down the emotional intensity. The goal is for her to stay in contact with whatever arises while processing the rape.

Going in and out of the experience of the assault also reinforces the person's knowledge that she is bigger than the trauma. The terrible images can be created and destroyed. The emotions can be felt and distanced from. The woman begins to regain control and perspective. The experience of processing a rape with EMDR isn't pleasant, but it does not take as long as the actual assault did, even if the person relives it scene by scene. However, everything does not necessarily resolve in one session.

At the end of the session, Laura checked with Dawn concerning her self-beliefs and whether there had been any change in intensity. Dawn said the feeling of powerlessness they had started with had dropped, although not much. It had gone from 10 to 7 or 8. Her feelings about her positive cognition ("I'm safe, I'm in control") showed even less movement, going from 4 to 5 (out of 7). Not spectacular results, Laura thought.

Their second session came a week later.

"How are you doing?" Laura asked.

"Okay. It's funny. Even though it hurt so bad last time, I want to get into it again and work on it. Something's telling me this is working."

"Is there some specific part you want to target today?"

"Taking a shower and they're watching me. For some reason, I think these guys were out there watching me when I took a shower. I always opened the bathroom window because there was no fan in there. Now I can't stand being in the shower unless I have my bathing suit on."

"Okay, let's start with that."

In this session, Dawn's negative cognition was, "They are watching me; I'm unsafe." The emotion she had was fear, and she felt it in her chest "like a screechy chill." She rated the intensity of her emotions at an 8 or a 9 out of 10. The positive cognition she wanted to have was, "I am safe; I am protecting myself," the truth of which she rated currently as very low, only 2 on the 1–7 scale.

The scene they started with was Dawn in the shower at her home in Colorado Springs; after just a few passes, she cried out, "They're watching!" She had gone back into the night of the rape, picking up the "movie" where she had left off the last time. This time Dawn's flashes of memory continued past the point at which the men left. She relived the aftermath of the attack: waking her housekeeper, who slept at the other end of the house; getting her wrists untied; running in her nightshirt to a neighbor's house; calling the military police; and when the police arrived, telling them that she wanted to cut off her rapist's genitals.

The second session proved cousin to the first: Dawn's body went through the attack again, her breathing shallow and rapid, her muscles rigid, her face contorted with pain. Halfway through, Dawn held up her hand in alarm and asked Laura where the bathroom was. When she came back, she said, "Sorry."

"Are you okay?" Laura asked.

"Yeah. I got so scared, I thought I wet my pants like I did that night."

"And?"

"I hadn't, but it was probably real close," Dawn said with a short but genuine laugh. Relief showed on her face.

Laura and Dawn did seven more sets that afternoon, for a total of fourteen. Toward the end, Dawn said during a pause, "You know, I'm sort of proud of myself; I got them to stop hurting Amanda. I talked them into letting her out of the closet and untying her hands." Dawn's sense of power was coming back. Dawn began to realize that she had done the best she could in the circumstances, that she had exercised all the power she had.

At the close of the session, the intensity of Dawn's fear had dropped from 8 or 9 to 2. Her belief that she was now safe had gone as far up as it could go, to a 7. Laura breathed a sigh of relief. With only one session to go, she had been hoping Dawn would show significant progress that afternoon.

At their last session, Dawn wanted to work on her intense fear of being touched and the memory of one of the men rubbing her thigh during the robbery. She had compulsively rubbed her own legs ever since the rape. This was another indication that the physical sensations that Dawn experienced at the time of the trauma were locked in her body. Of course, these sensations were not stored in the cells of Dawn's legs; they were stored in her brain, in the neurophysiological network that contained all the information (sensations, thoughts, and emotions) about the traumatic experience. This is similar to what happens when you stub your toe: It feels like the pain is in the toe itself, but the pain center is in the brain. Nerve fibers from the toe carry the signals of pain to the brain, which registers the local sensations. If the nerves from the toe were severed, no matter how many times you stubbed it, you would not feel any pain.

When it comes to a traumatic experience, the brain not only registers the physical sensations at the time but also can continue to do so. During EMDR, the person may reexperience the sensations at varying levels of disturbance because that information is stored in the brain and is stimulated by the processing. Once the person has completely processed the trauma, the memory of it is again stored, but this time it is stored without the painful physical sensations. They have been "metabolized" or "digested," and the person's innate health has reemerged.

Dawn identified the negative self-belief she had as a result of the rapist having rubbed her legs as, "I can't stand being touched." The feelings that went with it were fear, anger, and anxiety, all of which were associated with the sensations in her legs. She rated the intensity of the disturbance at a 10. For her positive self-belief, Dawn chose, "It's okay to touch or be touched," and she promptly rated the truth of this statement as a dismal 1 on the 1–7 scale.

After eleven sets, which involved more flashes of the earlier experience, mixed with sensations moving along her leg and hands, Dawn's fear, anger, and anxiety had dropped to a 4, which was an improvement but still far from the goal of 0. Her belief in the statement, "It's okay to touch or be touched," had risen to a 5 or 6 out of 7. Despite the relief on Dawn's face, Laura was uneasy. "I don't think Dawn is through with this," she thought. "I wish I could have another session or two with her." But the rigors of the study Dawn was participating in did not allow that. Fortunately, once EMDR jump-starts the information-processing system, processing doesn't necessarily stop when the therapy session ends. This means that people need to know what to expect afterward so they can handle it. It also means that positive changes can continue even if the work with the therapist isn't complete.

Ninety days later, Sandra Wilson asked each of the men and women in her study to come in for a follow-up interview. Dawn was delighted to see Sandra again.

"Things are great. No panic attacks. I'm sleeping well. I'm actually feeling restful. I'm working fine with the men in my unit. I even had a date with one of them at Christmas. My kids are doing a lot better. I'm calmer with them, less angry. More able to be close with them and to help them." Dawn had also completed a special training, gotten a promotion, and applied for a mortgage. Her family and coworkers kept asking, "What happened to you?"

"I knew I was getting better when I started joking about sex again," Dawn said with a grin. But her supervisors were cautious: They still briefed new members of the department not to touch or startle Dawn and told them where she kept her medication. However, Dawn had stopped taking her medication two weeks before starting to take part in the study, and she never went back on it.

The next step in Sandra's study was to do a fifteen-month follow-up to measure whether the positive effects of the EMDR had lasted. She contacted Dawn in December 1994. Dawn told her things were flat-out wonderful. "Much better than before the rape, even. I'm back to myself again plus some, because I'm a lot happier. My spirits are so high. I feel a lot better about life." Dawn said she was engaged to a man she had met at work when she first returned from Panama, and she was looking forward to another overseas assignment after her marriage. "My fiancé is black, and my family was stunned because they thought I'd never go near a dark-skinned man again. To tell the truth, I never thought I would either."

Dawn had also spoken publicly about the rape. "I wanted to do something about the fact that the Air Force gave me so little help when I was attacked. So I went before what they call the Diamond Council. It's all the first sergeants at Peterson and the neighboring bases. There are about thirty of them, and nearly all of them are men. I told them my whole story and how no one on base knew how to help me. Of course, this was my first public speaking on it, so I broke down crying.

"I told them, 'I don't want to see it happen to any one of your troops. You guys might care, you men especially might care, but how will you know what to do when something like this happens?' Then they asked me if I would be willing to go along when they get a report of a woman raped on base. I told them I was very willing. Now when they call me about someone being raped, I go to the hospital with them, take them to their first counseling session, do whatever they need.

"I also got Amanda some EMDR, and she's stopped having night terrors and wetting the bed. She'll talk to me now about what happened. Actually, she'll talk to anyone she feels comfortable with about it," Dawn said with a laugh. "It's stunned a few of her friends' mothers. Of course, Amanda doesn't grasp the concept of 'rape,' but she knows that bad guys broke into our house and hurt us." Life had returned to normal for the whole family.

The previous summer, Dawn had also agreed to talk to reporters about her EMDR treatment and her part in Sandra Wilson's study. It turned out that 84 percent of the PTSD victims who were treated no longer had that diagnosis after only three EMDR sessions.[15] Many of the women in the eighty-subject study had reacted as Dawn did and progressed beyond where they were before their trauma. Some of the women felt so empowered that they made major job changes or enrolled in college for the first time. No study of other methods to treat PTSD had ever achieved these kinds of positive effects. The results of this, the first large-scale study of EMDR therapy, were reported at a special news conference called by the American Psychological Association, and many newspapers carried the story.

When a correspondent from a national newsmagazine came to interview Dawn, the reporter broke down in tears on Dawn's living room couch when Dawn described what Amanda went through.

"Do you want to take a break?" Dawn asked. She felt badly that she had upset the woman. It was so hard to predict what people's reactions would be.

"How can you sit there so calmly and just tell the story?" the reporter asked.

"Because that's what it is now," Dawn said. "For both of us, it's just a story."

9

Laying Grief to Rest

Give sorrow words: The grief that does not speak
Whispers the o'er-fraught heart and bids it break.

—WILLIAM SHAKESPEARE

THERE IS AN ancient story of a bereaved woman who brought the body of her dead child to a holy man. She begged him to have pity on her and return her son to life. The master agreed to do so but only if she would bring him a mustard seed from a house in her village where death had not visited. At first, the woman was excited because the request seemed so simple. She went from house to house searching for a family who had been spared, but to her dismay, she came up empty-handed. Gradually, she came to understand the wisdom of the holy man, that death comes to everyone. Silently, she returned to claim the body of her child and, carrying him tenderly, buried him in peace.

While death reaches into every family, few things cause us greater pain than the loss of a loved one. Technically, a person traumatized by grief cannot be diagnosed with PTSD unless the deceased died a violent or unexpected death. But in the face of such sorrow, diagnostic labels have no meaning. Pain is pain, and EMDR is particularly useful for helping people lay their grief to rest, no matter what their symptoms, no matter how their loved one died.

One particularly stubborn reaction to death is a persistent feeling of guilt. We feel responsible for things said or left unsaid. We think back in anguish about the hurtful things we may have done. We revisit the deathbed in our minds or hear the cries of pain. All of these responses are normal after a loss, and they should slowly fade and resolve over time. Sometimes, however, the healing process gets stuck. When that happens, EMDR therapy can be used to help jump-start the system.

Grief does not confine itself to private losses. The lives of many police officers, firefighters, railroad engineers, and rescue workers have been heavily impacted by tragedy, including line-of-duty deaths.[1] Individuals who suffer in this way often feel responsible for what has happened and are left feeling rudderless by the shattering of their sense of control. If only they had been quick enough, they speculate, death could have been prevented. EMDR is often used to unlock this unreasonable thinking and emotional response. Likewise, EMDR is used for police officers who have seen a partner shot in the line of duty or who have had to kill someone themselves. These survivors are often deeply shaken and picture the horrifying event over and over again.[2]

Even medical personnel suffer the trauma of loss. A fifty-year-old man worked for seven days straight, covered in blood, in the medical examiner's office after the crash of TWA Flight 800. He was devastated with guilt because he felt he "couldn't get the bodies back to the families quickly enough in order to give them some closure." One emergency-room nurse was part of a medical team working on a baby who was badly injured in an auto accident. The baby died, and afterward the nurse was plagued with the fear that her own two-year-old child would be killed. She became fiercely and obsessively overprotective. During her EMDR treatment, she targeted the scene in the emergency room and reported that she saw the face of her child on the dead baby. As the eye movements continued, the superimposed image of her child's face lifted from the face of the dead child. She hadn't consciously known that the two faces were connected. Even if she had, she probably wouldn't have been able to do much about it.[3] Intellectual awareness and insight about our problems are rarely enough to resolve them and change our behavior. Change has to take place on an emotional level as well.

At times, someone's death (or suffering) can cause people who hear about it to experience what is known as *vicarious traumatization*. Even if they were not physically present, they can be strongly affected by the trauma, picturing the painful scene in dreams and having obsessive thoughts about the traumatic events. One policeman's wife, hearing about the death of her husband's partner, kept seeing her own husband lying in a pool of blood. EMDR has been used successfully to help people in these situations return to equilibrium.

In another case, an Israeli psychologist sought help because he thought he was going crazy. He kept having flashbacks and nightmares of being gassed in Auschwitz during the Holocaust, although he had not even been born at the time. It wasn't until the middle of his EMDR session that he realized his mind was simply replaying the old stories of his uncle who had died thirty years before. He had felt such empathy for him as a child that he had substituted his own face in the "remembered" pictures of the death camp. During EMDR processing, he shuddered and shook as if the experience had happened to him. Even though he was only vicariously traumatized, these disturbing sensations and emotions were locked in his nervous system for thirty years.

EMDR can also be used to help people who are bombarded by fear for their personal safety after they've suffered the loss of a loved one. Loss threatens our deeply held conviction that life is supposed to go on in a predictable, unchanging manner. Once we lose someone we love deeply, it's hard to feel safe ourselves. We all get by, day to day, with the illusion that we have a certain amount of control over the events of our lives. Loss makes us feel as though we have somehow failed. Many people start taking drugs and alcohol to stop the grief and fear, which only adds dependency and weakness to their spectrum of painful feelings. It also appears that drugs and alcohol, which may momentarily still the suffering, can interfere with the mourning process.[4]

At times, emotions are so buried that we don't realize the roots of our distress. But some of our greatest pain can come from the fear of reaching out to receive or of showing others our needs. We may try to push our pain away because we think we are supposed to or to help others get through theirs; however, this can just push the grief underground. There seems to be an important window of opportunity after a death. If we fail to concentrate on our own sad feelings, the pain may wall off, but it may not go away. Instead, the results of unresolved grief can show up as intense overreactions to related events in the future. For instance, a young woman threatened to break off her engagement when she learned that her policeman fiancé had been shot. During the EMDR session, she realized that she had not sufficiently grieved for her brother's death and was afraid of losing her future husband as well.

In some ways, EMDR appears to reopen the window of opportunity so that resolution can occur. It enables the person to begin to grieve and mourn in a protected environment, where she does not have to squelch her feelings or disguise them to protect someone else.

An excellent framework for understanding the bereavement process has been offered by psychologist Therese Rando.[5] She pointed out that the word *bereavement* derives from the same root as the word "rob." The expected and natural reaction to having something valuable unfairly and forcefully wrested away is to suffer from feelings of grief and victimization. During a grief reaction, the mourner naturally focuses on the loss with behaviors and expressions of pain and anxiety and with the wish to undo the death or believe it didn't happen. In uncomplicated bereavement, the person eventually enters into a second phase of mourning, actively concentrating on the internal and social needs that allow him to adapt to the loss and begin to develop a new sense of identity. During the third phase, the mourner learns to live in a healthy way without the deceased. Although the movement of focus from the deceased, to the self, to the external world is part of the natural healing process, the process sometimes becomes stuck. That is when EMDR can be used to help the healing take place.

The grieving process tends to benefit from the passage of time, but there is no easy answer to the question of how long a person should wait before seeking help. Someone with profound spiritual beliefs, and in the right circumstances, may see death as a release for the loved one. Others take months to stop blaming themselves—and the universe—for their loss. For still others, grief goes on and on. Aspects about the death interact with past experiences, and the pain doesn't heal over time. They feel as though life has stopped, except for the unremitting pain. A further complication is that the mourner may think this reaction is normal or believe that to feel less pain would be dishonoring the dead. But being bombarded by pain or being able to think of only the most distressing memories does not do the deceased, or the survivor, any justice. Survivors often try hard to handle grief in constructive ways, but sometimes talking about it, forcing oneself to "get on with it," or giving oneself more time is just not enough.

Some clinicians believe that to interfere with the grieving process, no matter how lengthy or painful, deprives the mourner of learning everything possible from the experience. But the truth is that time does not heal all wounds. If it did, there would be no need for the field of psychotherapy. If the healing is stuck and not progressing, using EMDR does not short-circuit the learning process; it merely speeds it up. As the processing takes place, insights emerge and patterns are recognized, but connections to the loved one remain. What gets left behind is the intense suffering that has prevented the mourner from thinking peacefully of the deceased. Once that peace is reached, he can reconnect with life itself.

Illustrating that point is the transcript of three sessions of EMDR with a mother who lost her child. Mia Russo's healing process, told in her own words as the sessions progressed, is representative of the natural sequence that unfolds for many people during EMDR therapy sessions.

～

Billy Russo was ten days short of his twelfth birthday when he was killed on a railroad bridge less than two blocks from his home in New England. The commuter train was traveling northbound at the allowable limit of seventy miles an hour when the engineer spotted two boys crossing the tracks ahead. One of them made it across, but the other stopped halfway and bent over, as if to balance a penny on the track before skipping away.

The boy didn't stand up or leap to the side. He stayed rooted to the spot, bent over and calling out to his playmate. Horrified, the engineer slammed on his brakes, blasted his whistle, and unable to stop in time, ran directly over the boy. As it turned out, Billy Russo wasn't being careless or mischievous. His black high-top sneaker had gotten stuck under a railroad tie.

The accident happened at four o'clock on a hot summer afternoon in late July. When Billy's mom, Mia Russo, got home from her day job at about quarter after four, she noticed a crowd down at the railroad bridge. She opened the front door of the three-story family house and went into her parents' first-floor apartment to find her son. Mia's retired father, who watched Billy when Mia was at her day job, told her that Billy had gone to play at his friend Jerry's. Mia stayed at her mom and dad's until five o'clock, then climbed slowly to the apartment she shared with Billy on the third floor. Mildly surprised, she found that her son had not yet come home. Usually she and Billy had supper together before Mia, a hard-working single mother of thirty-three years, went off to her night job as a cashier in her brother's liquor store.

By quarter after five, Mia started to worry a bit. Billy was usually right on time. She checked the second-floor apartment, where her brother and his family lived, then went to her parents' apartment on the first floor. Still no Billy. Mia decided to walk to Jerry's house to see if Billy was still there. On her way down the porch steps, she met her sister and sister-in-law coming in from doing errands. They told her they'd heard there had been an accident down at the train tracks.

Mia walked quickly around the corner to Jerry's house and knocked on the door. No answer. She pounded. Still no answer. She kept pounding. There had to be somebody in there.

Finally, the next-door neighbor came out.

"You know my son, Billy?" Mia asked. "He was with Jerry, but there's no one answering their door."

"They took Jerry in the ambulance," the woman said, her expression frozen.

"What are you talking about?"

"He passed out. He ran into the house and told his grandmother something and passed out. Then the ambulance came. I think you better go down to the bridge."

"But where's? . . ."

"Talk to the police. I don't know anything else."

Mia hesitated.

"Go, now!"

Mia headed for the railway bridge at a run. Somewhere in the crowd of emergency vehicles, police cars, neighbors, and rubberneckers, she found a uniformed cop. Trying to catch her breath and quiet her racing heart, she managed to get out a few words.

"I'm looking for my son. His name is Billy Russo. Has he been around here? Is he involved in this?"

In reply, the policeman carefully took Mia by the arm and started walking her to his squad car.

"Have you seen him? He's eleven years old with light brown hair and brown eyes. And big dimples." Mia's voice was strained and rising with every sentence. "His hair is thick and straight. He has long eyelashes and he's wearing green shorts, a green T-shirt, and black and white high-top sneakers. Where is he?"

Mia, now white with fear and hyperventilating, allowed herself to be helped into the back of the police cruiser, felt the slight jolt as the door slammed closed, then heard the door locks click into place.

Billy's funeral was held four days later. Mia was still in shock and was barely able to talk. Billy had been her whole life. Now she had nothing. No reason to work two jobs. No reason to get up in the morning. No reason to do anything. Mia blamed herself for Billy's death ("If only I'd been home . . . ") and her grief for her son was multiplied by the fact that although she had badly wanted another child, she had been unable to become pregnant for the past ten years. She assumed she would never have another child because she believed the surgery she had had for cervical cancer a few years back had left her infertile.

As the days went by, Mia's shock turned to grief, then depression. The only thing that got her to climb a little way out of the yawning pit of despair she woke to each morning was the terrible pain of the rest of her family. Billy had been the family favorite, and they were hard hit by his death, especially as it came just seven months after the death of Mia's grandmother.

One night, a week or so after the accident, Mia had a nightmare, the first of many, in which she was at the scene of the accident (where, in fact, she had not been permitted to go) and saw Billy's head, torso, and limbs strewn across the tracks. She woke up sobbing. A day or so later, a letter from the police department arrived, addressed to Mia's mother. Mia opened it by mistake. It was a copy of the police report on Billy's death, and it included a diagram of the accident scene showing precisely where each part of Billy's body had been found after the train had hit him. She was devastated. It was just like she had dreamed it.

The nightmares continued. In some, a train was chasing her; in others, she was looking at the accident scene with Billy's body parts. Mia went back to her day job at the warehouse, but she did her work like a zombie. She had crying spells. Her concentration was shot. She quit her night job. Eventually she moved out of her apartment in the family house because it reminded her too strongly of Billy.

Mia thought about the accident every day and kept asking herself *why*. Why would that happen to a little boy? A devout Catholic, she even stopped going to church for several months. Since losing Billy, her faith was severely shaken. On the night of the accident, a priest at the hospital where she was being treated for grief had come to see her. When he started talking to her about God, she cut him off. "Please don't tell me anything about God, because why would he take an innocent child in such a horrible way? I don't want to know anything about him. I don't even want to hear his name."

Mia's staggering pain went on for a year, and then it got worse. When the first anniversary of Billy's death came around, Mia was more distraught than ever at the loss, and her engagement, the only positive thing in her life, had turned sour. She and her fiancé were having loud arguments that involved jealousy, heavy drinking, and physical abuse. With Billy gone and her relationship on the rocks, she wondered if there was any point to going on. Over and over in her mind, she told herself, "If this is the way life is going to be for me, there's just no sense in me being here . . . no sense in me being here . . . no sense . . . "

About six weeks after the anniversary of Billy's death, Mia swallowed a massive overdose, about twenty times the recommended dose, of Ativan, a sedative she had been taking for anxiety. Her fiancé found her in time and rushed her to the hospital, where her stomach was pumped and she was kept for three days in the psychiatric ward. Then she was released.

"You don't really belong here," said the staff psychiatrist. "You're not a mental patient. It's just that you've been through a lot. You just have to learn to deal with it."

But Mia, now on disability leave from her job, had been seeing a board-certified psychiatrist every week. She had been taking Ativan as well as Prozac, the powerful antidepressant. The medications calmed her, but she didn't like the way she felt when she took them. She thought they clouded everything. She felt unable to concentrate and unable to think. In addition, she had decided she could not continue the psychotherapy. Even with her medical insurance paying 80 percent of the psychiatrist's fee, she was getting deeper and deeper in debt trying to come up with her 20 percent. She told her psychiatrist she couldn't keep coming, and he suggested she contact a therapist who was doing research on PTSD. She might be able to get treatment without cost.

Two weeks after Mia's suicide attempt, she started treatment with Dr. Steven Lazrove, a surgeon-turned-psychiatrist at the Yale Psychiatric Institute. Steve, who was trained in EMDR, was working with a small sample of clients with chronic PTSD to gather information on whether EMDR was worth investigating more seriously. If so, he would become part of a team that would design a large-scale, formal research project on the therapy. Mia had been referred to Steve with a diagnosis of PTSD, so she fit the requirements of his preliminary study. However, a number of senior investigators argued against including Mia in the study. They were worried that her symptoms (major depression, posttraumatic stress disorder, and suicidal impulses) were so severe that EMDR could not realistically be expected to make a difference and might be harmful. Steve disagreed. "This is real life. These are the people we're saying that we can help." Steve discussed the case at length with Mia's primary psychiatrist, and together they decided that it was safe to proceed with EMDR.

When Mia took a seat in one of the Institute's stark consulting rooms, Steve sat at a right angle to her, his chair less than a foot from hers. Mia and Steve had met the week before to go over the facts of Billy's death and Mia's ensuing problems. It had been a painful session for Mia. Now, they began with Mia's reading aloud the story of Billy's death as she had told it to Steve in their first meeting. She held her chin high and read slowly in a deep voice filled with pain.

When she was done, Steve asked her, "When you read that now, how disturbing is it on a scale of 0 to 10, where 0 is not upsetting at all and 10 is the worst experience you can imagine?"

"Ten," Mia immediately replied.

"Which part of the story is the most disturbing part; what really stands out?"

"The body parts."

"Do you have a picture in your mind of that?"

"Yes."

"When you picture that, what words go with it, words about yourself?"

"Terrifying, horrible, unbelievable."

"And what does that say about you?"

"Sometimes, I still can't believe it. I can't get rid of it from my mind because it's always there. I guess it will always be there. I always get the same picture in my head."

"When you see that picture, what do you believe about yourself?"

Mia's voice was barely audible. "Guilt. He was my responsibility regardless if I was working. He was eleven years old, and he was a block away, and he'd never been up there before."

"How would you rather feel?"

"It was an accident."

"Can you describe the emotion?"

"Pain in my chest. Emptiness, like a part of me was stolen, a part of my heart was stolen from me. My life was turned upside down."

Steve asked Mia to concentrate on the picture of the body parts and began the eye movements.

After the first set, Steve noticed that behind her smoky-lensed glasses, Mia's eyes were filled with tears. He handed her a box of tissues, but she didn't take one. Steve saw that she was using pure willpower to stop her tears and dam them up before they spilled over onto her cheeks. He waited for her to speak, but she said nothing.

"Just let what comes to mind, come to mind," Steve said softly. "Just see it and let it go."

They started a second set of eye movements. At the end of it, Mia was quiet for a long time, then said, "The picture would blank out, then it would try to come back."

"Shall we keep going?"

"Yes."

The third set of eye movements went on for a long time, perhaps two or three minutes. "What's going on?" Steve asked when it was over.

"The scene was changing. The part on the tracks was blanking out. I never was up there, but my mind was up there. It went to when I was in the police car afterward." The picture was beginning to alter. This was a good sign.

The fourth set was also very long. Mia spontaneously started to go through subsequent events chronologically, reporting a change of scene after each set. This often happens in EMDR sessions. As the information processing begins, the memory of the traumatic episode is able to complete itself instead of remaining stuck at the worst part.

"I was with my family . . . they were all gathered around at my mother's house, crying."

"Were you there?"

"I was there."

"Just go with that."

After the fifth set, Mia said, "I left my mother's house. I was at the funeral. I didn't want to get out of the car. Then I got out. I couldn't believe I was sitting there. When they brought the casket over, it had a picture of me and my son on top of it. I got stuck on that."

They did a sixth set.

"I was back at my mother's house. I went to the third floor and I was packing, packing my things."

They did a seventh set.

"I was at my job, doing the packing. I was back to work. People were trying to support me."

They did an eighth set.

"It was Thanksgiving. It was the holidays. Me and my son were supposed to have our first Thanksgiving alone, just me and him. But he wasn't there. Then it was Christmas and there were no gifts and there was no tree. It was just another day."

"That's pretty sad. Can you stay with the sadness?"

Mia nodded and they started a ninth set.

When it was over, Mia said, "I put flowers on my son's grave. Thinking he was never coming back." Her voice was still barely audible, her face wooden with the effort of holding back waves of pain.

They did a tenth set. They had been using the eye movements for twenty-eight minutes.

"I was holding him in a dream I had. Just holding him and asking him to stay, stay a little while longer. It really felt like I was holding him. But I woke up and he was gone. But it was so real, I was really holding him."

They did an eleventh set.

"I kept seeing trains again . . . I just keep seeing them and not being able to get up there . . . the trains . . . I keep seeing them, like in dreams. I just keep seeing them going by me real fast."

They did a twelfth set.

Now Mia unclasped her hands and gripped the arms of her chair. "A lot of things were happening. I was in church, having a mass for my son, lighting candles. I kept seeing him, though. I just kept seeing him. Very clearly. You can see him. My mind is not wanting to let that picture go."

"What's the fear if you let that picture go?"

"He'll be gone." How many of us have felt that way? Afraid that if we let go of the picture, or the pain, we will lose the person forever.

"Just stay with that."

After the thirteenth set, Mia said, "I took a little while to get by that picture. It just kept staying there. It wouldn't let go. Then I saw myself alone, walking alone. He wasn't with me anymore."

They did a fourteenth set.

"I was with Ray [her fiancé] . . . it went from being alone to being with him, and we were watching a movie, *Mrs. Doubtfire*. We were laughing. I felt happy. Some of the pain was gone."

They did a fifteenth set.

"I saw fences being put up . . . on the side where my son was killed. Everything's going out of my mind in order, like it was really happening. Everything came to mind in order, the way it was. I stopped at the fences."

"Are those fences there now?"

"The fences are there. They were put up in springtime . . . my head feels very . . . I got a headache. I gave myself a headache."

"When you go back to the original scene, how does it seem?"

"How does it seem now? Kind of vague now. I can still remember it, but it's fading."

Steve asked her to rate the intensity from 0 to 10.

"It's a 5."

"What stops it from going lower?"

"Part of it is still there."

"What part?"

"The body parts."

"Let's go with that. Just let it go. See what comes next."

They did a sixteenth set.

"It was the same picture. I was telling my son I couldn't help him. 'I can't help you. I can't put you back together.'"

"Stay with that."

They did a seventeenth set.

"I saw my son," Mia said in a broken voice. "And he said, 'You can't put me back together. God put me back together, because I'm an angel now. And he was all together.'"

"Stay with that."

After the eighteenth set, Mia sniffled and said, "I saw him up in the sky, with my grandmother. They were both up there, looking down."

"How did that feel?"

"Better."

"Stay with that."

They did a very short nineteenth set, after which Mia was silent for a long time. Then she said, "I asked my grandmother to take care of Billy, and she said she will. He's with her."

"What does that mean for you?"

"That he's being taken care of."

They did a twentieth set.

"He was saying he was okay. He was saying, 'Be happy, I'm okay.'"

They started the twenty-first set. As Mia was moving her eyes back and forth, Steve asked, "Does that mean it's okay to be happy?"

When the set was over, Mia said, "I told him I didn't want to be without him. It's hard to be happy without him. He was saying I have to try. I have to just try."

"Is that okay?"

Mia nods.

After the twenty-second set, Steve asked, "How is that original scene now?"

"Not bad. Like it happened, but . . . "

"On a scale of 0 to 10?"

"A 0."

"How do you feel?"

"I feel better."

"Close your eyes for a moment and feel how your body feels. What do you notice?"

"I feel relieved. I feel more comfortable, like a weight is lifted off of me. When I think about that the way I did before, it was really hard, it was really painful. But I don't see it like that anymore. The painful part is gone out of that."

"It's okay to try to be happy?" Steve asked.

"Yeah."

"Let's just close on that."

Then they did their twenty-third and final set of the day, one hour and eleven minutes from the time they sat down together. In this, the first of three EMDR sessions, Steve and Mia focused on the terrible way Billy died. As with most people in mourning, EMDR moved Mia through this aspect of her grief rather quickly. This happens because the mourner realizes that it does not matter how the person died. What's important is that the person is no longer there. The details don't matter. Following the protocol that Steve developed for working with complicated, painful bereavement, his next session with Mia would focus on the consequences of Billy not being there.

One week later, Steve and Mia met for their second EMDR session.

"How are you doing?" Steve asked.

"I was doing really well all week, but then just yesterday I saw a little boy who reminded me of Billy. Since then, I've been thinking about it again."

"When you think of the original scene now, how does it seem?"

"Well originally it was like 0 all week. I felt pretty good. But now it's like 2. There's something about the little boy . . . "

Steve felt that this was a really good sign. When people have done part of the work but they know there's still more work to do, they protect themselves until just before the treatment. Then all of a sudden something happens or they remember something else. It shows that they are preparing themselves to continue. He also noted that Mia's body language still said "depression" and her face was pale and expressionless, framed by two hanks of thick brown hair she had pushed off her forehead.

When they targeted that "2-level" feeling, what came up for Mia was not the picture of Billy's body parts that had haunted her in their previous session but being back at the fatal scene and fighting frantically to get up to the tracks to see her son's body while her family and the police held her back. As they did EMDR on that memory, a completely different image came up, and Mia began to cry quietly.

"I saw my son, his face. Very happy. Saw a smile on his face." Mia's own face softened. "I couldn't let go 'cause then he would be gone. He said, 'I'm leaving, I have to go.' Why did it have to be you? 'It just had to be that way. I have to go. I can't come back. We'll be together again.'"

"Can you let him go?"

"I don't know. I'll try, but I don't know if I could."

"Well, just stay with that, and whatever happens, happens."

During the set that followed, Mia started moving her lips as if silently talking to someone. At the close of the set, she wiped tears from her eyes.

"He was leaving, and he was angry at me for not letting him go. 'You have to let me go. You have to.' And he was gone. I couldn't see him anymore. But he was angry at me."

"What does that mean?"

"It means I have to . . . but it's hard to 'cause I have to live with it every day that he's gone. And he doesn't know what I feel. Maybe he really does. I don't know."

"Just stay with that," Steve said, and they started another set. While leading her in the eye movements, he added, "Mia, do you see any difference between letting him go and forgetting about him?" The purpose of this question was to help the processing along at a point where it often becomes snagged.

"No."

"Do you think that he'd ask you to forget about him?"

"No."

"Maybe he means something else."

They did another set.

"It does mean something else. It's really two different things. I could let him go and not forget about him, 'cause he'll always be there anyway."

Another set.

"He's saying they are two different things, letting go and forgetting. 'Don't forget how we were, 'cause you'll always have that. Nobody can take that away.' To remember him the way he was, not what happened to him. I really, I could let him go."

They began another set, during which Steve asked, "Does it seem okay this time?"

"Yeah, it's okay. He's gone now."

"And?"

"It's okay. He's gone in the sense that his body is gone, but he'll never be gone."

"That's right."

"As long as you're in my memory, you'll always be there."

"Could you go on with that?"

"Yeah. I could try my best."

"Stay with that," Steve said, and then he led Mia in a very short set.

"Seems like things would be different," she said.

"How so?"

"Different feelings about what happened. But he's still going to be with me, no matter what changes . . . jobs or moving or whatever. He'll still be with me."

"How does it feel?"

"Better."

"When you go back to the original scene, how does it seem now?"

"Kind of vague now. Now I don't even care to go up there [the tracks where Billy was killed]. I really don't want to. I want to not forget it happened, but forget how it happened. And he's gone just like anybody else who's gone. But he's not ever forgotten."[6]

"And how is it now, 0 to 10?"

"Zero."

"And how true is it that it was just an accident?"

Mia paused, then said, "Very true. Just an accident. It's not any different than my grandmother's death. She was very old."

"Your grandmother?"

"I believe she went to take care of Billy. She went before to take care of Billy."

"Is it your responsibility now?" Steve asked, to check on the progress. This is often one of the most painful sticking points.

"I can't . . . " Mia's voice faded away.

"Stay with that." Steve led a very short set.

"I did what I could for him while he was here. I really couldn't hang on . . . that's part of letting it go. He's not my responsibility anymore."

Another set.

"It's changed now. It's not thinking about all those things anymore. The guilt is gone. Everything's gone. It's just the way it's gotta be. Everything's gone." And now that everything is changed, we have to accept who we have become. Coming to this acceptance often means coming up with a new sense of identity. Mia could not define her life around being Billy's mother anymore. She had to come to emotional terms with what she needed to hold on to and what she would be able to let go.

"Is that something you can live with?"

Mia nodded and smiled very slightly.

"You could try?" Steve asked.

"I'll try."

Another very short set.

"I'll try to live with that and accept it that way. And try to move on."

"When you say 'try to move on,' what do you mean by that?"

"Try to go back to work. I don't know if I want to go back to that job. Being there is painful for me 'cause that's where I was when he was killed. Maybe I could do something else."

"Can you just hold that in mind and see what comes up?"

Another set.

"I don't see myself going back there. I've been watching children. I baby-sit for my nephews a couple days a week. Maybe I could do something like that. I feel better when I'm around children."

"Just go with that. Take a deep breath."

Another set.

"I see myself around children, my nephews, my fiancé's two little boys. I see myself around them. It's like another way of life, not taking care of Billy, but that responsibility, of caring for a child. Maybe adopting a child. [Mia had been told by doctors that she might not be able to have another child.] There are a lot of children out there that need parents."

Another set.

Mia smiles. "But I want them to be mine. And I don't want them taken away again. I don't know how I can make that happen, though. Maybe it's something I can work on."

"It's hard to know what's going to happen the rest of our life," Steve said softly, "when in one afternoon . . . "

"Right. If I did that, I could kind of still be the person I was. Maybe that's why my mind thinks that way. Because I raised a little boy by myself for twelve years—it's a very big part of my life—and that was taken away from me." This was Mia's longest response so far. "Maybe I could have that part back. Not through him, but through other children. I want to try to let him go."

Another very short set.

"He's gone. I can't forget him. He doesn't want me to forget him. He wants me to remember. I think I should try to do that, try to let go of that. Nobody could do that for me. That's the hard part. I have to do it.

"Well, maybe it's time for me to really try hard. I don't think I was trying hard before. I was still trying to hang onto things—anything I could that I felt was keeping him alive—but I can't do that anymore 'cause then he won't rest in peace. He's going to be disrupted. I need to work on that now. Letting him rest."

Another set.

"I keep seeing 'gone but not forgotten.' I just see those words in my head." Tears were now streaming down her cheeks, her hands still clasped tightly in her lap.

"Mia, there's nothing I can do to make it not sad. I think it's supposed to be that way, too. It's part of remembering."

"Right. I think it would be great if it wasn't sad, but there probably would be something wrong."

"Can you live with that? Is that okay?"

Another very short set.

"I think it will be okay."

"How true does that feel, from completely untrue, 1, to completely true, 7?"

"Completely true."

"Hold that in your mind." And to help strengthen the positive cognition, they did another short set.

"I felt like a weight was taken off my mind. I feel more peaceful, I think more than I ever did. I feel better about things."

"How does your heart feel?"

"It still hurts, but it's different. I think it will always hurt. It feels like an emptiness there. Nothing can fill it. No one can fill it 'cause that spot's for him. And I can keep all my memories there."

"Mia, does it seem like there's anything that's left undone from today?"

"No. I'm gonna stick with 'gone but not forgotten.' I'm gonna keep thinking of that . . . try to keep those thoughts with me."

On these words, the session ended.

When Mia returned a week later for their third (and final) treatment session, Steve noticed that she had a lot more color in her face and her hair was waved. She was also dressed in brighter colors, including a vibrant purple top. Steve viewed the final session of the study as an opportunity to find out if there was anything left that was still unresolved, any fears or negative beliefs that might block the completion of Mia's mourning and healing process.

"How have things been?" he asked.

"Okay. Pretty good. I've been keeping the thoughts I left with, 'gone but not forgotten.' And I try to keep it that way . . . I've had some painful days. I had a dream with Billy in it. He was sitting in a chair. Sometimes the dreams don't help."

"How is your sleep?"

"Better. The first scene [her son's body parts on the tracks] is almost kind of vague now. Before, every time I thought about it, it was magnified. It was really, really bad. It's not so bad now. I'm not stuck on that scene."

"What do you think you're stuck on?"

"I think just the death itself . . . not any particular thing, the train or the scene. I think I just have to, I guess, cry when I have to." Mia's arms lay on the armrests of her chair. As she talked, she moved her head and made facial expressions, something she had not done before. She also spoke in a louder voice.

"Were you crying last week?"

"Yesterday I did, 'cause of the dream. It was the first time all week. Before, I was crying every day.

"I can't change what happened. The death itself is always going to be there. I keep thinking, we all have to die sometime . . . I just want to live on earth and do my best and be a good person. 'Cause I know my son is in heaven. And if I keep thinking that way, I know eventually I will get to be with him. That's what saves me, thinking that someday I'll be there with him."

"You thought that before, in taking the pills, that it might be a way to get there sooner. [Steve is referring to Mia's serious suicide attempt.] Do you still have those thoughts?"

"Yes, honestly, a little bit, I do. But it wouldn't really be the right thing to do. Because you're not supposed to end your life like that. God would be very angry with me. I'd be hurting a lot of people. My family has had a hard time over it [Billy's death], too."

"How has it been going to the house [her mother's house, where she and Billy lived]?"

"Not too bad."

"You could stand it?"

"Yeah. But I wish my parents would move. It's painful there and it's painful for them, too. But it's not like an apartment where you can just pack up and go. They own it."

"If you think of the original scene, what do you get from 0 to 10?"

"Zero. I just see it a different way. Very vague. It was an accident. It happened. My son is not up there [on the railroad tracks] anymore. He's gone. My son is lying in the cemetery. So when I want to see him, that's where I go."

"If you try to bring it back now, what happens?"

"It's not that bad to think about, when I bring it back now. That pain that used to get in my chest is gone. The scene is real vague. Before, everything was real clear."

"If something in that scene still bothered you, what would it be?"

"The train, the people, me in the police car, no upset. Just his body."

"Do you want to try EMDR around that one thing?" Mia nods. "Bring it [the picture of Billy's body] to mind. What's the thought?"

"Sadness."

"What words about yourself go best with that picture?"

"I'm horrified at the thought of that. Disbelief."

"In our first session, you felt guilty. How's that now?"

"It's not there. I don't blame myself. Now I blame the two jobs I had to work."

"Hold that feeling of blame together with what's left of that picture. When you do that, what feeling do you have in your body?"

"It's really not my fault."

Steve held up his right hand, and they started the first set of their last session together. It was a very long one. Afterward, Mia was silent for about a minute.

"I see the blame going away, 'cause there's really no one to blame."

Another set.

"I just see us as being in an accident. When something's an accident, there's really no blame. 'Cause there was nothing done intentionally."

"How sure are you?"

"Completely sure."

Another set.

"I see it as being an accident and that's all. That's all it was. It was no one's fault."

"Not even yours?"

"No. 'Cause I was working, and even if I was home, it was just a block away . . . how could I know he would ever go up there? Maybe I blame the child who took him up there. But you can't blame a child."

A very short set.

"The blame is all gone." Mia spoke slowly, as if in a dream. "There's no one to blame, not even the little boy."

"What about work, jobs?"

"No. I had to do that. Whether he understood or not. I was supporting him, trying to get him everything he wanted. But I don't know if he really understood that, 'cause he didn't like me doing that."

"When you think of the whole event, what's still upsetting about it?"

"I do blame the railroad for not having fences up. My son was wrong for going up there, and they were wrong for not being sure their equipment was safe. It was an accident, but he was a child, curious. He wanted to know what everything was. A train was probably an awesome thing for a kid. 'Oh, wow, a big train!'"

"Can you forgive him for that?"

"Who?"

"Your son."

"I'm still . . . angry at him for that."

Being angry with the person who died is usually hard for people to admit—it can lead to more guilty feelings—but it is a completely natural response.

Another set. Steve and Mia were thirty minutes into the session.

"I can picture seeing him and telling him I am angry at him. He caused me a lot of pain and suffering. He never wanted that to happen . . . I just have to try to forgive him for that."

Another set.

Tears rolled down Mia's cheeks, and Steve handed her a tissue. "My son always used to say, 'I'll never leave you, Mommy.' . . . And I was thinking of that and that he was gone . . . he didn't want to hurt me, but it was his time to go."

"Can you accept it?"

"It's hard to accept it, but I could try."

Another set.

"I told him I will try to accept that he didn't intentionally want to hurt me. He would never have gone up there if he'd known what would happen."

"No more blame?"

"No."

"If there were a piece of blame left, what would it be about?"

"The railroad. It's a senseless tragedy . . . I guess the part about his foot still haunts me, because if he wasn't caught, he would have gotten out of the way. A woman was there and she saw him pulling at his foot. So he tried, but he couldn't."

Another set.

"I was wishing I could have been there to pull him out and ask the little boy why he didn't help Billy . . . but he was afraid to."

Another set.

"I could see my son. I was talking to him. He was saying, 'It wasn't nobody's fault, Mom.' He never really wanted to leave me. But I have to try to go on. That's what he keeps saying. It's better. I can feel that part. It's better."

"If you go deep, deep inside of yourself," Steve asked, "what keeps the statement 'he's gone' from being completely true?"

"I don't want it to be true that he's gone."

A very long set, maybe three minutes.

"I can picture . . . him gone . . . that's not the way life is supposed to be. You're not supposed to bury your children. But he really is gone. That's the bottom line. He really is gone and there's nothing I can do to change it but try to accept it, try to go on for whatever the rest of my life may be worth. Try to go on."

"Mia, if you go back now to the original scene, what's it like?"

"Like nothing. Like it happened but it didn't. He's gone and that's it. That scene can't hurt me anymore. I'm not gonna let it hurt me, because I can't change anything about it. Maybe it always bothered me before 'cause I pictured him in that scene. But I've gotten it into my head that he's not in that scene . . . I took him out of that scene and put him in heaven."

"If you let yourself think about all the events around that day, if you sort of play it in your mind, if you come to a part that seems upsetting, open your eyes and tell me what it is and we'll work on it."

Mia was silent for a long time, then she said, "Being back at my mother's house, after they brought me back from the hospital. Seeing my family the way that they were. [Mia's parents, her brothers and sisters, and their spouses and children were also hurting from Billy's death.] I was in so much pain at the time, but I wanted to take the pain away from them."

Another set.

"I told them I didn't want them to hurt. But they said they had to for a little while, they had to."

"Can you live with that?"

Another set.

"They told me it was okay for them to grieve, that it was a part of life they had to live through. But they were more concerned about me. My family was destroyed over that, my brothers and sisters, my parents, my nephews. There were times when I was really in bad shape, but I would comfort them. To this day, I think Billy helped me do that because I don't know where that strength came from."

"If you think of that scene now, being at your parents' house, how does it seem now?"

"Not too bad. Not as bad as it seemed before."

"Zero to 10?"

"About halfway."

"What stops it from going down?"

"The pain of it. Just the pain."

Another set.

"I can see my family and they're telling me they're okay. I guess they have their bad days. That scene is not as upsetting now."

"What words about yourself go with that?"

"I loved them very much."

"I wondered if you blamed yourself for their suffering."

"I did. I tried to take everybody's pain."

"Let's try to do that now, take on everybody's pain and see how that goes."

Another set.

"I think they needed to go through what they went through. They needed that. It's just a part of life and I couldn't take it away from them. You can't take the pain away from anybody else. You wish you could, but you can't."

"How does the scene seem now?"

"Very normal. They were doing what they had to do, and I was doing what I had to do."

"Zero to 10?"

"Zero."

"Reliving the events again, see where it's still stuck." By now an hour of their third session had gone by.

"Probably that I never really said good-bye to my son."

"Let's go with that."

Another set.

"I didn't say good-bye at that scene or on that day, but I remember the night before, when my son was going to bed." Mia paused, her voice choked with tears. "Every night, I would hold him and kiss him good night and tell him that I would always love him. And he said the same, 'I'll always love you, too.' And I never saw him that last morning; when I went to work, he was sleeping. So really, I did . . . my last words spoken to him and his words spoken to me were 'I love you.'"

A very long set. Steve's hand moved back and forth despite the tears now in his eyes.

"I really did say good-bye to him . . . that was the last time I saw him alive. Maybe it was kind of like a good-bye, but we didn't know it at the time."

"Is that okay?"

"It's okay."

Another set.

"I really did say good-bye to him. He reminded me of that night. And those were our last words. And I said good-bye when I buried him, too."

"How does that scene seem now, Mia?"

"Better. Much better."

"Is it okay for it to be that way?

"Yes."

Another set.

"I feel better about that."

"Go through for anything else that's kind of stuck or caught."

"No, I don't get caught on anything else. I think I worked out everything in my head, things that were bothering me, myself. And I found the answers to the upsetting thoughts. It doesn't have to bother me now."

This is an important outcome of EMDR therapy. Mia knew that she was responsible for the healing. Steve just assisted the process. As he told her at the end of their final session, "It was a privilege for me to be allowed to help you with that."

⁓

When Steve saw Mia for a follow-up session eight months later, he learned that she was doing well. She had broken off her troubled engagement, moved back into the family house, and started work again at the warehouse. She no longer felt the need to distance herself from the past. She was sleeping well and was no longer having obsessive memories about the tragic accident. And, to her delight, she was pregnant. The doctors had been wrong after all. When Mia came back to the Institute for her fifteen-month follow-up, she brought her new baby, Nicholas.

Steve asked her how she felt now about losing Billy.

"Even though it was really hard," she told Steve, "you just have to keep going and you can make it. You have to. Everybody's life is important." She told Steve, "Your life is just as important as your child's.

"I feel like God's given me a second chance," she told Steve with tears in her eyes. This time they were tears of joy.

⁓

The ripples of pain caused by Billy's death weren't limited to Mia and her family. Our lives intertwine in ways we rarely think of until tragedy strikes.

The engineer who was driving the train that hit Billy Russo was hospitalized for trauma afterward. When he was released, he went back to work. Five months later, on the eve of retirement, he died of a heart attack.

Even in the midst of her own pain, Mia felt badly for him. She wanted to tell him she knew it was not his fault. "I don't know who I felt worse for, him or me," she said.

Mia's compassionate reaction is unusual. "Most people you talk to, the first thing they'll say is, 'Why didn't you stop?'" says Jim Duque, a longtime railway engineer and union boss. But you can't stop a fast-moving train in anything less than half a mile. And you can't steer it. Absolutely nothing the engineer does or doesn't do can change the fact that his train is going to run over whatever appears suddenly in its path. An engineer can choose how to respond to the situation, but he cannot control it, and he cannot control the horror, grief, and guilt he feels afterward.

"All you can do is watch it happen," Jim recalls. "And you have no place to hide."

∽

In January 1973, Jim, then in his early thirties, was running the locomotive of a freight train hauling iron ore northward on a branch of the Missouri Pacific Railroad that hugged the western bank of the Mississippi. As his engine came around a sharp curve some twenty-five miles south of St. Louis, Jim saw to his right a boat storage area where several boats and river barges were moored. A driveway with a level crossing connected the small marina with a cluster of houses on the west side of the tracks. Following standard operating procedure for approaching a grade crossing, Jim reached up with his right hand and blew a warning on his whistle. Then he saw trouble ahead.

Just north of the crossing were two bridges, one for the road running north from the tiny neighborhood and one for the train tracks. But the road bridge was flooded, and Jim could just make out four small boys pushing their two-wheelers across the railroad bridge. They were about three hundred fifty yards ahead.

The moment he saw the kids, Jim put the train into emergency. Using his left hand, he shoved the train-brake valve to the far right, an action that applied the brakes on the locomotives and each car and put the engines in idle. With his left hand, he kept tugging urgently at the whistle. One of the kids had gotten his bike stuck on the guardrail. He was jerking it back and forth, trying to free it. Then, to Jim's intense relief, the kids heard the train coming. All four of them ran off the bridge, leaving behind the stuck bike. Thank the Lord, Jim thought. But too soon. One of the boys dashed back onto the bridge to save his bike.

Jim yanked the whistle in vain as he watched his 385,000-pound diesel-electric engine, traveling at fifty miles per hour and backed by nearly a half mile of fully loaded hoppers of iron ore, bear down on the boy and his bike. The last thing he remembers seeing is the seven-year-old child, looking for all the world like his own young son, running back toward his bike and directly into Jim's blind spot, the area immediately to the left of the cab. Then came the thump of the impact. And then Jim's mind went blank. The whole episode, from the time Jim noticed the kids to the moment of impact, had lasted only thirteen seconds.

When Jim recovered himself, the first thing he noticed was that the train had come to a complete halt another half mile or so down the tracks. The second thing he noticed was that he must have, at some point, manually disengaged the diesel locomotive's independent brakes. The valve controlling those brakes was now closed, signaling that he had overridden the automatic kick-in and disabled the secondary brakes. Jim's breath caught in his throat. Why had he done that? And when?

Then, recalling the thump of impact, Jim jumped out of the cab and started walking back up the line. He was going to tell the kid that it was okay, that he understood why the boys were on the railroad bridge. Because he had obviously creamed the kid's bicycle, he would tell him he was going to buy him another one.

Jim had trekked down the long line of freight cars for about three hundred yards when he saw one of the bike's tires under the train. He could go no further. He knew then that he had run over more than the bike, and when he got back to the cab, the conductor called and confirmed his worst fears. They had found the boy, and he was dead.

Back in 1973, what Jim went through was not thought of as "trauma." It simply went with the territory: You worked on the railroad, and you saw people get run over by trains. When coming off duty after the accident, a buddy told Jim, "Whatever you do, work tomorrow. Don't lay off tomorrow. If you do, you might not come back. Just work tomorrow and then take off whatever time you need. But work tomorrow."

Jim took his advice and went about his normal life. Except that it wasn't normal anymore. He started drinking heavily. Like many others, Jim used alcohol to stop the pain, but it was a temporary fix. Sooner or later, the pain came back. He was unable to sleep through the night, startling into consciousness every two or three hours. He had recurring intrusive thoughts and feelings about the accident and was haunted by the picture of that little boy racing back across the bridge. Whenever he heard of any train accident anywhere, his thoughts became obsessive. When he was assigned to travel that same route, he could hardly bear it. Crossing the bridge triggered heart-breaking flashbacks of the accident. He finally transferred to a different part of the railroad so he wouldn't have to cross that bridge again.

Jim's grief, including obsessive thoughts and heavy drinking, rode with him for the next nineteen years. His marriage fell apart. He remarried, but that union, too, ended in divorce. His sons grew up, and with every year they gained, Jim thought of that little boy: Had he lived, he would now be eight . . . nine . . . ten . . . fifteen . . . twenty-one . . . twenty-six. The guilt he felt was relentless. He wracked his brain trying to think of what he could have done differently. He never told anyone at work about the disabled secondary brake; he felt too guilty. Maybe if he hadn't released that locomotive brake, it would have given the boy the extra second or two he needed to get out of the way. Even though he knew intellectually that the one or two seconds wouldn't have made a difference, the way Jim felt about it, it was as though he had held the gun to the boy's head and pulled the trigger.

In 1990, Union Pacific (which had merged with Missouri Pacific) started offering peer support groups for employees who had been involved in what were now called *critical incidents*. Jim, who by then was in his early fifties and widely respected for his work as chairman of the local chapter of the Brotherhood of Locomotive Engineers, went to one of the first two-day training sessions for peer support counselors. The program was set up and run by Tim Kaufman, a staff counselor. As a licensed engineer, Tim understood from his own experience how difficult it would be for Jim to describe the vivid sights and sickening sounds and to share his feelings.

Tim opened the training by telling the small group of men and women, all of whom had been involved in at least one critical incident, to "leave their guns" at the door. "We are not going to talk union business or management stuff," he told them. "We're going to talk about critical incidents and what peer support is all about. You've already paid the terrible price of admission to this workshop by being involved in an incident. The price you pay to remain here is to respect every other person and his incident and to agree to strict confidentiality about what anyone else says."

Okay, I can do that, Jim said to himself. But I'm not going to tell it all. No way I'm talking about that brake being released. No way.

As people took turns telling their painful stories, the emotional level in the room skyrocketed. Reports of death, dismemberment, grief, and inevitably, soul-scorching guilt were put before the group. It was the first time in Jim's life he'd seen twenty men cry at the same time, and he was one of them. When it was Jim's turn to talk, he went ahead and told it all.

Later in the day, Tim introduced Roger Solomon, a psychologist then working for the Washington state police, to talk about EMDR therapy. Roger had been using EMDR successfully with patrol officers involved in critical incidents. Tim wasn't sure how his railroad people, generally conservative, skeptical, macho, and totally uninterested in flaky things like psychotherapy, would react.

"Please give EMDR a chance and hold your judgment about how goofy this may look," he told the group.

After explaining what EMDR was, Tim and Roger offered treatment to workshop participants on a voluntary basis. Jim Duque was among those who were willing. Privately, he was leery. He didn't know the program and he didn't know Roger. But he'd agreed to try it, so try it he would.

Roger and Jim decided to target Jim's intrusive image of the little boy running back across the tracks to save his bike. The emotions Jim felt were sadness and guilt, summed up by the words, "It was my fault he died." His positive cognition was, "I did the best I could."

Roger started the set.

The first thing that came into Jim's mind at the sight of Roger's moving fingers was the thought, "Well now, this is a joke." Then things started to happen. By the third left-right pass of Roger's hand, Jim had begun to relive the accident, moment by moment. He was back in the cab of the locomotive, blowing the whistle, spotting the kids on the tracks, putting the train into emergency, then seeing the child climb back onto the bridge. Next he heard the sound of the impact, but this time his mind didn't go blank. He was acutely aware of everything around him, including the sight of his left hand on the handle of the train brake and his right hand pulling the whistle.

In a flood of relief so intense it was almost joy, Jim knew that the boy had not died through his negligence. He knew he had not disabled the secondary brakes until after the accident. He couldn't have; he hadn't had a free hand to do so. Jim felt his whole body straighten as if the guilt had been a physical burden he was no longer carrying.

Roger, still moving his fingers back and forth, saw Jim's serious face lighten and tears come into his eyes. The expression on the face of the big man was one of amazement, relief, and happiness.

"For all these years, I've had a doubt that if I hadn't done that, shut off that brake valve, maybe that boy would be alive today. But it's not true. I didn't do that until after the accident. I did the best I could. There wasn't any more I could have done."

Later that year, Tim gave Jim a call to see how he was doing. Jim said he was sleeping well and had gotten his drinking under control. He admitted he still had thoughts of the accident at times, but the picture of the boy no longer haunted him. He was also offering peer support for other railroaders involved in fatal accidents. More than anything else, he wished he could help prevent the careless, senseless tragedies. "Maybe it would help," he said, "if people understood that there's another human being driving that train."

10

Breaking the Iron Grasp of Addiction

> History, despite its wrenching pain, cannot be unlived,
> and if faced with courage,
> need not be lived again.
>
> —MAYA ANGELOU

THERAPY OF ANY kind is a way for an individual to begin to reclaim control of past experiences and learn to process pain in a healthy way. But too often a person's first impulse in the face of pain is to escape suffering rather than confront it. For instance, people with PTSD try to commit suicide eight times more frequently than those in the general population.[1] It is not surprising, therefore, that people who have experienced trauma are more apt to abuse drugs and alcohol.[2] It is estimated that three-quarters of the general public will experience an event that could cause a traumatic response sometime in their lifetime. Is it any wonder, therefore, that chemical dependence is achieving epidemic proportions?

EMDR therapy goes beyond quieting the pain. Although few formal studies have been completed, there are numerous published reports of the success of EMDR in clinical work with alcoholics and drug abusers (see Appendix B). It can rapidly pinpoint and reprocess the underlying causes of the distress, whether traumatic or otherwise; often one of the reasons for the addiction can be traced to childhood events.[3] Children who have been victims of crimes or physical abuse or have witnessed violence are at higher risk of later substance abuse, as are children who have suffered from dysfunctional parenting including psychological abuse, such as neglect or verbal assault. Those children grow up without the appropriate foundations for self-esteem, and they often are drawn to different forms of drug abuse to find relief.

Especially at risk are children who grow up in chaotic environments provided by withdrawn, traumatized, or insensitive parents, who themselves may have been alcoholics or drug abusers. In these instances, family life is dominated by alcohol or drugs, and the children are often left to fend for themselves. As they try to maintain a sense of order by normalizing, denying, or excusing their parent's substance abuse, these children also experience an ongoing sense of abandonment and the lack of safety. These children understand that they may, at any moment, become an object of abuse or may be called on to protect or "save" the parent. Even though the child may have no basis for comparison and therefore considers the situation normal, the negative experiences can have a devastating effect on the psyche and personal development. To maintain a place in the family, the child has to give up an independent sense of self and take part in the deception and dysfunction. The terrible cycle of trauma sets in motion a lifelong struggle.

In EMDR treatment, substance abusers reprocess the past as well as present situations that cause them disturbance. Distress becomes a call to be aware of the environment and take action, not to try to escape it. Clients learn coping skills for the future: how to handle stress without using drugs or alcohol and how to resist current triggers to substance abuse (the sight of a whiskey bottle, for example). In addition, EMDR is used to address the person's internal triggers, such as adult feelings of inadequacy stemming from the original trauma, which in turn can exacerbate the substance abuse.

Although there may be a genetic susceptibility to addiction for some individuals,[4] heredity is not destiny. Substance use is based on an interaction of heredity with past or current experiences.[5] Whatever has been learned can be changed. It may not be easy, but what has been experienced can generally be reprocessed. Even when there is a genetic component, EMDR clinically appears to be an effective option. In those cases it is especially important to mitigate other factors.

Again, EMDR should never be used in a vacuum but rather as a part of a system designed to make the client feel safe and supported. It works best when it is used in conjunction with counseling groups that provide a nurturing atmosphere, such as group therapy, Alcoholics Anonymous (AA), and Narcotics Anonymous (NA). In these groups, a person's feelings of isolation are replaced with a sense of community. When one person shares his painful experiences, many others can identify with his thoughts and feelings, even if the details of their own experiences may be different. Group members are able to feel a sense of connection and compassion they may not have experienced in years, if ever.

∽

Not all drug abuse starts at a hot party or in an unlit alley. For Amy Kuwabara, it started at a hospital in Kansas where she was a young nurse in the obstetrics-gynecology department. Amy loved her work delivering babies, but as a newcomer with no seniority, she was assigned to the night shift, and the hours were miserable. Having difficulty falling asleep during the day, Amy soon ran herself down. One day she overheard other nurses talking about taking sleeping pills to adjust to rotations from day shift to night shift. Amy decided to try the pills too and found that getting them was easy; the hospital stocked them by the palletful. They worked. Over the next few years, Amy used them occasionally to get to sleep; although they gave her a pleasant feeling, she took them only on an as-needed basis.

In 1987 Amy, who was born and raised in Hawaii by Japanese parents, left Kansas to sign on as a travel nurse, working a series of three-month stints at hospitals in different states. Amy's assignments took her to southern and northern California and Alaska. She liked the work and, always a loner, didn't mind not having enough time in any one place to connect with her colleagues or establish intimate friendships. Amy had never been comfortable in social situations, and at twenty-six, she had had only three dates in her life.

In some ways, travel nursing suited her all too well. The situation was chillingly familiar, at least on an unconscious level. As a child, Amy had felt like the outcast of her family. She remembered sitting out on the porch one night, waiting to see how long it would take for her family to notice her absence. They never did. Now, the role of outsider in other people's territory brought back her childhood feelings of overwhelming loneliness and isolation. Alone on her nursing posts, this pain resurfaced, and she turned to the one source of happiness she could get her hands on: pills.

The drug was named Stadol. It was a synthetic narcotic that not only blunted Amy's emotional pain and put her to sleep but also made her feel good. Amy was amazed; she had no experience of feeling that well. Tempted to experiment with other painkilling drugs the hospital stocked, such as morphine, Demerol, and Phenergan, she reasoned that other people in pain took drugs and felt better. Why not her?

In less than a year, Amy's sporadic drug use was no longer enough to keep the lid on her painful feelings. In fact, the drug-withdrawal cycle only added to them, causing the addiction to take on a life of its own. First, Amy developed symptoms of chronic fatigue syndrome, although she was never diagnosed with it (they may actually have been drug-withdrawal symptoms), and she was hospitalized for two weeks for depression and suicidality. The psychiatric staff tried to work with her, even prescribing an antidepressant, but nothing made a dent in her pain.

When she was released, Amy, now twenty-seven, decided to move back home. She took her old room in her parents' house in Honolulu, found a full-time nursing job, and tried to live a normal life. Despite her recent bout with chronic fatigue, Amy's parents expected her to take full responsibility for her adolescent brother and sister, do the laundry, and cook certain meals. It felt to Amy like it had when she was fourteen. Both her parents were working then, and she was going to school and completely responsible for her toddler sister and infant brother. Amy didn't say a word to her parents about having been hospitalized for depression; any discussion of mental health problems was taboo in her Japanese family.

Once again employed as a nurse, Amy started signing out Stadol from the locked narcotics cabinet whenever she needed it. She "needed" it more and more frequently. One night, Amy convinced herself that she needed the narcotic because her feet hurt from working so much. At other times, she just needed relief from the hell that was her inner life. Amy was starting to experience those intensely painful feelings again, the feelings (compounded by withdrawal) that seemed to come from out of nowhere. The smallest incident would set her crying. If she was at home, she would run to her room and sob into her pillow, just as she had done as a child.

Given the way Amy was raised, nursing had seemed to be the ideal career for her. The oldest of four, she had been responsible for the other three children early on, even to the point of being blamed for their transgressions. She was also supposed to be stoic, never showing sadness or anger. (If she did show her feelings, her father would get enraged and repeatedly hit her with his fists, kick her, or thrash her with a wooden hanger. It wasn't just a whack or two; these were beating sessions.) Amy's mother simply ignored her. Neither parent ever praised Amy, no matter what she did or how well she did it. Both parents made it clear that she was "a mistake," that they were hoping for a boy. This uniform demeaning treatment left Amy feeling invisible, unimportant, and isolated. As a nurse, she continued to focus on the needs of others, receiving little or no praise.

It wasn't long before Amy was using Stadol regularly, either taking it in pill form or shooting it into her muscles several times a night to get the quick high that would free her from the relentless discomfort and put her to sleep. A year and a half later, Amy's hand got caught in the cookie jar.

The hospital opened an investigation into why so many of their narcotics were disappearing. Amy knew she wasn't the only one stealing drugs—other nurses and doctors did it, too—but her name was on the list as having signed out more narcotics than anyone else. The hospital authorities called her in and told her she had to get treatment or they would fire her and she would most likely lose her license. Amy agreed to get help. She loved her work with new mothers, and more important, she could not imagine surviving the shame of losing her license. It would dishonor her parents; she would have to kill herself.

In November 1990, Amy was suspended from her job and started three months of intensive outpatient treatment. She saw a counselor once a week, went to counselor-led group therapy once a week, and attended AA meetings three times a week. The group meetings were nearly unbearable for her. They took her back emotionally to her experience with the only other group she'd known, her family. To Amy, being in a group meant leaving herself open to severe criticism, rejection, and physical abuse. When she arrived at her first AA meeting, Amy was intimidated by how dressed up everyone was. When the speaker announced that it was break time, she stood up and ran out. Her heart was racing and her fingers had gone stone cold. The AA group had become a trigger for the feelings of fear and pain that were embedded in Amy's childhood experiences.

Even while she was in the treatment program, Amy continued to use drugs. She *liked* using drugs. They made her feel better. Because she couldn't get any Stadol, she took sleeping pills. One day she found cough syrup with codeine in her parents' medicine cabinet and found that it worked quite well. Later, her brother got some Tylenol with codeine and Amy helped herself to that.

At the end of the three months, it was apparent to the hospital authorities that outpatient treatment was not working for Amy. A counselor on staff recommended that she go to an inpatient program especially for women. She had no choice but to agree if she wanted to keep her nursing license.

Amy was sent to a women's treatment center in a Catholic hospital and assigned a room in the former nuns' quarters. Every morning someone came at six-thirty to get her up. When it was time for her to go to an AA meeting, someone else would drive her there and back. There was no way she could get drugs, so Amy became clean and sober by default. She had a few physical withdrawal symptoms, but nothing unbearable. However, her deep-seated fear and distrust of other people still blocked her road to recovery.

At the treatment center, Amy was required to go to group sessions five days a week with two counselors who used confrontation as a way to help addicts face their problems. They immediately spotted Amy's holier-than-thou attitude—"I am a registered nurse and everyone else here is on welfare"—and confronted her. Amy admitted to having an attitude, but she said nothing else. How could she? She knew she needed help, but she didn't know how to ask for it.

About six weeks into the program, one of the group counselors lost patience with Amy and read her the riot act. "You can't go to the meetings anymore. You have to sit outside in the hall until you learn to ask for help." Dejected, Amy dropped onto the bench in the hallway. She didn't know what to do, so there she sat, ever the outsider. A day or two later, Amy was asked to leave the program.

Amy managed to get readmitted a week later. She had stayed off drugs and gone regularly to AA meetings during that week, and the counselors were willing to give her a second chance. Ten days later, Amy left of her own accord. She hated the restrictiveness of the treatment center. On the plus side, although she was still on suspension from her job and now living on welfare herself, Amy was now clean and sober. She desperately needed to stay that way to keep her license, and she knew she needed more than AA to do it. That was when she got a referral to Dr. Silke Vogelmann-Sine, a psychologist who specialized in using EMDR for substance abuse.

Amy walked into Silke's office on August 5, 1991; she was now thirty-one. During their first session, Amy told Silke about her history of drug abuse and her current situation. She said the sight of medicine bottles triggered her urge to use drugs. Silke asked Amy about her family and her childhood. Then she spelled out the conditions under which she would be willing to work with Amy. They were tough: no drug use, regular AA attendance, working with an AA sponsor who would help her stick to the program, and doing psychotherapy with Silke once a week. Amy's heart sank, but she consented. The treatment plan that Silke set up for Amy was designed to help her stay off drugs, always the first plan of action in any form of substance abuse therapy; however, there were deeper reasons behind the specific prescription. When Silke listened to Amy's story, she saw that one of the biggest obstacles to Amy's recovery was her lifelong distrust of other people. Silke hoped that requiring Amy to work closely with an AA sponsor would give her the "training wheels" she needed to learn how to relate to another person. In working the Twelve Steps of AA with the help of her sponsor, Amy would have to open up and share her feelings, even at the risk, which was terrifying to her, of being criticized or rejected.

Another, more immediate implication of Amy's perennial distrust of others was that before she could make any significant progress in therapy, she would have to feel safe with Silke. This became the major objective of Silke's first few months of psychotherapy with Amy. Beyond that, therapy would require Amy to unlearn the key lessons her childhood had taught her, lessons that were not only inaccurate ("You are worthless") and inappropriate ("Don't take risks") but almost malevolently self-fulfilling.

As the first weeks of therapy went by, Amy kept her commitment to Silke and stuck to her treatment plan (although she still hated group meetings). It would take courage for Amy, because of her early training, to cross the bridge from the austere, chilling world of her childhood to the emotional and unpredictable world of adulthood. One big problem was that Amy's early childhood perceptions were true. It had been dangerous for her to show her feelings. If she did, she would be beaten. The safest way to deal with that reality was to find a way to wall off the feelings so they didn't show. In therapy, the way to freedom was to allow her feelings to emerge, but all her fear and danger reflexes were mobilized to prevent this.

In PTSD the inner state experienced during the traumatic event is apparently locked in the victim's nervous system. Some patients even use the intonations or demeanors of a child when speaking of their childhood experiences. Present-day dangers bring up the same painful feelings even though the man or woman is three feet taller and thirty years older than when the abuse occurred. In an EMDR therapy session, as the memory is targeted and activated, the original physiological state can manifest clearly and then be resolved. Fortunately, time is not an important factor in the EMDR treatment, so that even events from long ago can be processed effectively. However, the patient must be willing to allow the processing to occur. Amy first had to learn that it was safe to do so.

Because of Amy's childhood experience of neglect and abuse, Silke had to conduct the case as a form of long-term psychotherapy. Although EMDR is capable of causing rapid changes, it is important that it, like any therapy, be customized to the needs and readiness of the individual patient. Amy's negative beliefs about herself ("I'm worthless") and her attempts to cope (taking drugs) were not the result of an isolated traumatic event that could be rapidly targeted with EMDR; they stemmed from the very fabric of her childhood. Even when numerous events in a person's life have given her similar negative messages, however, several representative events can be targeted with EMDR. The positive results then generalize and spread to the other memories, creating a fabric of a different hue and pattern. Silke knew that she had to move slowly, making sure that EMDR didn't trigger in Amy an avalanche of bad memories and an ensuing rush back into the suffocating but comforting arms of addiction. It would be important to wait until Amy had sufficient support, through either her relationship with Silke or the AA network, to see her through the rough spots. It was going to take some time.[6]

One day in October, Amy became newly traumatized. Hospital investigators had called her at home and told her they were pressing charges against her for stealing drugs. She became overwhelmed with fear. Although the usual mode of EMDR treatment is to start with earlier memories first, when dealing with substance abusers, it is often necessary first to provide relief from the pressures of present stressful situations. Silke thought that this present-day event would be a good target for EMDR. She explained the procedure, and Amy agreed to try it. When Amy brought the investigation to mind, what she felt was, "I am bad, I am an outcast, I am useless." What she wanted to feel instead was, "I was sick; I can cope with the situation." Amy rated the truth of her desired feelings at a 2 on the 1–7 scale. She rated the anxiety she felt about the investigation at a 10 out of 10, the most anxiety she could imagine feeling.

When they began the eye movements, Amy found that if she concentrated on following Silke's fingers, she couldn't concentrate on the target. Although this happens with many EMDR clients at first, Amy responded to the difficulty with self-blame and fear of failure. Silke encouraged her simply to keep her eyes moving. Eventually, Amy managed to stop crying, but her mind was still a blank. She couldn't keep the investigation in mind. Silke continued to lead the eye movements.

Then, as if something in her heart had cracked open, Amy started sobbing aloud. Tears coursed down her round cheeks. She felt like she was falling into a bottomless black hole. "I want to hide in my room," she cried in a tiny high-pitched voice. Her childhood state was being triggered in earnest. "I don't want anyone to see me. I want to die. What will my parents do if I get convicted?" When her tears had stopped, Amy said that these were the exact same feelings she'd had when she first heard about the investigation. "I thought that if I just didn't deal with it, it would go away."

Slowly, as the eye movements continued, Amy began to shift from the "nooooooo!" of pain to the "oh" of dawning awareness. She realized that the hospital investigators were making her feel the same way she felt as a child: rotten, unwanted, and worthless. In another set, Amy recognized that when she felt that way, she got an overwhelming urge to use drugs to overpower the painful feelings. As the processing continued, she spontaneously shifted to a more positive perspective: that she was weak when she stole the drugs and was unaware of the full impact of her actions. The perspective of a healthy, aware adult was achieved once the childhood fear was processed.

By the close of their first EMDR session, it was clear to Silke that although Amy had made a connection between her upbringing and her response to the investigation, she wasn't ready to pursue this connection. However, in this session, she was able to define a course of action. First, Amy would call a lawyer, and second, she would start talking with her AA sponsor every day until the case was resolved. Then she and Silke applied EMDR to an image of taking these steps to make sure Amy felt ready for them.[7] It was necessary that treatment take place on many levels: education, abstinence and assertive skills, and recognition of danger cues, to name a few.

The second time Silke and Amy used EMDR processing, they focused again on a specific present-day problem. On the day of the session, Amy came into the office crying and near panic. Her whole body shaking, she told Silke she felt an overpowering urge to use drugs. What set off this emotional chain reaction was a disagreement Amy had had with her AA sponsor, on whom she had learned to depend for support. The sponsor had found out that Amy was taking a narcotic-like pain medication that had been prescribed for her following abdominal surgery. She had accused Amy of using drugs again. Amy had been shocked. True, she had not thought to ask her doctor for a nonaddictive painkiller, but Amy thought her sponsor was being unfair.

Amy and Silke targeted her feelings about "my sponsor betrayed me" as a 10. It only took a few sets before Amy's mind made the link between her sponsor's response and the way her father had accused her unfairly as a child. Again, Amy wanted to run to her room and barricade the door so no one would see how bad she felt. As the sets continued, Amy recalled other upsetting incidents from her childhood that shared the same theme of betrayal. For each of these old memories, Amy and Silke continued doing sets until Amy was no longer upset about them. Then Silke asked Amy to bring back to mind the conflict with her sponsor, and they started doing sets on that encounter again. After several passes, Silke asked, "What do you get now?"

"I think my sponsor is too rigid," Amy said.

"Okay, stay with that."

Another set.

"I ought to tell her how I feel," Amy said.

Another set.

Silence. (Putting her feelings into words was not Amy's strong suit.)

Another set.

Silence.

Another set.

Silke asked, "Amy, what do you *want* to think about this?"

"That I did the best I could. That it was an honest mistake."

"Okay, hold that in mind." Silke led another set, then asked, "Why was it an honest mistake?"

"I didn't realize I should tell my doctor about my addiction problem."

This was the step Silke had been waiting for: It was the beginning of a plan of action. "What would you say to him?"

"I have an addiction problem."

"Okay," Silke said, "picture yourself telling your doctor and follow my fingers."

Another set.

Silence.

Silke asked, 'What do you get now?"

"That feels fine. He understood."

"Anything else you want to say to him?" Silke asked.

"Maybe to ask that next time he gives me a nonaddictive painkiller."

"Hold that in mind." Another set.

"How is that?"

"Fine."

"How about your sponsor? What will you do about her?"

"I will tell her I made an honest mistake."

Another set.

Silke says, 'What if your sponsor doesn't agree with you? How will you cope with that?" It was important to make sure that Amy could withstand the disappointment and rejection that could occur.

"I don't know," Amy replied and looked away.

"Can you picture yourself telling her?" Amy nodded. "And her disagreeing?" Amy said nothing.

"Follow my fingers."

Another set.

Silence.

Silke asked, "What do you get now?"

'Well, she still disagrees. But that's her problem."

"Anything else?"

"Yes. I will tell her I am going to keep my original sobriety date."

And so the sets continued as Amy slowly constructed and committed herself to a practical, step-by-step plan of action to cope with her situation. Her anxiety had dropped from 10 to 2.5. She felt her desired belief ("I am worthy; this is my sponsor's viewpoint; I can manage the situation") was mostly true (5 out of 7). Amy felt that it was okay that her belief did not feel one hundred percent true, because she still had to get through the confrontation with her sponsor. After all, this was her first try at confronting anyone.

Overall, Amy had made progress she could be proud of: She had recovered from intensely painful feelings without the numbing solace of drugs; she had done some successful problem solving about how to respond to her sponsor's accusation; and she had noticed once again that feeling victimized in the present was linked to the low self-esteem she had developed in childhood.

In the course of the next six months, Silke and Amy alternated weekly talk therapy sessions with EMDR processing sessions targeted on Amy's current problems. They did four EMDR sessions in a row targeting different aspects of Amy's continued urge to use drugs, which appeared to be triggered by the sight of bottles of medication, an obviously destructive trigger if Amy was to regain her position as a nurse. (In all types of drug use, the associated paraphernalia can, through conditioning, become a potent trigger to use of the drug.) Amy identified the emotion behind these urges as anxiety, and she rated it at 8.5 out of 10. Her thoughts when triggered were, "I need it; I want it; I am vulnerable. I can't cope without drugs." This response in turn triggered feelings of shame about still wanting drugs: "I've been clean for so long, how come I can't stop having these feelings?" According to EMDR theory, of course, the reactions were locked in her nervous system. No amount of insight or cognitive determination was sufficient to cause them to go away. Amy was caught in a cascade of painful reactions: The sight of medicine bottles triggered obsessive thoughts of wanting drugs, and recognizing that she wanted drags triggered feelings of self-loathing and despair that she would start using again. The despair made her want the drugs even more. Her desired belief was, "I can handle my feelings; I can manage situations adequately."

In the first of these four sessions, Amy said she did not want to face the pain from the past and confront difficult situations. She was conditioned to believe that she would fail because experiencing any feelings at all was in direct contradiction to her parents' most vehement teachings. She also said that she was not used to receiving attention and caring from others, which was beginning to happen now that she was starting to heal, and it frightened her. The session closed with Amy doing eye movements and imagining that she was talking to the childlike part of her that was so scared. "I'll be there with you, you know. I'll help you manage it. We can handle our feelings." Amy was beginning to recognize that, as an adult, she could be more in control.

The third EMDR session on Amy's triggers switched quickly out of the present and into the past. Amy's responses started with, "Drugs make me feel so good; I have no worries." Next came, "It's an escape, like from loneliness." Then, "Friends haven't been there for me in the past." These opened the door to Amy's memories of childhood, and Silke led Amy in sets of eye movements while Amy talked about her extreme loneliness and the time when she was seven years old and left alone at home when she was sick. Weeping, she said her parents saw her as the strong child, and her mother thought she could cope with being alone. That set the precedent for the rest of her childhood. Whenever she was sick, she stayed home alone. Her sister insisted that her mom stay with her, however, and her mother did. Amy never said a word.

In this session, Amy also processed a lot of the physical abuse by her father, which she had felt was her fault. Amy's sadness was nearly overwhelming, but she was able to keep doing the eye movements until she reached a place where she could say, "I am a good person. My father is the dysfunctional one." This evolution of a healthy perspective for most childhood abuse victims has revealed itself over thousands of EMDR sessions. The first stage involves the recognition by the client that she is not to blame for the abuser's actions, an important developmental stage that allows separation from the perpetrator. The second stage is an awareness of being safe in the present. As long as the physiological responses of the abuse are locked in the body, there is a sense of current danger. Although a person may intellectually realize that her perpetrator is sick, dead, or in another country, the childhood terror state can remain. Finally, the third stage involves the recognition that the abuse is in the past and that the person has reclaimed her ability to choose what happens to her in the future.

Over the course of the next eight or nine months, Silke met with Amy about once every ten days and used EMDR to remind Amy how to cope with situations that might trigger her desire to use drugs (for example, call a friend or her new sponsor; use a self-control technique; immediately leave the presence of the physical trigger) and to have faith in her own ability to handle painful feelings without using drugs. In August 1992, a year after she had started working with Silke, Amy came to Silke's office in crisis. She had awakened from a nap the previous day and suddenly remembered that she had been molested once by an uncle when she was in the eighth grade. Amy had known about the molestation before—in fact, she'd reported it at her intake interview when she was hospitalized for depression back on the mainland—but she had put it out of her mind. Now it was back, and her feelings of being dirty and worthless were overwhelming her.

Amy's lonely upbringing made her a prime candidate for substance abuse. With a history of molestation added to that, she had the deck further stacked against her: Sexual abuse victims are more likely than the general population to develop a psychiatric disorder and more likely to become substance abusers.[8]

Amy told Silke that since remembering the molestation, she had desperately wanted to use drugs; it was the only way she knew to stop the flood of painful feelings. Silke asked her if she would try processing the memory with EMDR. Amy agreed.

The target they used was Amy lying in bed and being touched. Her emotion was fear, and she rated it as a 10. Her negative belief based on the incident was a familiar one: "I am vulnerable; I am a victim." What Amy wanted to believe instead was, "It's over; it's in the past." She rated how true that felt to her in the moment as 1.5 on a scale of 1–7.

As soon as the eye movements began, Amy started sobbing, and she continued this deep sobbing throughout. Feelings of fear, victimization, and abandonment flooded her in every set.

After the opening set, Silke asked, "What do you get?"

"I'm scared," Amy said, rocking back and forth with her arms clasped over her stomach.

Silke led another set.

"What do you get now?" she asked gently.

"I'm scared, noticing him. What he's doing there. He's not supposed to be there." More rocking.

Another set.

"I still see him there. It's as if he is going away."

Another set

"I woke up. My clothes are up and my tummy is exposed. My chest hurts." Deep sobs continued to shake Amy's body.

Another set.

"I feel shock. Disbelief. How could something like this happen? What did I do to cause it?"

Another set.

"I didn't have anyone to talk to. Nobody was home. I could not talk to my parents about it. . . . I had nowhere to put it. Nobody to talk to."

Another set.

"Nobody was there. Nobody was home. There was nobody to talk to."

Then, as Amy's time was almost up, Silke helped her to close down the scene and put her feelings away into an imaginary container. The painful feelings would stay there until their next meeting, Silke said, when they would take the lid off and work on them again. The session concluded with Silke using EMDR processing to reinforce some healthy coping strategies (such as calling a friend or sponsor) in case the painful feelings came back. First, Amy did eye movements on the positive belief, "I now have people who can help me." Then Silke asked her to pair the scene of the molestation (and her feelings of abandonment) with that belief.

Another set.

"What kind of support do you need in order to cope with this situation?" Silke asked.

"Calling my [new] sponsor or talking to my AA home group," Amy said.

"Hold that in mind." Another set.

"How's that?" Silke asked.

"Fine."

"Is there anything else you can do?"

"I could call a couple of my girlfriends."

"Okay, picture yourself doing those things," Silke said, and she led another set. Again, Silke was giving Amy "training wheels" to help her learn how to cope with the bad feelings instead of giving in to the urge to use drugs. By the close of the session, Amy's fear had dropped from a 10 to a 6.

Amy came back the next day. Her fear had dropped a little more, to a 4.5. She told Silke that she still felt like a victim, but that she *was* a victim and there was nothing she could do about that. It had already happened.

As they began processing, the fear declined, and Amy's feelings started to move from grief to anger. "What is he doing in my room?" she said during one set. "I want to push him away."

Another set.

"He's still standing there. I'm scared . . . I brought a picture of him." Amy looked through her oversize straw purse. "Here." The photo showed two men, both Asian Americans, standing for a formal portrait. Their faces were intent and serious, their suits slightly old-fashioned.

"Which one is he?" Silke asked.

Amy closed her eyes and shook her head. "I can't look at it."

"Is he on the left or the right?"

"I don't know. I don't remember." Amy's whole body was tensed, every muscle ready to withstand attack.

Silke led a set.

"I'm scared. Maybe he'll do something violent."

Another set. Amy started weeping.

Silke led more sets until Amy had calmed down.

"Can you look at the picture now?" Silke asked.

Amy nodded. "He's the one on the right."

"How upsetting does that original scene feel now, from 0 to 10?" Silke asked.

"Six point seven."

Another set.

"How could he do this?" Amy said angrily.

Another set.

Amy began talking as if her uncle were in the room. "How could you do this?" She clenched her fists into balls.

Another set.

"What do you get now?" Silke asked.

"Nothing."

"Take a look at the picture. How does it feel now, from 1 to 10?"

Amy paused to consider. "Three point five."

Another set.

"He is a sick person."

Another set.

To close the session, Silke asked Amy to pair her belief, "he is a sick person," with the photo. The next time Silke checked, Amy's fear had dropped again, this time to 1.5. Color had come back into her face.

At their next session, Silke checked on the level of Amy's fear about her uncle. It was at 1.2.

Amy reached a milestone in her recovery from drug abuse in December 1992, when she was able to go back to work full-time as a nurse. She continued to see Silke once every three or four weeks, but she rarely had fear-of-relapse crises. Gradually, using EMDR therapy, Silke helped Amy explore the family connection to her problems: her low self-esteem, her fear of relationships, her habit of withdrawing and isolating to avoid criticism or abuse, her extreme sensitivity to rejection, and her three-plus decades of denying and repressing her feelings.

Even more gradually, EMDR helped Amy become able to *feel* the feelings she had bottled up as a child. She got angry. She got sad. She got heartbroken. And she got determined to heal. With this, Amy began to shift, to move, to grow. She came to realize that it was not the world that she had always been so afraid of; it was her parents. She came to respect deeply the little girl who had the courage to survive the emotional abandonment by her mother and the unceasing rage and hatred of her father. In early 1995, Amy finally moved out of her parents' house into an apartment.

Now, five years after starting psychotherapy, Amy is still working as a labor-delivery nurse in Honolulu, but she is taking psychology courses to see if she would like to become a psychotherapist. She says she is tired of being treated like a second-class citizen by the doctors in the hospital. She sees Silke as needed, still goes to AA, and has joined a support group for nurses with addiction problems. Amy has remained clean and sober, one of only three women from her inpatient program who have achieved this. The other twelve are using again.

Not that the urge to use never comes up. In January 1996, Amy called Silke in crisis. A doctor had prescribed pain medication for her bursitis, and she had taken four Vicodin tablets. They made her feel high, and Amy was terrified she would relapse. Silke gave her an appointment for that afternoon. They met and agreed on a plan. Two hours later, Amy returned, the bottle of Vicodin gripped in her right hand. Together, Silke and Amy walked to the bathroom and emptied the contents of the bottle into the toilet. Amy flushed it.

⌇

The goal in doing EMDR therapy with a substance abuser is to touch into and process the negative emotions that are perpetuating his or her addiction. Most alcohol and drug abusers feel they don't fit in or belong anywhere because they are different, in a bad way, from everyone else. Twelve Step programs can give them a foundation of support and renewal, but as one AA member put it, "To get to the other side, to peace and serenity, some things have to be processed. And sometimes you need help to do it. Alcohol, or drugs, is the symptom; it is not the problem."

What about the people who get clean and sober but can't stay that way? Relapse into substance abuse can ambush a recovering addict even if he is fully committed to abstinence and has been sober for a long time. Some of the most common warning signs of relapse are the inability to think clearly, memory problems, mood swings from emotional overreaction to numbness, sleep disturbances, problems with physical coordination such as being clumsy or accident prone, and extreme sensitivity to stress. These symptoms often appear from six to eighteen months after the addict initially achieves sobriety, although they can crop up as long as two years after. They tend to surface when the person is experiencing a lot of personal stress.

All recovering addicts experience some of these symptoms at some time. Some handle the symptoms without relapsing. Others relapse once or twice but work through what caused the relapse and eventually reach recovery.

But some proportion respond to these distressing symptoms (all of which get worse without treatment, especially the mood swings) by using drugs again (and again and again). The cycle of addiction is set back in motion, causing additional pain, confusion, and frustration to the addict and her loved ones, pain that she may then "medicate" with yet more drugs or alcohol. This condition, called *chronic relapse*, shows a promising response to EMDR treatment.

⁓

Ross Birrato started doing drugs when he was twelve, shortly after his grandmother died and left him alone in the big house with his father and grandfather. Ross's parents had divorced six years earlier. His father had won custody of Ross and had prevented the boy from seeing his mother. In fact, Ross never saw or heard from her again: Any letters, cards, or presents she sent were destroyed unopened. When, at age twenty-one, Ross started searching for his mother, he found out she had died the year before.

Even when Ross's grandmother was alive, it hadn't been much of a home for the boy. Although Grandma thought he could do no wrong, Grandpa thought Ross, like his father before him, could do no right. He told the boy he was stupid, useless, rebellious, and insignificant. He was the disappointing son of a disappointing son. When Grandma died, Ross's grandfather told him it was his (Ross's) fault.

Ross's grandfather was a socially and professionally prominent man. A Lebanese immigrant, he had come to the United States as a young man and worked his way up from the shipyards to Golden Glove boxing to his current position as a successful dentist and church leader. Behind all these achievements was a controlling, power-hungry perfectionist and a sadist. He did extensive dental work on his young grandson, filling cavities, making crowns, and doing root canals—all without benefit of anesthesia. Grandpa always turned off his hearing aid before he started drilling. "I am a painless dentist," he used to brag. "If I didn't hear it, it didn't hurt." But hurt it did, terribly. Ross used to cover his mouth with his hands to make his grandfather stop. It didn't work. To this day, the backs of his hands bear scars from cuts made by the high-speed drill.

What of Ross's father during all this? Greg Birrato was a narcissistic and emotionally empty man. Once again in his parents' house, he stepped back into the role of mom's precious boy. He treated his son as if they were brothers. Actually, he treated Ross as if Ross were his *older* brother. Ross, in a vain attempt to win his father's love, threw himself into his role. He became the responsible one, the caretaker, and the people pleaser, doing whatever he could to fill the needs of his father and assuage the temper of his grandfather.

As Ross grew, so did his involvement with drugs. Smoking pot grew into taking speed. Doing a little drug dealing to pay for his habit grew into running a ten-thousand-dollar-a-week operation with seven "shops" (houses or apartments that were rented, furnished, and staffed) dealing cocaine and marijuana. Ross figured he could avoid the most common pitfall of all dealers, taking out all the profits in goods, by selling drugs he personally didn't use. But drug addiction doesn't yield to intellectual strategy. By the time Ross was in his early twenties, he was not only seriously dealing but also seriously drugging.

At this time, he got busted for carrying five ounces of cocaine. He went without a struggle; it was a fair bust. Ross was convicted, but he never served time. Half of the white powdery evidence had disappeared before he came to trial, which meant that he would be tried on a first-time charge in county court rather than federal court. The judge suspended Ross's sentence and put him on three years' probation.

Getting busted threw the fear of God into Ross. He packed up his apartment and moved to a suburb on the far side of town to start a new life—clean, sober, and legitimately employed. The first day he was there, he installed formidable security locks on his doors and windows, a ritual he would later repeat in every place he moved into. He got a job as a private-duty nurse and found he was effective with psychiatric patients. He also became a psychiatric patient himself.

Ross had started having psychotic episodes during which he would lose touch with reality. He would have delusional thoughts that sent his anxiety level through the roof. Sometimes he could ride it out, but other times he had to be hospitalized. He was diagnosed with manic depression (today called *bipolar disorder*) with a strong tendency toward the manic side, meaning that he suffered from periods of extremely high energy (marked by lack of sleep, rapid disconnected thoughts, high-risk activities, and feelings of grandiosity) that alternated with episodes of deep, dark, unmitigated depression. Although bipolar disorder is caused by a chemical imbalance, it is believed that stress added to that condition can result in psychotic episodes. Of course, Ross's severe drug abuse may have produced symptoms similar to those of all these conditions; therefore, it is hard to know whether the diagnoses were appropriate. Nonetheless, to treat both the bipolar disorder and the psychotic episodes, Ross was prescribed three powerful medications. These included lithium carbonate, which he took in substantial doses daily to help control his manic episodes.

Ross didn't succeed in staying off drugs, despite having moved to a town where he didn't know any drug dealers or associates of drug dealers. He found a connection anyway and started taking speed again. Then he did some penny-ante dealing to pay for his habit.

In his late twenties, Ross once again drew the line concerning his addiction. I'm better than this, he told himself. I just can't do this to myself anymore. He stopped using speed for a while and then started again. Every time Ross stopped, he found he could go for about a month before he'd relapse again. Then he met Hal and began the longest and stormiest relationship of his life.

Ross had been sexually active with other boys from the time he was seven. At first, things with Hal were good. They were in love. They were both using. About a year into their relationship, Hal asked Ross what he wanted for his birthday. Without thinking, Ross replied, "I want to be clean and sober." They went to a drug rehabilitation clinic, got a good counselor, and got clean. Ross still had occasional relapses, but nothing he felt he couldn't handle.

Whenever Ross stopped taking drugs, his psyche's internal strategy for avoiding emotional pain fell apart. Before sobriety, whenever he got very stressed or anxious (which could mean a psychotic episode was coming on) and started free-falling into a sickening feeling of powerlessness, he would run out and get a bag of speed. That little bag, he knew, would take him on a ride for twenty hours, and maybe those bad feelings would be gone when he got back. Once clean and sober, Ross had to find something to take the place of speed in his internal balancing act, something that would nourish and calm him and make him forget about his pain. He switched to food. Already a big man (the kind of big that got him mistaken for a bouncer in nightclubs), he started putting on pounds. He gained seventy pounds over the next couple of years, which was dangerously taxing to his diabetic body.

His relationship with his partner, which had worked less and less well the longer they were together, developed some serious cracks in it. They fought.

They didn't talk. They did petty things. (One day Hal polished Ross's antique sterling silverware with steel wool.) They slipped into the roles for which their childhoods had tailored them. Ross became his lover's caretaker in a vain attempt to win love. Hal also had diabetes, but his was more serious; he was deteriorating rapidly.

One night, Ross drove to the county psychiatric hospital in a blind panic and begged them to admit him. He had been feeling a major psychotic episode coming on for about a week, and he didn't think he could stave it off any longer. His anxiety was skyrocketing, and his mind was starting to shear off in a thousand directions at once. In addition, he was nearly out of medication. At the hospital, he was given a tranquilizer and a list of local counseling centers, and he was sent home.

Luckily, the psychotic episode did not occur. Even more luckily, Ross made an appointment at one of the clinics. It would prove to be one of the more ironic events in Ross's life that the hospital's uncaring attitude resulted in his finally getting the help he needed.

Ross was thirty-six years old and weighed 340 pounds when he met Bob Kitchen, a marriage, family, and child counselor from Hayward, California, who was a specialist in addiction and relapse prevention. Ross told Bob his history of manic-depression, psychotic episodes, and addictions, and the two men agreed to work together. After they had done five sessions of talk therapy and established the trust and personal connection necessary in any kind of therapy, Bob told Ross about EMDR therapy and asked if he'd like to try it. They could start by targeting something small, like a recent incident with his partner in which Ross had felt his privacy had been invaded.

"Fine," Ross agreed, ever upbeat. "Let's do it."

"Before we start," Bob said, "I want to caution you that it's possible you may have urges to relapse after EMDR because we are stirring up old things, old feelings. You may be triggered by what comes up and you may really want to use again. That is unusual, but if it happens, it doesn't mean you're a bad person. I want you to be ready just in case that urge comes up."

This caution is vital for anyone in EMDR treatment for substance abuse. As soon as the disturbing memory is targeted, it can trigger the person's primary coping mechanism: using drugs or alcohol. Understanding that this is an automatic physiological response can help the person avoid self-blame. This is vital because self-blame will only intensify the downward spiral.

Bob and Ross started EMDR by targeting the interaction with Hal. However, as Bob put it, "With EMDR, whatever it is you say you want to work on, you're going to work on what you need to work on." For Ross, that first eye-movement session opened a door straight into his childhood. A memory of his father came up, from the days when Ross, then a teenager, and his father lived in a small apartment and shared a bedroom. Ross still played the role of people pleaser and caretaker, and it still didn't make his father love him. Hal, he suddenly saw, reminded him of his father. They had the same narcissistic qualities and the same emotional emptiness that made any real relationship with them impossible.

As treatment continued, EMDR kept taking Ross back to his childhood. He and Bob did several sessions on the appalling physical and emotional abuse his grandfather had perpetrated on him under the guise of dental work. The terror that Ross experienced in reliving these events during EMDR processing was staggering, as was his anger about it. It became clear to Bob that Ross's grandfather, dead these twenty years, played a critical role in Ross's life today, providing the root of his addiction and perhaps his manic-depressive swings as well. Now it was Ross's task to dig up a lifetime of buried feelings and to stay sober while doing so. Ross began to see that he had been using first drugs and then food unconsciously to keep a lid on his fear and anger and to console himself for his pain.

Bob watched Ross heal week by week, impressed by the man's stamina and determination. But he was waiting for something else to happen. During an EMDR session about six months into therapy, it did.

Ross had come in feeling that a psychotic episode was coming on. He was feeling very anxious and stressed, and as he discussed this with Bob, neither could find anything current happening in Ross's life to account for it.

"Okay, Ross, try this," Bob said. "Go back to the first time when you felt this anxious." He paused. "What do you get?"

Ross was silent for a full minute, then spoke quietly. "It was when the men broke down the door."

"How old were you?"

"Five."

"What happened?"

"It was before the divorce, and my mom had taken me away from Dad. We were living in different apartments; we moved around a lot because we knew Dad was looking for me. One night, my mom woke me up and started to get me dressed. 'Be quiet, be quiet,' she said. 'We have to leave.' She kept looking out the window, and she was very afraid. Suddenly, two men kicked in the door. One of them came in and the other stood in the doorway. I couldn't see his face, but his body was outlined by the light in the hallway. Before I knew what was happening, he came in and threw a pillowcase over me, dragged me to his car, and threw me in the backseat. Then he drove away. He never said a word the whole time."

"What happened after that?" Bob asked.

"Well, I remember him pulling me out of the car. We were somewhere like in a garage; I remember how cold the concrete was on my feet. I was still in the pillowcase; I hadn't even tried to get out of it. I was paralyzed, helpless. The man never said a word, but I knew I was going to die and there was nothing I could do about it. I don't remember anything after that. Except that I was okay. But I couldn't go back to my mother. I was put in a foster home until the divorce."

This type of memory was exactly what Bob had been expecting. The previous year, Bob had read about a study showing that many addicts who repeatedly relapse have had some kind of life-threatening experience in their history or an experience that they had perceived as life-threatening.[9] These experiences set off a tidal wave of intense anxiety and unbearable feelings of powerlessness. To avoid these feelings (and, therefore, in the logic of the automatic connections, to avoid dying), the recovering addict would do whatever it took, even go back on drugs after years of sobriety.

Looking back at the many men and women Bob had treated for chronic relapse, this theory seemed to fit; therefore, he decided to start working with addicts by looking for the life-threatening experience in their past and targeting it with EMDR. He was astonishingly successful. Over the years, he found that 80 percent of the chronic relapsers he treated were able to stay clean and sober after EMDR. This included most of the drug abusers and all of the alcohol abusers he had treated. The only addicts who continued to relapse after treatment with EMDR were people who were still using amphetamines or amphetamine-like drugs. According to recent research, this finding might have something to do with a metabolic abnormality of the orbital frontal cortex that prevents the information processing from actively taking place.[10] Fortunately, Ross had been clean for a while.

Bob and Ross decided to target the kidnapping blow by blow, just as the events had unrolled that night thirty-one years ago. The sets started with

Ross's mother pacing the floor and repeatedly looking out the window. When it got to the part when the men kicked in the door, Ross began reliving the event, having all the physical and emotional sensations he'd had at the time. Terror zinged through his body.

"One of them is in the room and the other is on the threshold," he told Bob. "I know I am going to die."

Ross's heart was pounding; his breathing had gone shallow; and the paralysis he'd felt that night had seized his thirty-six-year-old body. Ross couldn't move a muscle or utter a sound, but his mind was racing. What was happening? Who were these men? Would they hurt my mom? Why did they break the door?

Then Ross suddenly recognized the second man, who was still silhouetted in the doorway. The shape of his business-like felt hat, his small stature, and his classical boxer's build were unmistakable. The man was his grandfather.

Now crying, Ross kept following Bob's fingers, as he began to move step by step through the succession of emotions associated with the grief process: denial ("That couldn't have been him"); depression ("How could he do that to me?"); anger ("I could kill him for doing that"); bargaining ("If I had been a better kid . . ."), and finally acceptance. His body kept pace with these feelings, and there were a number of dramatic moments when Ross had spontaneous physical releases of body tension. In one of these, his shoulders moved as if he were throwing a punch without lifting his arms: His right shoulder came forward while the left went back, releasing the back muscles.

For Ross, recognizing that his kidnapper was his grandfather was like finding the key to a code.[11] So much of his life suddenly made sense, he thought, from the benign to the bizarre. Of course, I install security locks on every door and window every time I move into a new place, he reflected. Of course, I'm afraid my partner will betray me. Ross saw that the seeds of betrayal had been sown very deeply in him by his grandfather. Circumstances in his adult life could easily trigger these feelings. Most important of all, Ross recognized that this event was another taproot to his lifelong anger, an anger so out of control that one time he picked up an ex-lover bodily and threw him through a wall and into the next room.

By the time Ross and Bob finished doing EMDR on the rest of the kidnapping event, Ross made what proved to be a major and seemingly permanent shift in his feelings and attitude. Looking back at the time, after three years, Ross said, "It's a shame that it happened, but it wasn't my fault. I really didn't have anything to do with it, so I don't have to pay any more dues to it. I had so much anger behind it. I had always been a really angry person, but that wasn't who I wanted to be. I really didn't know where the anger was coming from."

Three months after doing EMDR therapy, Ross was doing so well that Bob suggested he talk to his prescribing doctor about adjusting the level of his medication for bipolar disorder.

"Oh, that," Ross said. "I stopped taking them two, three months ago."

When bipolar disorder is diagnosed, it is considered an organically based condition and is treated with lithium carbonate to maintain the neurological salt balance needed to keep a person's emotions on an even keel. Therefore, the years-long remission of Ross's symptoms seems to indicate one of two things. Either processing his early trauma restored the chemical balance Ross needed to deal with present-day stressors, or the symptoms of trauma can convincingly mimic aspects of what are assumed to be organic conditions. In either case, for Ross, the result was a sense of freedom.

Ross continues to work with Bob on the aftereffects of his childhood, but the list of things to tackle is getting shorter. Ross has stayed off drugs. He has had no more psychotic episodes (despite having dropped the medication), and his manic episodes have ceased. He has also lost more than one hundred pounds and his diabetes has gone into remission.

"I have a new way of dealing with things," Ross says. "I work them through. I see that stress is only temporary, and if I deal with it now, I don't have to get back on the merry-go-round with it later."

Ross ended up deeply grateful to the psychiatric hospital that refused to admit him. "Actually, they did me a service. If I had gotten hooked into that system, I'd still be there today. Now I feel like I have a life. I may not be completely in control yet, but I know that's what I'm working towards."

"Working it through" is not done only on an intellectual level. The goal of EMDR is to work things through on all levels so that the person's "knee-jerk responses" are naturally healthy ones—intellectually, emotionally, and physically.

The Final Doorway:
Facing Disease, Disability, and Death

It is never too late to be what you might have been.

—GEORGE ELIOT

AS WE GO THROUGH LIFE, we usually think of ourselves in terms of our intellectual or physical capacities. In some cases, our identities perch precariously on a single salient fact: "I am a lawyer," "I am a runner," "I am a painter," "I am a carpenter." This fact becomes our anchor, the one sure thing we know in a chaotic and rapidly changing world. What happens, then, when the painter loses her eyesight or the carpenter's hands are crippled by arthritis? What happens when the lawyer contracts cancer and is too ill to practice? Suddenly the person has to face not only the loss of control that physical disability brings but also the death of the old identity. What happens when the body we took for granted no longer obeys our commands or the simplest movements cause us pain? I have seen numerous times in working with clients that such a loss can result in emotional and psychological consequences that mirror the symptoms of PTSD.[1] Fortunately, EMDR can help mobilize all the person's resources during a confrontation with disability, disease, or even death itself.

When Richard Webster consulted psychiatrist David McCann, he was trapped in the shattered remains of his life. The victim of a devastating mining accident in the early 1980s, he suffered the loss of both his arms, was badly scarred over his face and other exposed areas, had become deaf, and

needed prosthetic shoes to walk. For eight years after the accident, he suffered daily flashbacks and nightmares, which he described as a living hell.
Richard described to David how he had been lowered thirty feet into an
eight-hundred-foot mine shaft when a gas explosion enveloped him in a ball
of fire. Richard explained that every night as he tried to sleep, he would feel
as if his scalp was burning and would become engulfed by an overwhelming
sense of fear. Television programs showing accidents or explosions would
trigger intrusive thoughts of his traumatic event and feelings of depression.
Every year at the time of the anniversary of the explosion, his symptoms
would become worse. Only forty-one years old, Richard needed twenty-
four-hour-a-day nursing care.

During their first EMDR therapy session, David and Richard identified the target. Richard envisioned himself being consumed in a sphere of
flame, recalled the thoughts he had had ("My God, I'm on fire!"), and felt
the adrenaline rush of fear. During the first set of eye movements, Richard
thought, "I'm a dead man," and felt himself gasping for air. As the processing
continued, his initial images and sensations blurred, and he vividly remembered himself looking down, as if outside of his body, watching himself in
flames on the ground, surrounded by the rest of the crew. Richard recalled
the feeling as his protective suit burned and melted on his skin; he remembered his tearful plea, "My God, do something to help me!"

Suddenly the scene shifted to the memory of another near-death experience, when he had gotten caught in an oil-drilling rig. All he could think
of at the time was, "I'm going to die." Then spontaneously, as the processing
continued, Richard felt himself floating on clouds and heard the words "I'm
alive" reverberating calmly in his consciousness. "I think I understand now,"
he said through his tears. He explained later that, although he was not a
religious man, he knew in that moment that "there are other dimensions in
this universe."

By the next week's session, all of Richard's symptoms had disappeared.
His new goal was to be as independent as possible. For the first time in eight
years, he started taking care of himself and his home, going eight hours each
day without any nursing assistance. He said that because of the EMDR session, "a boulder was lifted off me." The next month, using prosthetic arms,
he passed his driving test and drove around town feeling like he'd been "pa-
roled from prison." Richard said he had had enough of "you'll never be able
to function normally" and declared that there was now no limit to what he

would be able to do for himself. Three months later, he drove off on his own to visit his hometown and enjoy the solitude of a leisurely trip through a national park. One year later found him actively helping other amputees and serving on the board of a program that helps children who need prosthetic limbs.

Two years later, Richard described his EMDR session as follows: "It was an amazing experience that defies imagination. I concentrated on the most terrible things that had ever happened to me, and it all went away. The treatment made me look deep, very deep, into my own existence. Now I see very clearly the fragility of human life and what it means to me. I'm more attentive to my feelings. I treasure each and every moment of my life." In many ways, Richard is an icon for a saying I hold very dear in the context of EMDR work: "It's not what happens to you that matters; it's how you deal with it."

Although physical complaints should certainly be evaluated by the appropriate physicians, EMDR therapy has also been used successfully to assist people with many types of illness and somatic response. In some cases, EMDR clinicians have found that the cause of the person's physical pain is a traumatic memory that has been stored in the nervous system. For example, one man came in to deal with a driving phobia that had bothered him for years. As he processed the memory of a car accident, his back and shoulder went into a spasm, causing the same pain that had sent him to a chiropractor almost weekly for years. During EMDR he remembered that the first time he had experienced this pain was during the accident, in which he had been broadsided on the right. As the treatment progressed and his memory of the accident was processed, his right shoulder completely relaxed. He was never bothered by the spasms (or driving phobia) again.

In between physical problems that are purely psychological in origin (such as pain stored in memory) and physical problems that are purely organic (such as amputations), there is a spectrum of conditions and illnesses that seem to be caused by an interaction between the physical and the psychological. Psychoneuroimmunologists have found the course of many diseases, including cancer, is impacted by the interplay between a constellation of factors including genetics, the environment, and psychological factors.[2] This doesn't mean that people are to blame for their disease, but it can mean that a sufficient amount of stress of a specific nature can have a negative effect on physical health. EMDR therapy can be used to alleviate much of this stress.

Any event can be an opportunity for growth. Richard came away from his EMDR session having transcended the physical limitations of his accident in a way he'd never dreamed possible. For cancer patients, regardless of their prognosis, EMDR can provide a doorway to understanding. Every person's experience of life-threatening disease is unique, but each of us has the potential to work through the pain and the places we are stuck.

One woman, when faced with a mastectomy for breast cancer, was horrified at the thought of her body being ravaged. Until she processed her fear, she was immobilized. She could not even understand the options presented to her by her physician. She used EMDR to help her choose a type of treatment and arrived at the calm understanding that she was much more than her body. She realized that she had a lot to live for and that the person she was would always shine through.

Another woman was terrified of cancer surgery. In her EMDR session, she recognized that she was less afraid of the operation itself than of what would happen to her husband and child if she were to die. During EMDR she realized that she had already given her family a strong foundation; if she died, they would make it through. After she recovered from the operation, she became less controlling and more at peace.

A third woman was diagnosed with a virulent and always fatal form of cancer. Her husband of many years had left her, and she feared dying alone and in pain. During EMDR processing she saw herself surrounded by her parents and the family members who had gone before her and declared, "When I die, I'm going to die with dignity." Talking about this experience later, she said, "It was all right. I didn't have to hurt anymore . . . someone was holding my hand." She took charge of her life and became an inspiration to all who knew her.

We will all die sooner or later. When faced with it, we have choices. We can cherish the time left or lose it in lamenting. If we can retain any common sense or spiritual principles, the choice seems clear; however, fear can triumph over logic or faith. Fear can separate us from our most firmly held beliefs. Therefore, in dealing with disease and the possibility, or certainty, of death, targeting the fear itself is one of the most constructive uses of EMDR.

⌒

When Jan "Johnny" de Groot, age sixty-five, was diagnosed with prostate cancer in November 1988, it was a disease that wasn't much talked about.

It would be more than seven years until *Time* magazine put prostate cancer on the cover of its April 1, 1996, issue and announced, to the horror of the public, that one in five men in the United States could expect to get it. The article said that Bob Dole, General Norman Schwarzkopf, and actors Jerry Lewis and Sidney Poitier had had the disease. By 1996, prostate cancer had overtaken skin cancer to become the most common type of cancer in men in the United States. The average age at onset was seventy-two.

In 1988, even the medical profession was not as alert or informed about the dangers of prostate cancer as it is today. In fact, Johnny de Groot's doctors at the huge health maintenance organization he belonged to didn't discover the cancerous tumor in his prostate until it had reached Stage D,[3] the final stage before death.

Johnny's prostate cancer had already metastasized; it had spread beyond the walls of that walnut-sized sex gland to all the bones in his body, with the odd exception of his lower legs. It was too late for radiation or chemotherapy. The only thing that the oncologists could do was to slow the spread of Johnny's cancer cells by cutting off the flow of the male hormone testosterone, which stimulates their growth. The procedure, called an *orchiectomy*, is the surgical removal of the testicles. It is followed by hormone therapy to stop the remaining production of testosterone, which is also manufactured by the adrenal glands. Johnny entered this course of treatment.

Johnny was a quiet, restrained man, whom his friends described as "superdependable" and "supernice." A native of Holland, he was an engineer by training and by nature, and when he was young it had always been assumed that he would join the prosperous family business in Delft when he completed his degree. His older brother would inherit it, but that was all right with Johnny. It was traditional.

World War II changed all that. Johnny was eighteen years old and studying engineering in Amsterdam when the Nazis invaded Holland on May 10, 1940. He was able to stay in school, but he loathed the German Occupation. Periodically, he was forced into hiding when the Nazis did a sweep for young men to fuel their war machine. The five long years of the Occupation were a nightmare that Johnny would never forget or, until the end of his life, talk about.

After the war, Johnny felt differently about his beloved Holland and could find no reason to stay. His adored mother had died of a brain hemorrhage when he was four, and his father had immediately married the family's housekeeper, whom Johnny had loathed, as had his brother and two older sisters. (The second Mrs. de Groot had made a deep and enduring negative impression on Johnny, a dynamic that was to come out during EMDR processing.)

At twenty-five, when he had completed his engineering degree, Jan de Groot left Holland. He joined the Dutch Merchant Service, saw the world, and learned he loved to travel. In the early 1950s, Johnny emigrated to the United States. He settled in New York City, took a job as a draftsman with an optical company, and earned his citizenship papers in 1956 at age thirty-three. His liked his new homeland and adapted to it well. He had to modify his first name; Americans seemed unable to say "Jan" (pronounced *yon*), so he changed it to "John," which quickly became "Johnny."

In the winter of 1957, Johnny met Martha on a ski trip. She worked as a probation officer in New York, and the two of them hit it off immediately. Martha was intrigued by Johnny's European formality, his charm, his kindness, and his maturity; he was seven years her senior. Before the end of the year, they were married.

Their marriage was a happy one, affectionate although not passionate. Johnny left his job; the couple moved across country; and he started his own business, a Midas Muffler franchise. They also started a family, consisting of two daughters on whom Johnny doted. However, Johnny's business was not a success. He was forced to sell it a few years later and take a temporary job with the U.S. Postal Service as a letter carrier, a drop in status and income. As a result, Martha, who had been a full-time mother, returned to work as a probation officer and later trained to become a psychotherapist.

Johnny was sixty-five when he learned he had prostate cancer. He had recently retired from what had turned into a twenty-year stint with the Postal Service and relished having plenty of time for sailing and working on his twenty-four-foot boat moored in the Berkeley Yacht Harbor. He also was an avid skier, enjoyed puttering around the house and garden, and had recently taken up playing the piano and flute. Although Johnny's cancer was advanced, he didn't feel, look, or act like a man with a terminal illness. He was physically fit and led an active life. He wanted to stay that way. It was in this spirit that Johnny decided to seek psychotherapy; he thought there might be something in his personality that was contributing to his illness.

I met Johnny in late May of 1989. We spent our first session together going over his history and talking about his current state of mind and his marriage (both of which, he said, had deteriorated since he was diagnosed six months earlier). The operation had left him permanently impotent, and he was having obsessive fantasies about people in his life dying, especially Martha. He found that he was becoming short-tempered and more anxious about little things, a typical response to being diagnosed with a catastrophic disease.[4] It seems as though all of a person's resources are focused on keeping down his fear of the future, and he has no patience left for the little difficulties of daily life. Even people who have always been known as sensitive, nurturing, and "nice" experience sudden flare-ups of anger.

Johnny and I talked about his disappointments and regrets, which he summed up in the statement, "I can't succeed." I explained EMDR and suggested we might use it to address that belief in our next session. He agreed, and I asked him to bring in a list next session of any past or present beliefs he associated with "I can't succeed." At the next session, Johnny pulled open a neatly folded sheet of paper and said, "Okay, I am afraid to succeed." Pause. "I might lose my wife." Pause. "It's hard to get in touch with my feelings. Happiness is dangerous. I don't want to listen; this is a very common thing throughout my life. I don't want to listen unless it's a really fascinating subject. Maybe it relates to my stepmother; I was turning off my stepmother." Pause. "I can't get myself to play the piano or the flute. I really feel stalled, and yet I think I might love it if I do it. Weird."

Although Johnny was over sixty years old and had been through psychoanalysis when he was younger, he was still inhibited by messages from his childhood. Although we targeted his feelings about the cancer and the current situations that made him upset with Martha, much of his present stress and feelings of lack of worth stemmed from his family of origin. Like many cancer patients, Johnny had a problem expressing anger. We approached this issue through working with his fantasies of people around him dying.

"What happens with the death fantasies?" I asked.

"Not clear. They go so fast. Then I feel sad, depressed. They come up when I feel or want to feel bad. I think of Martha dying."

Hearing this, I decided to use EMDR to probe for the crucial elements of his clinical picture and rapidly defuse as much pain as possible. Because Johnny could die at any time, we didn't have the option of a long-term approach. I decided to start his innate processing system going on a variety of targets and focus in on them individually later.

"Go back to a time when you thought you'd be better with her dead."

"We were skiing," Johnny replied immediately. "We had a good time; it was at a national competition. But I couldn't find my way to a place, and she got very peeved. Said I was stupid. It happened in a large crowd and was very embarrassing . . . I got peeved about it. She really showed her annoyance with me. I couldn't get her to see my point of view. Things were really rubbing the wrong way there."

"When was this?"

"About 1984." Even though this incident had happened five years before, it still rankled. Unexpressed feelings have a tendency to do that.

"How are you feeling now?"

"Very annoyed." Like many cancer patients, Johnny couldn't identify his feeling in the moment as anger. Sometimes these patients can do it in retrospect, but often the feelings are identified as "upset" or "annoyance." They generally blame themselves for the feeling, and they certainly don't express it. Many cancer patients can't remember ever raising their voice in their own defense, as an adult.

"Where do you feel it in your body?"

"My stomach."

We did a set.

"It's still there."

Another set.

"My reaction to it was wrong. Instead of getting angry at it, I could have made a joke out of it. That's where I feel I failed." Johnny's inability to express anger was linked to early experiences that taught him it was dangerous to feel.

"How about the anger? What is wrong with feeling anger?"

"Nothing . . . anger is associated with heavy stuff. This comes from when I was very young, six or eight; I wanted to kill my stepmother. I might do it if I ever let go, so I could not be angry."

"Let's go back to the feeling, 'I can't be angry.' That's associated with your stepmother?"

"Yes. My brother and sisters felt the same. I used to think during the war, how come a bomb doesn't drop on her, but on good people? I wanted to get away from her, but as a kid you can't get away."

"Think of your stepmother. Where do you feel it?"

"In the belly."

We did a set.

"She was always bitchy and complaining."

Another set.

"It got me very angry. Instead of killing her, I wished she died somehow."

Another set.

"Wanting to do away with someone."

"Instead of trying to push her away," I said, "bring up your stepmother."

"I've never talked about it before, this memory. I was at the breakfast table, had just sat down, and my stepmother was standing up next to me. She was really bitchy, yelling, 'Put your socks in the hamper!' Very angry. She kept hammering at me. My father interceded. She ignored him. Kept yelling. Father told me, 'For God's sake, please leave us. Get out of the house. Leave us!' I hadn't done anything really wrong."

"How strong is the feeling?"

"Nine to 10. In my lower guts and solar plexus."

We did a set.

"It was so long ago," Johnny said, "and she couldn't help it anyway." The pain was softening, but there was a long way to go.

Another set.

"I feel better, but it's still so deep in me. I remember so vividly; it's deep into my life. Martha dying or somebody dying [like his mother had when he was four], it's a 5, in my upper chest."

Another set.

Johnny said to me, "I feel something that feels like worms at my sides and lower back. My older brother walked out of the house when he was seventeen." Thoughts of his stepmother, death, and his sense of failure were all intertwined.

We did a set.

"I can't be as successful as he is, 'cause my dad won't let me. Why didn't he send me out? My mind is as good as my brother's. Too bad I wasn't sent away. It would have helped."

"How do you feel now?"

"I wish she hadn't existed. A 4. It's still there, the upset. In my lower belly."

Another set.

"He succeeded to get out of the house, and I can't succeed to get out of the house . . . it was about success. I thought I could be successful, but it was out of the question. I was too little. I didn't even ask. There's still constriction in my upper chest."

"Get into that upper chest and the constriction that feels like 'I can't succeed,'" I told him.

We did a set.

"Seven. I don't deserve it."

"Stay with that feeling."

Another set.

When we stopped, Johnny paused for a long time, then said, "I'm here now. I can shift the past aside, set this aside. It's my past. I feel much better."

Another set.

"Good . . . good . . . good. My chest and upper body are better. Still a little dizzy. She was a damn poor soul. Pathetic, just pathetic."

Another set.

"I couldn't do anything about it. I might have felt in the early days that there was something wrong with her. Fantasy, forget it!" Johnny ran his hand over the thinning hair on his scalp and cupped the back of his neck, his thoughts returning to the present. "My wife, she has other things, just like I have other things. There are probably a lot of other ladies that squeeze out the toothpaste wrong. My complaints are just little things."

"Think of your mother. What do you get?" So much pain of loss had to be locked in those memories.

"First a funeral party. Second, no, this must have been first, I remember she was lying in the living room on the couch and she was very sick. My dad paid a lot of attention to her. He told us about how sick she was. Then I see her on her deathbed. I see that vividly. She was a loving and caring person, and she had some white salve on her nose. Father said, 'Why don't you ask her for a few pennies to go next door to the apothecary and get some licorice?' I did, and she gave me a few pennies. But she could barely talk. She just looked at me."

"Where do you feel it?"

"In my chest and throat."

We did a set.

"I want to cry. I can't cry, so I feel sad and depressed instead; it's a better way out. In the old days, it was, 'Don't cry, it'll go away.' Crying was not acceptable. I feel constricted. Now I feel a tingling sensation." Anger, sorrow, fear—all the emotions it was not all right to feel—can come back to haunt us for years to come.

Another set.

"It's also important that you look at me, pay attention to me. I somehow have the feeling that people didn't look at me when I wanted attention."

"How do you feel when you think of your stepmother now?"

"Sad. She died."

"Bring up 'I can't succeed.'" Without processing that belief, there was little hope that Johnny could learn to enjoy the days he had left, let alone try to heal the cancer. I decided to continue probing different aspects of the fear while setting his processing system in motion. Knowing that I might not have the time to deal with each pertinent memory completely during our sessions together, I decided I would have to rely on his innate system to move the healing along outside my office.

"My mother. I can't make her better. But I can't get away from the house. I can't get attention. When I got older, I was really revolting. I threw stones through windows, wanted attention. I wanted attention forever."

Another set.

"I can't succeed in getting attention. I need help. I don't get the help and I don't get the attention, so I can't succeed."

Another set.

"In general, I feel better."

"Go back to 'I can't succeed,'" I said.

"The piano playing and the flute. It's ridiculous. I can't get myself to do it."

Another set.

"I can't succeed in enjoying myself. I can't be happy under those circumstances . . . I cannot show or feel my happiness in success 'cause the purpose of feeling depressed and trying to get attention would be lost. I'd never get it. If I ever was going to get it. I'm feeling bad. I feel embarrassed to want people to help me, teaching me the piano . . . I want to tell the person I need help. All the time. I don't need one lesson now; I need a lesson every day! Six hours! It's too hard to do it on my own. To be successful and happy, that would defeat my purpose of getting attention!"

"How does that feel?" He seemed delighted as he came to these emotional truths. The web of his life and the forces that drove him were becoming clear as the pain subsided.

Johnny laughed. "It feels good!"

"How do you feel now when you bring up 'I can't succeed'?"

"It's ridiculous, but it's also the truth. I've been sure all my life that it isn't possible. It goes so far back . . . to grammar school. First grade . . . I had to do it over. All my friends went to the next grade, and I had a new class."

Another set.

"If I try to succeed, I will do it wrong. That's very common. I generally overcome this, but I know it's there. I feel sort of dizzy and amazed again."

"Now what happens with 'I can't succeed'?" Every time I asked the question, I triggered the stored information and linked it to his information-processing system.

"I cannot succeed in playing the piano. I cannot succeed in playing the flute. I cannot succeed at school or at work or with my parents."

"Where do you feel that in your body?"

"At the lower gut level."

Another set.

Johnny laughed but said nothing.

"Again, 'I can't succeed.' How does it feel?"

"Silly! Silly not to be able to succeed. Unless you don't want to succeed. Do I want to succeed? Hmmmm."

"What happens if you imagine succeeding?" It was time to give him some positive homework to do.

"It feels really good . . . I can't really deal with it . . . it defeats the purpose."

Another set.

"I really like to play, and I can see myself playing well."

"Try to imagine playing the piano this week. Take it step by step and follow my fingers."

"Well, I go into the room," Johnny said, his eyes closely tracking the movement of my hand. "I sit down at the bench, open the piano . . . " He paused, as if to let it sink in. "Then I get out the music and place my hands on the keys."

The set continued.

"I *can't* enjoy myself. Nobody can listen to me . . . but it feels good and I think I would like to try."

"What stops you?"

"I don't want to do it. It's scary."

"Where do you feel it?"

"In my lower belly. I might succeed, and that's threatening."

"Feel the threat," I said neutrally.

And we continued.

In later sessions, Johnny and I worked directly on the memories and present circumstances that distressed him. In addition, we devoted time to a visualization we had worked on. Carl and Stephanie Simonton, two pioneers in the field of psychoneuroimmunology, worked extensively with cancer patients and became interested in what allowed some patients to lead longer and more vibrant lives than others, even though they had similar diagnoses.[5] The Simontons decided that the difference lay in how the patients thought about themselves. They suggested that patients identify an image that allowed them to feel their immune system was stronger than the cancer. For some people, it can work to have their immune system seem like a powerful army and the cancer cells as a weaker enemy. Because some people are pacifists, however, I found it works best if clients come up with an image that feels good to them. For some people, it has been an image of the heart of Jesus radiating light into their immune system.

Probably because of his engineering background, Johnny developed an image of electricity crackling through his body and destroying the cancer cells. We used EMDR to enhance the image and paired it with the positive cognition "my immune system heals me." The combination gave him a sense of control and mastery. He knew there were no guarantees, but we were mobilizing all his potential resources. He tried it in my office and then used it at home and reported back to me. "I see a flow," he said, gesturing from head to toe. "A spark going through the bones. I fantasize that the white blood cells are doing this spark. I am doing it six times a day. I take it very slowly, head, cheeks, shoulders, arms, torso, knee joints, legs, toes."

Johnny had a total of four EMDR sessions, and according to Martha, he lived out his life with a freedom of expression he had never known before. She found Johnny distinctly different following EMDR, more affectionate, livelier, and more communicative and outgoing with her and other people. He started enjoying the piano, and he was no longer afraid of failing. He and Martha traveled widely in those last few years, visiting Thailand, China, France, Spain, and Alaska and going white-water rafting on the Colorado River for thirteen days. Johnny also spent three months sailing from California to Alaska with friends. Those friends noticed the change in Johnny, too. No longer did he have to be Mr. Nice Guy and try to please everyone.

He had become much more assertive. He told each of them that he wanted to be called by his correct name, Jan, and he taught them how to pronounce it properly. "He reclaimed his true identity," Martha says.

Jan kept up the practice we had worked out, which sandwiched his visualization of electricity zipping through his body to kill the cancerous cells between two periods of repeating his positive cognition while doing eye movements. In late 1991, Jan's doctors told him the tumor in his prostate had shrunk, and he came home jubilant.

"Martha, I think I've got this thing licked!" he told her with a smile.

But the cancer was still in Jan's bones. In January 1992, Jan entered a high-stress family situation that rapidly took its toll. By May he noticed that his body was weakening, and he consulted his doctor. The prostate cancer had now spread to his liver. Jan decided on one last trip, this one to his native Holland, where he rented a houseboat and took it through the canals for two weeks. Afterward, he spent a week with his family before returning to the United States. He knew he was saying good-bye for the last time.

Once home, his pain increased. By late June, his mind was beginning to go. Jan de Groot, age sixty-nine, decided to end his life by taking medication he had bought for that purpose in Holland. Jan had had a marvelous three years since his EMDR treatment and wanted to choose his own manner of death. He went peacefully, with Martha by his side.

�

Many cancer patients have found different ways to use EMDR to regain a sense of personal control and to get through the medical experience itself. For example, after Donna was diagnosed with breast cancer, she was unable to sleep for three nights. She would wake up at three o'clock in the morning, her mind racing in fear. She asked a therapist to use EMDR on an as-needed basis to help her get through the ordeal. Their first target was Donna's fear, "I'm going to die." During the session, Donna emotionally connected with her spiritual beliefs, and the phrase "I'm not ready to die; I want to live" took on a powerful resonance within her. This is an important step for many cancer patients, whose problems often trap them in feelings of helplessness, spoiling their quality of life and possibly compromising their immune system.

The second session targeted Donna's feelings of being overwhelmed, as many cancer patients are, not only by treatment issues and pain but also by the other obligations in life that must be put on hold: business demands, the needs of others, and so on. EMDR helps patients put their present issues into perspective and makes it easier for them to find solutions by helping to still their anxiety and fear.

Next, Donna used EMDR to deal with her reaction after the mastectomy. Although at first she couldn't bear to look at herself in the mirror, as EMDR therapy proceeded she learned to cherish her body again and came to feel at peace with her changed appearance. Donna's doctor was amazed at the speed of her recovery, and she went back to work four weeks later; however, her psychological healing wasn't complete. Donna had not used EMDR to prepare herself emotionally for the surgery, and she discovered the consequences of that weeks later. Stuck in traffic one day while driving to work, Donna was overcome with feelings of danger and feared imminent death. Later, during EMDR processing, she realized that these feelings were directly related to events that took place on the day of her surgery. She remembered saying good-bye to her husband with the fear that she might never see him again or that she would wake up disabled, paralyzed, or brain damaged. This was not the first time she had a serious physical problem. Twenty years before, she had nearly broken her neck and needed a spinal fusion. The cancer surgery had reactivated all the unresolved pain of that trauma as well.

⚏

As frightening as cancer is to many people, few diseases strike us with as great a sense of terror as AIDS. The AIDS epidemic was so frightening, many of us wished we could ignore its existence. However, there was no way for Hugh Rodgers to put AIDS out of his mind. For the past three years, Hugh's longtime partner, Brady, had suffered the inexorable symptoms of AIDS. Brady was Hugh's life. The two men were very much in love and had been happily and fully committed to each other for nearly nine years. They had bought a house together, reveled in raising a puppy, and like many other couples, shared their hopes and dreams for the future.

Brady, seven years older than Hugh and the strong one in the relationship, had consistently underplayed the severity of his symptoms. He got away with this because, at the time, neither Hugh nor Brady had ever known anyone who had died of AIDS. They had no idea what they were headed for.

Their ignorance lasted until the day in late 1992 when Brady insisted on going into work despite having a fever of 103. On the way, his mind wandered and he slammed into another car. No one was injured, but Brady's Porsche was destroyed. Brady never drove again, and he did not return to work. Hugh convinced him it was time to take his disease seriously.

Even with Brady cooperating, things got difficult. One day he passed out while taking a shower. Another morning, Hugh went to say good-bye before leaving for work and found Brady struggling to breathe, his face purple. Brady was conscious but unable to think, function, or speak. Hugh called an ambulance and sat by Brady's side en route to the hospital, where Brady was diagnosed with cytomegalovirus (CMV), a viral infection of the blood.

Hugh was committed to caring for Brady at home, although it was tough to do while working in his high-stress retail job. Over the next twelve months, from late 1992 to late 1993, Hugh watched his partner metamorphose from an intelligent, decisive, and dynamic businessman to someone who had the cognitive skills of an extremely ill five-year-old. At first, Hugh did not recognize the AIDS dementia caused by HIV infection of Brady's brain cells, but the dementia got worse and worse. Some days Brady couldn't think clearly enough to answer Hugh's simple questions: "What are you feeling? Are you hurt? What can I do?" Brady mumbled at Hugh in frustration and then slammed his hand down on the counter. Brady couldn't speak coherently, and he knew it.

The last straw for Hugh came one afternoon when he arrived home to find Brady wedged between the couch and the coffee table, flailing his arms but unable to get up by himself. Hugh could see that Brady must have been in that position for several hours, for he had urinated on the carpet. Brady clearly didn't know where he was or what had happened to him. He was completely lost. The sight of his lover reduced to this state broke Hugh's heart, and he began to cry. While cleaning Brady up, Hugh decided to hire someone to stay with Brady during the day; he would continue to do the rest. He tried to get through the period, using denial and the pressures of business to suppress his fear and grief. He focused on the practical side of things: fixing breakfast and lunch for Brady before he went to work, getting home on time, being sure Brady took his medication, and organizing friends to come in occasionally so he could have a breather.

That was only half of the problem, however. Hugh had been eighteen when he met Brady and they started to date. He had recognized that he was gay in his early teens, but he had never been sexual with anyone. When they wanted to make love for the first time, Hugh asked Brady if it was safe. Brady convinced him that it was. The truth is, it wasn't.

In 1988, when Brady started showing symptoms of AIDS, Hugh had himself tested. He learned he was HIV-positive with a T-cell count in the low 500s.[6] Hugh was put on the drug AZT and told to start bolstering his immune system immediately by taking very good care of himself: eating right, getting enough rest, exercising, and getting rid of any stress in his life. In late 1993, five years after this diagnosis, Hugh's life was more stressful than ever. Watching Brady dying day by day, inch by inch, was heartbreaking. What made it even worse was the role reversal AIDS had forced on them as a couple.

In late 1993, when Brady became bedridden, it finally sank in for Hugh that the end was coming. Their loving and stable relationship, which had always given them the faith that they could handle whatever life dealt them, had lost its mainstay. Now Hugh's world had collapsed, and he felt like he was drowning. One day in mid-November, Hugh rushed off the sales floor of his shop and closed himself in his office. His heart was racing, and he felt like he couldn't breathe. A call to the doctor resulted in a quick appointment and a prescription for anxiety medication, neither of which did anything to affect the cause of Hugh's attack.

It was at this point that Hugh heard about a psychological study offering four free treatment sessions to men who were HIV-positive or had AIDS. The study was run by Donald Weston, a psychologist who worked closely with the gay population in Portland, Oregon, and who was interested in the possible stress-relieving (and therefore life-extending) effects that EMDR might have with men and women who had AIDS or HIV.

Donald's study required four ninety-minute sessions. In the first of these, Donald asked each subject to answer the same six questions about how he personally saw himself, his present life, and his future regarding the fact that he had AIDS or was HIV-positive. Although this was not the traditional EMDR approach, it allowed Donald to track, in a controlled fashion, how EMDR processing affected the person's emotional pain regarding his negative beliefs and how effectively the person evolved a positive set of counterbeliefs. The person's responses to these questions would serve as the targets for EMDR.

The first time they started processing with EMDR, Donald helped Hugh work on his image of himself as an HIV-positive person. Hugh felt if he could take care of himself, he would not get sick. Deep down, however, as he watched Brady's disintegration, he experienced an overwhelming sense of fear and pain; he felt as though he was seeing his own death. In addition, he was angry at himself for having HIV. As they started processing, his SUD was a 9. After three sets, Hugh started crying. "I'm only twenty-six years old. AIDS began long before I was around. Brady had it before I knew him."

"Stay with that." A fourth set.

"I can take care of him, but it's not my fault."

A fifth set.

"I can take it one day at a time. If he needs something I can give, I'll do that. I can't worry about what I couldn't do in the past for him. I feel at peace, relaxed. My shoulders lost their tension right after I cried." Hugh paused, then tilted his head to the left and asked, "Is this supposed to work so fast?"

"Stay with that." A sixth set.

"It feels good. I can be responsible for what I can do to help Brady. I'm not responsible for being HIV-positive."

A seventh set.

"It feels good. I like this."

For their second target, Donald asked Hugh, "Do you have an image or picture of the HIV virus in your body?"

"It's a yellow color. It's like when they showed a picture in health class of a drop of blue food color in water." Hugh sketched the shape with his hands.

"What words describe what you say about yourself as a result of this image?"

"I try to keep it separated; I cut clean water from the color. I feel like I'm in the water and I'm fighting to get air, but I can't. I come to the surface and never quite get enough. Something's holding me down. It feels overwhelming."

"What would you like to be able to say about yourself?"

"I would like to feel I'm not drowning. I would like to accept what I have so I can enjoy my life day-to-day and not worry about the inevitable result of this disease."

"Where do you feel it in your body?"

"In my neck and shoulders," Hugh said. He rated its intensity at a 10.

When Donald started the eye movements, Hugh's first response to Donald's questions was, "Nothing."

A second set.

"Nothing."

Another set.

"I feel like I'm drowning. I can't get enough air."

Another set. Hugh started crying again. He was concentrating on all the bad things: his life, Brady's life, his work. It was like seeing his life flash before him but only the bad parts. Then suddenly his feelings shifted, and he smiled. The pain had been short-lived. Hugh had let his mind go wherever it wanted, and he felt light. It was curious. He wasn't soaring like an eagle but zooming through things at his normal height. It was not strenuous but peaceful.

"What comes up for you?" Donald asked.

"I see a light at the end of the rainbow. I'm not drowning anymore. I can swim. Now, I'm in a life raft. I can look down through the clear water and see the yellow covering the bottom."

"Stay with that." A fifth set.

"I'm looking through the water, and it is all clear. It's like the yellow is in my peripheral vision. I can look around. I haven't been able to look around me and see other things in a long time."

Another set.

"I can smell flowers. I feel the air, and I see what is around me."

A seventh and final set.

"I feel like I can live every day smelling flowers, feeling the air, and seeing what's important," Hugh said.

Hugh related this experience two years later with these words: "Grief, frustration, despair, anger, anxiety, everything I was dealing with every day came out in that two minutes. Then the good kicked in, and I started a kind of daydreaming and thinking about the positive; it was like running twenty-five miles, being exhausted, and then all of a sudden someone opens the door to heaven for you. All of a sudden the exhaustion was gone."

During the next session, the two worked on Hugh's belief that he hadn't lived up to his potential. After the third set, Hugh started crying. "There's so much I want to do . . . I haven't accomplished all I want to."

Another set.

Hugh shifted in the chair to straighten his spine, then said, "I've accomplished a lot. I'm only twenty-six. I have a list of good accomplishments."

A fifth set.

Hugh's face broke into a broad smile. "I was on the life raft. Now I'm on a cloud. It's like I can smell the flowers and feel the air up here. I'm looking down on my accomplishments, and the wind is blowing me along to new doors that are opening. I have time to do things I want to do."

Another set.

"I can't believe this. It really feels good."

Another set.

"I really have accomplished a lot in my life, and I feel good about the things I've done."

The eighth and final set.

"Yeah, it's really all right."

"How intense is that feeling now?"

"It's a 3. You really made it safe for me to cry. I haven't cried about what is happening." As Hugh later put it, the sessions were opening up a new path. "Instead of looking at the negative all the time, it made me instantly see the positive. It wasn't in the background anymore; it was the forefront. I could see the negative, but I could live with that. I felt like I was going from being debilitated to functioning again. And it made me determined not to give up."

Donald and Hugh spent one session working through Hugh's sense of his future and his fears of being sick. During EMDR processing, Hugh saw himself overcoming physical problems and opening the door to the sun and wind. Finally, they targeted how he would cope with all that would need to be done if he were to be dying. As they proceeded, Hugh's mind returned to Brady.

"I started to feel the loss of everything. Brady and I were supposed to grow old together and be sixty-five. I'm having to get rid of everything because I'll be gone soon."

A tenth set.

"I feel better. It's a picture of moving stuff out, and I remembered my pictures. I've got my pictures."

Another set.

"More importantly, I've got my memories. I can take those to sleep with me.

Several sets later, Hugh said, "I've thought about how wonderful it was and it made sense; it's over. What happens next?"

Another set

"I miss Brady. When I pass away, if there's any way, I'll find him."

Another set.

"I can hear Brady. We are in a park, and he is calling my name. I can't see him, but I'm going to find him. I feel relaxed again. It's not over. It's just that the scenery has changed."

Another set.

"It feels good. Everything bad was part of our life, but it didn't change who we are or change our lives. AIDS is just one of those things in our life. Brady's sarcasm and his sense of humor are part of us. It was fun."

Another set.

"I feel like I see the big picture, and the plague is a small part of my total life. Every time we had problems in our relationship, we worked them through. We'll work this out. We'll make it."

The next week Hugh defined the significance of HIV in his life: "It gives me a challenge. I don't see it as 'it's not fair' or 'it's not right.' How I got it doesn't matter; it's a challenge." After doing EMDR, Donald and Hugh used the rest of their time that day simply to talk. Hugh told Donald that his employees had been commenting on how much happier and more relaxed he seemed at work. As for Donald Weston's study, Hugh's ratings of his negative feelings were all at 0; his ratings of the truth of his new positive beliefs were at 7, the top of the scale.

Two months later, Brady died quietly at home. Several weeks after that, Hugh came in to see Donald again. He was troubled by something he had done after Brady died, afraid it was sick or weird.

"He was there, Brady was there . . . and then he was gone. Then I . . . " Hugh said haltingly, "I climbed onto the bed next to his body and just held him."

"That's not sick or weird," Donald told him. "That's love."

At the time this book was written, Hugh was still hard at work and feeling well. It had been nine years since he had been diagnosed HIV-positive. His T-cell count had been holding at 700—close to normal—for nearly two years. His gift shop had come in eleventh out of approximately eight hundred in an excellence study by the chain's management, and he had gone back to school, earning a 4.0 grade point average his first semester. Hugh did volunteer work for three nonprofit agencies and let a friend cajole him into entering a poem—the first he'd ever written—in a statewide contest called the Governor's Award. It won first place, and Hugh got to hear the governor of Oregon read his poem aloud to an audience of twelve hundred. Hugh is an eloquent spokesperson with a deep understanding, an understanding that echoes clearly for so many who have passed through the shadow of death.

Visions of the Future:
The Global Reach of EMDR

The significant problems we have cannot be solved at
the same level of thinking with which we created them.

—ALBERT EINSTEIN

A MIDDLE-AGED WOMAN is estranged from her father and has rejected his overtures her entire life. She tells her therapist that because her father abandoned her when she was a child, she wants nothing to do with him now. But during EMDR processing, she recalls the specifics of the day he left. She realizes that it was her mother who ordered her father out of the house; he had not wanted to go. Witnesses corroborate the story, and the woman joyfully reconciles with her father.

How many people are suffering because they have fallen victim to the fallibility of memory? What can EMDR reveal about how memory works on a physiological level? These are the kinds of questions that have surfaced in response to the reports of the rapid results seen with EMDR therapy.

Each new application of the therapy leads to new questions. In scanning the last twenty years of EMDR practice, the central questions that arise for me include the following: What can be learned from EMDR physiologically, psychologically, and socially? What scientific investigations and practical applications come next? What can we learn about the relationship of mind and body? How far can we progress when our fears and barriers are removed?

∽

As cases pour in from all over the globe, it has become clear that there are many more common denominators among people and societies than there are differences. The fact that EMDR therapy shows predictable and rapid results when the appropriate protocols and procedures are used indicates that cross-culturally we share physiological responses that can offer a window into the human mind and potential.

As a goal for future studies, it would be wonderful to see the implications of different EMDR protocols explored. We could learn a lot about how the brain organizes memory and experience. For instance, during my first eighteen months using EMDR, I worked with people who had been traumatized at an earlier point in their lives: maybe a year, maybe a decade or more. None were in the immediate aftermath of trauma. Then I met the victims of San Francisco's Loma Prieta earthquake in late 1989. Less than a month earlier, their houses had collapsed, their children had been injured, and their pets had disappeared. The very ground they walked on had rumbled, rolled, cracked, and split wide open. It was no wonder that many of them felt that nothing and no one could be trusted anymore. When I started working with these victims, I used the same EMDR procedures as with my previous clients. I would ask the person to identify the most upsetting moment of the quake, such as when the chimney collapsed and nearly buried him, and hold that in mind while we did the eye movements. After that incident had been desensitized, I would ask him to bring to mind a second upsetting scene from the quake, such as having to jump out of a third-story window of a burning building. On the basis of experience with my previous clients (those recovering from distant traumas), I fully expected that this second, related scene would be reprocessed, too. I was wrong. This time there was no generalization from one branch of the traumatic memory to the other. We had to work on each distressing scene separately.

This finding told me I needed to modify my EMDR protocol when treating victims of recent trauma, but it also suggested new information about the brain. Why didn't one remembered scene from a recent trauma link up in the mind with other scenes from the same event? Were the different moments of a horrendous event somehow stored separately in the brain at first? It appeared as though some period of time was required for the different incidents of a single trauma to consolidate fully in memory into an integrated whole. This was doubly curious because my quake clients could easily describe in sequence the events that had befallen them. In other words, some important neurological connections (including time sequence) had been made, but others had not.

This discrepancy offers neurobiological memory researchers special access to the hidden recesses of the brain. A better understanding of exactly when memory consolidation takes place could be ascertained by determining at what point the EMDR procedure for healing recent trauma (treating each scene separately) is no longer required for the client's complete recovery. The need to use different protocols in treating recent versus long-ago trauma has been borne out in EMDR treatment all over the world, whether it be with a child afraid to leave his home after a major brushfire in Australia or a Long Island woman who developed a flying phobia and couldn't visit her family because she was haunted by images of a bloody ocean and body parts after the crash of TWA Flight 800.

Another potential area of future research concerns how a person's associations to a particular memory differ before and after EMDR treatment. For instance, I worked with one woman whose father died of cancer in a nursing home. In the two years since his death, she had been living with a "black cloud" over her head, seeing only the picture of her beloved father dying painfully among strangers and herself powerless to do anything about it. Although father and daughter had been close and had many happy times together, anytime she tried to think of him or was reminded of him, only the "black cloud" images would arise. We started her EMDR treatment by focusing on her memory of her father lying in bed in the nursing home. When this scene was worked through by processing, I asked her to think of her father now. What came up was the time she was at home with him at Christmas and they were having a good time.

I have seen this kind of shift from obsession with a bad memory to an effortless remembrance of a positive memory in innumerable clients who were grieving. In another case, I worked with a ten-year-old girl whose father had committed suicide. The only thing she could remember about him was how he looked on his last day (which was a fantasy, because she had not been there) and how he looked in the months before his death: sitting around in a ratty bathrobe, surrounded by empty beer cans. After she focused on those images and processed them, I asked her to think about a different time with her father, and she remembered a camping trip they'd taken. This memory did not cause her any grief. The same thing happened when I treated her brother. It consistently appears that clearing out a recurring bad memory makes room for the person to recall heartwarming good memories. Ongoing clinical observations such as these have numerous implications for the study of the neurophysiology of memory.

✍

Another area for future study concerns the different ways memory of events and physical sensations are stored. Sometimes, chronic pain and ongoing physical distress can be successfully treated with EMDR by targeting the initially disturbing event. For instance, a therapist in Russia reported working with a thirty-one-year-old man in a Moscow hospital who had chronic headaches and unpredictable bouts of depression. The man's sleep was disturbed by constant nightmares, and he felt hopeless about the future. He had been troubled with these symptoms since his army unit had been sent to Chernobyl in 1986 to try to minimize the consequences of the nuclear power plant disaster. After he was demobilized, his financial situation was bleak, and he developed various physical symptoms that were attributed to different illnesses. The man's sense of futility increased when he was given neither psychological nor physical help by the authorities. Now, ten years later, he was afraid of dying of radiation poisoning as a number of his friends had. He had maintained himself on antidepressant medication for the past ten years.

During EMDR therapy, the man targeted a representative memory of his traumatic experience at Chernobyl. He had been leaving the shelter at the power station to complete the next task in removing the radiation from the surface. When the man recalled that moment, all he felt was fear, attached to a sensation of radioactive particles penetrating his body. Later, these intrusive feelings recurred any time he left the shelter to go to a work site. During EMDR, he processed his feelings of helplessness and despair regarding his present problems, including his depression about his sexual dysfunction and his feelings about his wife. Through successive sets, he moved into a determination to do something about his situation, and the thought emerged that "those radiation particles might be in my imagination only." After the EMDR session, he reported a feeling of elation and made no further mention of headaches. The next day, he stopped his medication and talked of possibly resuming work in the collective farm where he had previously worked. He gradually improved and was discharged from the hospital. Future studies of EMDR might help us determine why some memories have such negative physical effects.[1] (See item 13 in "EMDR Therapy–Evaluated Clinical Applications," in Appendix C, for the many articles dealing with EMDR treatment for medically unexplained symptoms.)

Sometimes we cannot determine what the initial event was that caused the person's physical problem. Such was the case for a one-and-a-half-year-old girl in Buenos Aires, who was brought to see a therapist because she could not defecate, sometimes for as long as ten days at a time. This problem had caused a distention of the colon, which had started seven months earlier, and she was now facing an operation to correct it. The situation was also causing serious problems in the child's growth. When all attempts to solve the girl's problem had proved unsuccessful, her parents consulted psychiatrist Graciela Rodriguez, one week before the operation. Graciela focused on the girl's present physical discomfort using EMDR with alternating auditory tones, snapping her fingers on either side of the child's head as she spoke to her. During the session, the girl asked to be taken to the bathroom. The doctor went with her, all the while using the tones to dispel the child's fears and reprocess her feelings while she made a successful effort to defecate. The next day, the parents called to say that the girl was doing well. The operation was canceled, and the child has had no more such problems since then. This case leads one to wonder how many other medical problems might be handled by psychological interventions such as EMDR.

An important case in point involves a thirteen-year-old girl named Tina, who was dropped off at the organization Forjar in Bogotá, Colombia. Forjar is an agency that helps abandoned children who have AIDS or cancer. Tina's leg had been amputated, and EMDR therapist Linda Vanderlaan was called in to help because Tina was hysterical with phantom limb pain, a condition in which the surgically removed limb feels present and the patient is in intense discomfort. Using EMDR, Linda and Tina targeted the sensation of pain; soon the pain eased, and the girl dropped off to sleep. The next day they used EMDR again, and the phantom discomfort moved though cycles of pain and into prickly sensations of electricity before disappearing. Tina went through feelings of trauma and loss, first for her "abandoned" leg, and then for her mother, who would be gone for at least a month. Unfortunately, as some of the children at Forjar have found out, the parents sometimes do not return, and that fear has to be processed, too.

During Tina's EMDR processing, she worked through her shock ("I can't believe my leg is gone") and her grief that she could not get up and play with other children anymore. After further processing, she exclaimed to Linda, "I'll walk again!" When Linda tentatively asked, "How are you going to do that?" she was rewarded by Tina's simple explanation, "I'll walk again with a prosthesis, of course." Tina began interacting with the other children, and within the week she was happily showing off her new earrings. A follow-up visit nine months later found her still pain free and preparing for her new prosthesis.

In addition to demonstrating the return of this young girl's self-esteem and the physical relief she obtained, the case also opened up questions about the use of EMDR therapy with phantom limb pain. The pain sensations are apparently stored in memory because of the trauma that injured the limb and/or because of the operation. To date, EMDR therapy has been effective in eliminating or substantially decreasing phantom limb pain in approximately 80 percent of the cases evaluated in published articles.[2] To date, there are no medical cures for phantom limb pain; perhaps further EMDR therapy studies will shed some light on the matter and bring needed relief to those who are suffering. Given the many accident victims and war veterans affected by this problem, such research is highly recommended.[3]

Sometimes, physical distress in the present is caused by the unsuspected memory of a past event. For instance, a British woman in her thirties was in health-threatening gastric distress because of prolonged overuse of antacids to prevent nausea. She was dependent on the medication because the very idea of becoming nauseated was horrifying to her. Her intake history revealed that she also suffered from symptoms of PTSD caused by sexual abuse. Her therapist decided first to use EMDR therapy to try to relieve the stress that was causing her to take the antacids. During EMDR processing, the woman recalled an incident in school in which the child next to her had vomited and some of it had landed in her hair. She remembered running out of the room screaming. After this memory was processed, the woman's need to use antacids disappeared; she was no longer concerned with becoming nauseous. What is noteworthy here is that the central cause of the client's physical distress was a small "t" trauma. Although processing also defused her reaction to the sexual abuse, which she now thought of as "in the past," the abuse was not the primary cause of the problem. It is vital that we stay open to the possibility that the causes of disturbances and self-destructive behaviors are not earthshaking events that have been branded into memory. The events can be fruitfully processed nonetheless.

∽

Clearly, the interconnectedness of memories can enlarge some of our most common fears and have a negative impact on present behavior. Ad de Jongh, an EMDR therapist who is also a dentist, tells the story of Claire, a forty-year-old woman in the Netherlands who suffered from a dental phobia. When Claire was eight years old, she was sent by herself to the dentist, where she understandably felt alone and anxious. When the dentist started drilling, she became frightened and started to cry. When she tried to get up, the dentist became angry and tied her arms to the dental chair. He started drilling again, and she had a panic attack.

After the dentist let Claire go, she ran back to her house crying for her mother. Unfortunately, her mother reprimanded her for being childish. Claire avoided dentists for decades after that, but her fears worsened. After the birth of her first child, she started to experience panic attacks that gradually became more intense and more frequent. She started to avoid situations involving crowds, such as large stores, and enclosed places such as buses and elevators. A year of behavioral therapy provided no relief from these symptoms, and she stopped going to the sessions. Three years later, after watching a program about dental anxiety, Claire applied for treatment in a dental-fear clinic. Because she had avoided dentists for more than thirty years, her dental health had greatly deteriorated; she had only five teeth left.

When Ad and Claire were preparing to use EMDR therapy to treat Claire's traumatic memory, she revealed that the most upsetting part of the event was not what happened in the dentist's office, but rather the confrontation with her mother, who demanded that she stop acting childishly. Just thinking about this scene provoked the highest possible level of anxiety on the SUD Scale, a 10. Her desired positive belief, "I can control myself," was rated only at 2 on the VOC Scale. During EMDR, Claire realized her mother's pervasive frailties and fears of dental treatment and then thought of how beautiful her own children's teeth were. By the end of treatment her sense of control had increased, and after the EMDR session, she felt competent enough to go shopping for the first time in years. Although Claire's primary goal was healing the dental phobia, her panic attacks and agoraphobia disappeared as well. An additional session focused on the panic attack she had

had after the birth of her first child. When the session ended, she reported feeling peaceful. A two-year follow-up visit showed Claire to be free of panic attacks. She had completed dental work, wore a beautiful denture, and had found work as a shop assistant in a local supermarket, one of the places that used to terrify her.

It is interesting to note that Claire's target for the EMDR treatment was her mother's reaction rather than the dentist's actions. This fact raises another series of questions. Is there a crucial window following a traumatic event during which nurturing and support from a loved one can help to alleviate the suffering and during which the opposite reaction can cause even greater pathology? Furthermore, were the fears of losing control that Claire associated with her mother so extreme that the birth of her own child triggered similar panic because Claire herself was now inextricably linked to the mother role? How often are phobias and panic disorders caused by complex memory interconnections? How many disorders identified in long-term psychoanalysis as based on complex role identifications can be treated in a focused manner by EMDR therapy?

It is clear that, as traumatizing as physical pain and disease might be, the lack of family support can be even more devastating. Sara, another Colombian child, was eleven years old when she was diagnosed with cancer. She underwent treatment for a tumor on her cheek that was the size of a large grapefruit. When I met her, her face looked like a death mask to me. Her color was gray, her eyes seemed dead, and she had a black mark on her face where the chemotherapy had scorched away the tumor. Sara lived about a hundred miles from Bogotá, and her grandmother, who was the head of her family, had decreed that Sara could no longer live at home because of the danger of "contagion." This is not an uncommon reaction in such rural areas. The ignorance of the disease process breeds fear, and ailing children are often abandoned. Sara had to remain in Bogotá to finish chemotherapy, and it was unclear whether or not her grandmother would let her return home.

Dr. Pablo Solvey, who had traveled from Buenos Aires to help me teach EMDR therapy in Colombia, worked with Sara for about twenty minutes using alternating hand taps. First he asked Sara to remember happy times to give her a "safe place." Then he had her tell him her story while he continued to use the hand taps. He asked her to remember the worst part of her ordeal, which she identified as her mother leaving her, and concentrated on processing that thoroughly with her. Sara smiled after a while and said maybe her mother would come back sometime. He had Sara concentrate on the positive things in her life as he continued the processing. When I saw Sara the next day, I could scarcely believe my eyes. In the place of the withdrawn, silent child I had seen the day before was a smiling, chattering young girl. She even draped her arm over my shoulder when I sat next to her. The reports I heard a month later from an amazed Forjar staff said that they could not believe the change in Sara. She seemed to have broken through her sense of isolation, and reports years later indicated that she continued to be outgoing instead of depressed and withdrawn.

ᦥ

Stories from around the globe show a clear link between unprocessed trauma and feelings of isolation. Sometimes the depression and isolation become so intense that suicide seems the only answer to the person in pain. Fortunately, EMDR therapy often offers a way to help even the most troubled minds. Reports have come in from a number of residential treatment centers throughout the United States and Canada on successful applications. One representative example, reported by clinical director Lew Hamburger, involves Cynthia, a sixteen-year-old girl who had been sexually abused and had made multiple suicide attempts, using razors, knives, pills, alcohol, and a pistol. In addition to suicidal attempts, she had homicidal urges, stating, "I'm the type of person who wouldn't hurt anyone, and suddenly I wanted to beat the crap out of somebody just because they were walking down the street."

Cynthia's history of sexual abuse caused this teenager to believe that men "were going to take me somewhere and hurt me." She also hated and wanted to hurt all females because, as she put it, "they betrayed me. They weren't there for me when I was raped. I hated them because it seemed their biggest problem was what to wear or when to go shopping." Feeling disconnected from those around her, believing that no one could help her, Cynthia often went into a "depression spiral," in which she didn't care about eating, sleeping, or living. "The more depressed I got, the harder it was to get out," she said.

Years of conventional counseling and hospitalizations had failed to alleviate her suicidal depression, yet just two months of EMDR treatment enabled Cynthia to process her most vivid traumatic memories and led to a rapid transformation of her condition. She worked on eight memories, including being locked in a room and sexually assaulted by a cousin; being taken away from her mother after her parents' divorce and seeing how sick her mother became; and being date-raped by her boyfriend. After EMDR, Cynthia's therapist told me, "The attractive, bouncy sixteen-year-old woman with the radiant smile that glowed from a block away as she neared the office on January 17th was a stunning change from the disheveled 'wreck' who shuffled through the door on November 24th." Cynthia had reversed the effects of years of abuse, trauma, depression, and anxiety that had resulted in three recent hospitalizations for suicide attempts. She at first had appeared distraught, hopeless, and convinced nothing worked (including the psychiatric drugs she'd been taking). The psychiatrist who referred Cynthia for EMDR treatment said that he did so because "nothing else has worked. You might as well try the hocus-pocus." He reported that after six sessions, she "bounced into the office, announced that she felt just fine, thank you, and began a new life that included a return to school, relationships with males and females, and . . . behavioral and thought changes that have been steady and improving."

Even among young children, isolation and depression can breed high-risk behavior and violence. For instance, in San Francisco, a six-year-old was arrested for attempting to kill a one-month-old baby. Living in an economically depressed area and raised in a troubled environment, the boy claimed he "had to kill the baby" because the baby's family had "looked at him the wrong way." In England, a toddler was stoned to death by two ten-year-old boys. In Chicago, a five-year-old boy was murdered by being dropped out of the window of a high-rise building by a ten-year-old and an eleven-year-old. Although the economic and social realities leading to criminal behavior and despair have to be addressed, how much of this pain can be treated by psychological interventions before violence erupts, compounding the problem and perhaps ruining all chances for a healthy life? EMDR treatment within adolescent offender units appears to prevent the slide into prostitution, addiction, assault, and depression that characterizes this population. Perhaps the same would be true in treating younger children who are at high risk. Could EMDR be employed preventively in programs throughout areas populated by people at high risk for violence?[4]

⁓

Each act of violence indelibly affects many lives. Social and legal reforms are important, but we have to approach the issue in any way possible. Sometimes the systems we depend upon can fail us and cause even more trauma. Ricardo Wiggs's experience is a prime example. Happily married for five years, Ricardo and his wife were shot by a stalker. Sharon died; Ricardo was unable to save her. Trusting in the judicial system, Ricardo gave his eyewitness testimony. The same day that he assured his young daughters that Daddy was going to "get the bad man who shot Mommy," the jury brought in a verdict of not guilty. He recalls, "At that point, it was as if all twelve people loaded the shotgun and fired it at Sharon and me again. The verdict made no sense. One juror stated that because it was raining the night of the shooting that maybe I didn't clearly see the shooter. I told them in the courtroom that I was shot inside my home, not outside, so the weather had nothing to do with it. . . . Maybe I should have shown the jury the grapefruit-sized hole in my right arm to convince them I was shot. I can't understand it. . . . What more evidence do you need to convict than an eyewitness identification?"

The scenes from this event played over in Ricardo's mind day after day. Anger, loss, betrayal, and despair pushed him into psychotherapy. Feeling hopeless, he took care of only the bills essential to his family. He began to channel his pain into presentations at training workshops for police recruits and speaking engagements to promote victims' rights. It wasn't enough. As he put it, "Although my community service meant the world to me, I was not moving forward. A certain song, movie, related news event, or a friend will often throw you back for whatever reason without warning. You are living the experience again."

Four years after the shooting, Ricardo began treatment with therapist Nancy Davis, who diagnosed him with PTSD. As he put it, EMDR treatment released him: "My thoughts of hope for the future are returning. I can say that beyond a shadow of a doubt, I am clear and free of my trauma prison. I don't have to remember every detail the first minute I awake. I choose to remember if I want to . . . I no longer hide under the Jekyll-Hyde mask. No longer am I physically reacting to flashbacks. I don't grab my arm in psychological pain. I don't view the appearance of my arm as a badge of dishonor for not saving Sharon. I gave the best effort I could that night, and I don't even know if I could match it in the future. All I know is I am alive and I can help others." He is ready to start a new life "free from sadness and pain."

This kind of work with EMDR poses many questions. Foremost, is it possible to develop EMDR programs to help victims of violent crime reclaim their lives more quickly? Some individuals have speculated that getting rid of the pain might be counterproductive or ethically questionable. They worry that it will diminish the victim's sense of outrage and make him less socially responsible; that it will deprive him of his innate fight-or-flight response that might protect him when threatened by violence in the future; or that it will make him too forgiving of the perpetrators of crime. Clinical work with EMDR has indicated that these fears are groundless. Artists who have used EMDR to process their traumatic losses have reported enhanced creativity as they found themselves more open to experience. They have not stopped painting, although they may have begun to use different colors. Combat veterans have reported that they still have their "edge" when they need it. Losing the pain did not take away Ricardo's desire to advocate for victims' rights; it enabled him to be more effective at it.

Can victims worldwide learn that it is all right to go from victim to survivor to thriver? Honoring the dead, our losses, and our experiences is a natural consequence of the events that will not be forgotten, even if we accept help to put the past in its proper place. Healing doesn't take away the commitment to change. As Ricardo put it, "There was a Ricardo Wiggs before this all happened, and I want to make it clear that I'm back and in control. I look at it this way: I've had what you might call a rough paper route, but I still deliver the news."

In the same way, Linda Crampton, who suffered in the Oklahoma City bombing, helped pass an antiterrorism bill. Dawn Baumgartner, the Air Force sergeant who was raped in Panama, now provides support to rape victims and educates officers concerning how to respond to women in the military who have been assaulted. Railroad engineer Jim Duque offers peer support to other railroaders who have been involved in line-of-duty deaths. Don Heggie, an Australian bomber pilot shot down in World War II, mobilized hundreds of combat veterans to reclaim their lives after his own treatment. We can learn from the pain and be motivated to help others without being stuck in it.

Most poignant are the questions raised by the case of a nine-year-old girl who was stabbed thirty times and left for dead, allegedly by a neighbor who was a registered sex offender. Her doctor was quoted in the newspaper as saying, "In her physical recovery, she'll be up and around in a month or two. As for her emotional recovery, I can't say." His is a natural response, given the history of psychological treatments. But do we have to continue separating the physical and psychological consequences of trauma? Doesn't

EMDR show us that the mind can heal at the same rate as the rest of the body? Perhaps we can incorporate refined psychological interventions into a follow-up regime after a trauma to prevent long-term disturbance.

A case reported in New York City supports this goal. A little girl was brought in to therapy for disruptive behavior. The therapist investigated the home setting and found that the father, who was working hard to make ends meet, was often irritable and angry with the family. Although he was not psychologically minded, the father agreed to do an EMDR session on his anger. During the eye movements, he remembered his own childhood and realized that he was reenacting the way his own father behaved. The next week he reported, "The only things I ever felt toward my children were angry or numb. Now I feel such caring for them." How many families could be helped by this kind of intervention?

Some have claimed that when families have been raised in a certain way for generations, nothing can alter the pattern. With EMDR we have the opportunity to investigate whether change is possible. From the Mideast comes the report of a seventy-year-old French-Egyptian woman who had been depressed for most of her life. She sought the help of a therapist, who used EMDR to help her reprocess an event that occurred at age three. She recalled her mother placing her younger brother in front of her and then going behind him like a coach, saying to him, "She's only a girl, go on, beat her."

"When I heard that," the woman said, "my whole world tumbled down; the stars and moon fell down . . . shattering." She realized during the EMDR session that, as a consequence of this event, she had "always been subservient." After processing both her grief and her anger, she asserted, "I've never wanted to be a boy. I'm proud of being a woman." Her depression lifted, and she was able to stop her medication. She said, "When I started, I was down on the ocean floor; now I've surfaced."

Once again, this case shows that even events that took place more than sixty years ago can have a stranglehold on a person's life. It also shows that these events can be fully reprocessed. In addition, what does it tell us about the effects of what many might consider to be a cultural norm? In many countries, females are considered second-class citizens—but does the fact that this is a centuries-old cultural belief mean that it is not potentially traumatizing? Can EMDR help cut through negative acculturation itself?

One of the problems is that some people feel they do not deserve help. They believe that because they could not live up to their own highest expectations, they should be feeling miserable. Often people are debilitated by guilt about things over which they had no control. Jacob, an Israeli war veteran, was blown out of his car when a terrorist bomb exploded on a Jerusalem bus. He awoke and saw what seemed to be a soldier with his eyes closed lying in the remains of the bus. Desperately, he tried to reach and help the soldier. He yelled to the soldier to move, and using every bit of his strength, he dragged himself toward him but collapsed. He awoke a second time and saw burned body parts all over the area. He collapsed again and awoke to find himself in the hospital. Only later did he realize that there must have been another explosion while he was unconscious.

Jacob had always been a success, a powerhouse of energy. He had been through war and had seen people killed around him, but something here was different. Although he was apparently uninjured, he suffered in the aftermath of this experience from chronic and intense headaches. He couldn't sleep at night because of recurrent nightmares concerning the soldier. Consequently, he would turn on the TV and radio, waking up his family, in order to get the image out of his head. He had uncontrollable episodes of anger and jumped at loud noises. This man, who had lived through several wars without fear, became afraid to go near buses. Every day he experienced flashbacks, which were the same as the nightmares, and he couldn't get the image out of his mind. He couldn't understand his reactions, lost his self-confidence, couldn't concentrate, and was in danger of losing his business.

Desperate because of impending financial disaster, Jacob sought help and was referred to Gary Quinn, one of the few therapists practicing EMDR in Israel at that time. During the EMDR session, he targeted the image of the soldier and the negative cognition, "I am helpless and weak." Jacob's anger and fear started at a 9 out of 10 on the SUD Scale. By the end of the session, his SUD was at 0 or 1, and his desired belief, "I did the best I could, given the circumstances," had risen from a 3 to the top of the scale, a 7, in validity. The ever-present headache that had started at the time of the bombing was gone, and he was able to concentrate again. As he put it, "I came in a broken man, and I walk out my old self." Once again, we see how the person's rational knowledge, that he had no control of the situation, could not become accessible until the event was sufficiently processed. How many ways can people become stuck at an undeserved level of responsibility and guilt? The spectrum appears endless. Do incidents have to be dramatic and obvious before we decide to get some help jump-starting our own information-processing system so that we can move beyond our feelings of shame and weakness?

Unfortunately, some of us have come to believe that if we continue to "reason" with ourselves or if we have enough faith, the problem will be resolved. The truth is that being unable to process one's own suffering has nothing to do with intelligence, personal strength, fortitude, or spirituality. Insight is not the cause of change but a manifestation of change. We can see in EMDR that one's unprocessed feelings are at the core of the problem. We can have intellectual understandings that have no impact on the emotions or on physiologically driven negative behaviors. People of the highest order and intelligence can eat too much, drink too much, overwork, or hurt others because of their level of pain. Knowing the reason is not the same as healing.

✍

One of the other questions opened up by EMDR is, how much impact can the resolution of personal trauma have on the causes of war itself? Although political, financial, and social causes exist, it appears that the hatred and anger born of previous assaults inflame the desire to wreak further vengeance. Do the horrors of one war beget the seeds of the next? When the EMDR Humanitarian Assistance Programs sent American therapists into the Balkans to train local mental health professionals in EMDR, they were told by a Croatian psychiatrist to make sure we also sent training teams into Serbia. "The killing won't stop until the pain stops," she said.

"The pain" was devastating in many ways. The stories from the war that got the most press worldwide involved massive bloodshed, refugees, and the horrors of sanctioned rape and "ethnic cleansing." But the everyday suffering of the civilians also took its terrible toll. When the EMDR therapists arrived, they found that apartment residents in Sarajevo had taken turns guarding the entrances to their buildings at night to prevent snipers from slipping in to shoot from their rooftops. Surgeons were working in emergency rooms without power or heat because the only alternative was to let the patients die. To drive in Sarajevo during the war was to risk your life; power outages meant there were no traffic lights to regulate the frenetic drivers dodging and accelerating rapidly to avoid sniper fire. Car crashes were so frequent they rated a mere 3 on the 10-point SUD Scale.

Death was a daily companion as men, women, and children witnessed the killing of family members. Quite simply, most everyone had lost someone dear to them, often in terrible circumstances. In Sarajevo, some people's families had been split down the middle when they were forced to declare themselves either Serbs (Eastern Orthodox), Croats (Catholics), or Bosnians (Muslims), a distinction few had declared or even thought about much before the war. Mixed marriages broke up, as did extended families. Friendships ended, too, as people were literally being shot at by folks they had known for years: neighbors, family members, and colleagues who had chosen the other side.

As the EMDR therapists worked with the Bosnian clinicians they were training and spoke with others in Sarajevo, they found that what most deeply affected these people was not the constant danger to themselves from rockets and sniper fire, but the danger to their children. Many agonized over the decision of whether or not to send their sons and daughters away to get them out of the besieged city or whether the kids would be safer under the protective eye of their parents. One man worried that he might not be able to rebuild his relationship with his adolescent son. "I've already lost three years with him. He's not the same kid I sent away. He's turning into a man, and I've missed valuable time that I can't get back." He also recalled how dangerous it had been to get him out of the city. "I was so busy packing and planning and making the arrangements. We took him down to the car, and just before the car drove away, there was a moment when we realized we might not see each other again. We both recognized it at the same moment and touched our hands flat against the car window."

The children of embattled Sarajevo were overwhelmed, too. One young boy who grew more and more afraid the longer his mother was away at work was equally terrified to tell her so: She might decide to come home early, and if she were killed on the way, it would be his fault.

In the EMDR sessions that the American therapists did with their Bosnian counterparts, two themes emerged: helplessness and survivor guilt. Living in a city that for forty-eight consecutive months had been shelled and riddled with small arms fire left all feeling utterly helpless to protect themselves. Stepping out of one's house was dangerous; not stepping out was dangerous, too. The people who survived these dangers often felt deeply ashamed that they were all right: "My problems aren't so big; I know a whole family that was wiped out."

We saw through the global reach of EMDR that the pain was not one-sided. Twenty-three-year-old Dimitri, a Russian soldier who had been pressed to serve in the Balkan conflict, came to an EMDR therapist in Moscow for psychological help when he read in the newspaper that one of his fellow soldiers had shot and killed all the members of his own family before turning the gun on himself and committing suicide. There seemed no explanation for the killing.

Dimitri's girlfriend told the therapist, Pavel Lushin, that when the young man had returned from the war, nobody—not even those who had known him well before—could recognize this changed man. He was full of anger and irritation toward the government and local authorities, who pretended that all the Ukrainian soldiers had participated in the conflict voluntarily. He was also uncontrollably angry at those who irritated him, often confronting anyone who crossed him in any way. His old friends avoided him.

Dimitri started to become aware that he was dangerous to other people only after reading about the incident involving the fellow soldier. At that point, he began to wake up in the middle of the night sweating and in fear. He reported a recurring dream of being pressed down by something squeezing his blood out of him. He also said that his fists were always about to clench. If somebody did something wrong, he had a strong desire to knock him down or shoot him.

During the EMDR session, Dimitri exclaimed that he had had no choice in the matter. When asked to explain, he described himself and the other soldiers standing in a row and being asked to volunteer. He had agreed but, he said with tears in his eyes, "They had beaten me up the day before, calling me a sissy." The therapist asked, "It was better for you to be ready to die than to go through that again?" "Yes," Dimitri whispered. At the end of the next set, Dimitri said, "That was my choice . . . nobody can call me inferior now." After the EMDR session, he reported a sense of emotional resolution and of stability.

That military experiences, including both major and minor trauma, can have a profound impact is an undeniable fact. But how widespread are the effects? It is striking that the language Dimitri's friends used to describe his personality after returning from the Balkans was almost word-for-word what hometown neighbors said of Timothy McVeigh, the perpetrator of the Oklahoma City bombing, when he returned from Desert Storm. They said they couldn't recognize him; he was angry with the government and seemed to be a completely different person from before. How many untreated, potential perpetrators are there walking the streets? Dimitri became scared enough by the newspaper report about his fellow veteran's multiple murders to come into treatment. What disaster might have resulted if he had met up with others who shared his hatred and his views, the way Timothy McVeigh allegedly did? Would there be a town in Russia suffering from the same consequences as Oklahoma City?

One of the most painful things about the 1995 Oklahoma City bombing was the way it shattered the sense of safety and community that people who lived there had cherished. There had been nothing to predict a major terrorist act. This was not New York or Los Angeles. This was the heartland. Before the bomb, Oklahoma City, with its one million residents, was a big town with a small-town attitude, a 1950s kind of place where people knew each other, went to baseball games, and shared potluck dinners.

The reality is that there is no such thing as "it doesn't happen here." Pain, loss, sorrow, injury, and sudden death can happen to any one of us at any time, anywhere. Whatever the cause of a tragedy—a terrorist attack, a hurricane, or a car accident—there is a person in the middle of it who is just like you and me. No one is exempt. In Oklahoma City, even the rescue workers, doctors, ministers, and counselors who responded to the emergency were traumatized by the magnitude of it. The sight of tiny body bags—nineteen children were killed—hit caregivers especially hard. In addition, most of the rescue efforts were in vain. Even the rescue dogs, unable to find survivors after the first day, grew lethargic and depressed. Workers tried to cheer them up by lying down in the ruins so the dogs could "find" them.

Whether the victims seen by emergency-relief EMDR therapists were citizens of Rwanda, Colombia, or Sarajevo, the message is clear: We all share the same capacity for destruction and for growth, as well as for pain and for healing. At the time of the Oklahoma City bombing, the covers of many newsmagazines showed the body of one-year-old Baylee Almon cradled in a fireman's arms. She became an icon of the devastation in Oklahoma. To Linda Crampton, however, Baylee was much more than a picture on a magazine cover. She was the little girl whose hair she had patted in the elevator the day before the blast. The memory of Baylee was the target of Linda's second EMDR session as she tried to deal with the terrible guilt that lay hidden behind her mental blackout of the bombing. Baylee had died in the bombing, but not immediately. Linda thought that if only she had turned left when she got out of the apartment building and gone down to the bomb site, she could have saved Baylee—found her before the firemen had and kept her alive somehow. By the close of the EMDR session, Linda realized she could not have done anything to help Baylee, and she described almost feeling the presence of the child fluttering around her shoulders and forgiving her. Linda's teeth grinding stopped, but there was more.

In her third and final EMDR session, her anger poured out: anger at Timothy McVeigh; anger at the deaths of her friends and neighbors; and anger at the loss of her home, her community, and her security. In the wake of anger came compassion for those who had lost their loved ones or their limbs or bodily functions like sight, speech, and the ability to walk. But there was still more. Linda's compassion turned to commitment. Eventually, Linda joined the Oklahoma attorney general's task force to help pass the federal antiterrorism bill, which she had the pleasure of seeing President Clinton sign into law on April 24, 1996. Linda, like so many others who have suffered, became imbued with the desire to make her tragedy useful for others and to prevent it from happening again. The desire to serve the common good and heal suffering has motivated the countless volunteers who have treated trauma victims through the many EMDR humanitarian assistance projects worldwide over the past twenty years. Unhealed trauma can have devastating, long-lasting effects on individuals, families, and societies.[5] Thousands of EMDR clinicians have dedicated themselves to stopping the pain by working with both local and international EMDR associations.[6] As with the Oklahoma City project, these clinicians provide pro bono EMDR therapy after natural and human-made disasters (see Appendix A).

EMDR may also show us that one way of stopping tragedy is to target the trauma that underlies potential violence before it breaks to the surface. Of course, perpetrators must be held responsible for their actions, but it seems eminently better to fix the problem than merely to fix blame. Such a stance was taken by Reverend David Price, an EMDR therapist at Bowden Institution, Canada's largest federal prison. He has reported that the majority of the prison's population are sex offenders and that the most difficult are the pedophiles, who are often thought to be untreatable. When a small number of pedophiles were to be released in ninety to one hundred days into the community without supervision, he decided to try EMDR with three of these men. They had been active participants in sex offender programming during this as well as previous incarcerations. Each of them had a history of sex offending and a pattern of repeating their crimes, on average, three to six weeks after being released. Reverend Price chose to work with these particular men because all three had taken responsibility for their crimes and had a spiritual relationship to a "higher power." It was important for the EMDR work that all had identified their "crime cycle," a process that involves mapping the events that trigger the heightened emotions and the thoughts and behaviors that progressively build and culminate in the criminal behavior.

One of the three, Sam, processed the traumatic memories associated with his nine triggers. As Reverend Price put it, "A major breakthrough occurred in Session 4. Sam recollected a repressed memory of rage. His sister, eight years his senior, would threaten and actually destroy his favorite toys if he did not perform sexual acts with her. Only nine years old, Sam had buried his rage, shame, and confusion over his sister's behavior for years. Sam participated in fourteen EMDR sessions over a two-month period and, like the other subjects, was followed after his release. Sam reported that his old thought patterns were gone and that even though he was harshly treated by his peers, he felt a sense of strength, peace, and control.

"I have maintained a biweekly telephone follow-up with Sam," Reverend Price reports. "He has experienced rejection, abandonment, shaming, as well as ridicule and denial of employment. In his untreated past, any one of these events would have caused him to isolate and progress to his offending cycle. To his delight, none of these emotional and behavioral patterns has emerged. Instead, Sam has established a positive support group, utilizing self-management skills he has learned. He keeps working at finding employment and made voluntary connections with the police. He is even working with the police to help set up prevention programs for parents and children. He reports no rage at society or self-loathing. He is gradually developing an appropriate relationship with an adult of his own age. He has been in free society for nine months, crime-free. The other two men report similar results." Since then, a published pilot study of EMDR therapy with pedophiles reported positive results in 90 percent of the participants.[7] Some of these positive effects were assessed through physiological testing of deviant arousal. The study participants took responsibility for their actions and no longer viewed children as sex objects. These positive results remained at one-year follow-up. Imagine how much suffering could be prevented with widespread effective treatment.

The learning and transformation process is not limited to healing pain. EMDR can be used specifically to enhance performance. It is a hallmark of EMDR treatment that negative imagery, emotions, and beliefs become diffuse and less valid, whereas positive images, emotions, and beliefs become more vivid and valid. Because of this capability, EMDR can help people learn the skills necessary to take important first steps and to continue with progressively greater achievements. We help clients to create images, such as those used by Olympic athletes to learn how to execute the perfect dive, and to combine them with the positive beliefs necessary to achieve their goal. The use of EMDR to give the client helpful "templates" for appropriate future action has proved so successful that many EMDR clinicians are now working as "coaches" with athletes, musicians, and executive officers of major corporations to achieve peak performance. As a matter of fact, various champion athletes have already benefited from EMDR treatment by winning a number of medals. The accelerated learning that takes place with EMDR is not limited to going from dysfunctional to functional behavior. The learning can also go from functional to exceptional. How far can any of us go if we process old memories of failure or humiliation and open the pathways of our brains to the potential of high achievement?

శ

One of the reasons for writing this book was to explore the fabric of the mind—to show the common denominators that link us all as a species. In all the cases reported in this book, the clients' psychological responses made sense, given the interaction between their upbringing and the special circumstances of their life. Underlying this truth is a beautiful fact: Our nervous systems respond in similar ways. Although the content of our experiences may differ, we are all linked by certain commonalities simply because we share the characteristics of a flesh-and-blood body. Because the brain is part of the body, we all share principles of mind and character, too.

I hope that one fact is clear from the stories presented here: Diagnosable psychological problems are merely extensions of experiences we have all had. We have all felt stuck. We have all overreacted to situations. We have all had problems in our lives that we could have used some help with. And we all have areas we may need help with in order to break through ordinary functioning and excel. Emotional pain and problem behaviors are understandable, reasonable responses to unfortunate circumstances and pressures.

We are more than our automatic responses. We can observe them, judge them, accept them, or suffer because of them. We can live in misery and accept our despair, or we can choose to do something about these responses. Although we have seen in this book that the automatic reactions of our mind and body are governed by cause and effect, there is a part of us that is distinct and healthy. The part of us that observes the misery is the part that can choose to reach out for the help needed to change. It's the part that brings us into therapy, or reaches for a self-help book, or cheers when the hero shows great nobility in a movie. It's the part that tells us who we could be if we weren't afraid. The thing to remember is that some of the fears we all face are merely earlier life experiences that are locked in our nervous system. This book has revealed how they can be released: how we can learn what we need to know from these experiences and discard the rest. Once we have done this, we can choose our actions rather than being propelled by automatic *re*actions.

This book is everyone's story. You may see yourself in these pages or perhaps a neighbor, friend, or family member. Remember that our innate core of health blossoms forth when given the chance. We readily accept this principle when it comes to our physical health, and it's time we also came to expect it concerning our psychological well-being. The brain is a part of the body and is governed by comparable laws of cause and effect. When we feel physical pain, our bodies flinch in response. Our minds have similar automatic reactions to external pressures and experiences. Some of these responses are life-enhancing and serve us well; others are not, but they can be changed. As we observe the process of healing that takes place in one person's mind, we see the reflection of our own potential for healing. Perhaps we can also see a ripple effect that might lead to the eventual healing of us all.

APPENDIX A

CHOOSING A CLINICIAN, AND FINDING AN EMDR THERAPY ORGANIZATION

Choosing a Clinician

EMDR is a form of psychotherapy that is recognized worldwide as effective in the treatment of trauma and other disturbing life events. The eight phases of EMDR are designed to ensure that the client's emotions, thoughts, and body reactions evolve into a healthy state (see www.emdr.com/what-is-emdr). There are numerous procedures for each phase and specialized protocols for different problems. The cases you have read in this book were provided by well-trained clinicians using the EMDR reprocessing procedures that have been tested and validated by research. It is important that the clinician you choose does the same.

Make sure that your therapist has taken a course that is approved by the EMDR Association in your region. The organizations below maintain lists that you can use to find a therapist in your geographic area. You should check credentials, since some clinicians may have unknowingly taken substandard training. For instance, in the United States, some training courses being offered are only one-third the length of the approved courses.

EMDR therapy should only be administered by a licensed (or supervised) clinician specifically trained in this form of therapy. Take time to interview prospective clinicians. Make sure that he or she has the appropriate training in EMDR (basic training is a minimum of six full days, with additional supervision) and has kept up with the latest developments. As with any form of therapy, while training is mandatory, it is not sufficient. Choose a clinician who is experienced with EMDR therapy and has a good success rate. Make sure that the clinician is comfortable treating your particular problem. In addition, it is important that you feel a sense of trust and rapport with the clinician. Interview as many as you need to find one who is knowledgeable and feels good to you. Every treatment success is an interaction among clinician, client, and therapy.

Here are five important questions to ask a prospective clinician:

1. Have you completed the training approved by the EMDR professional organization (see below)?
2. Have you kept informed about the latest protocols and developments?

3. Do you use the full eight phases and standard protocol as taught in approved training sessions and as validated by research?
4. How many people with my particular problems or disorder have you treated?
5. What is your success rate with comparable clients with these problems?

EMDR Therapy and Training Resources, North America

EMDR   Institute

The EMDR Institute has trained over 70,000 clinicians in EMDR therapy since I founded it in 1990. It maintains an international directory of Institute-trained clinicians for client referrals and trains only qualified mental health professionals according to the strictest professional standards. Training authorized by the Institute displays the EMDR Institute logo. It is now one of many training organizations approved by the EMDR International Association (EMDRIA).

For further information on training or a referral, contact the institute by phone: (831) 761-1040; fax: (831) 761-1204; email: inst@emdr.com; mail: PO Box 750, Watsonville, CA 95077; or website: www.EMDR.com.

Soldier Center

Soldier Center is a treatment and training center located near Fort Campbell, Kentucky, and Clarksville, Tennessee. The center specializes in EMDR therapy with military personnel, veterans, and their families. Treatment is available weekly and as five- and ten-day successive day programs. Many referrals from military installations and veteran self-referrals from across the nation utilize the successive-days program. Grants and pro bono services are available for veterans with no resources. Soldier Center also maintains a roster of EMDR-trained clinicians with a military specialty in various parts of the country.

EMDR basic and advanced approved trainings focused on military and veteran issues are provided on-site and as well as contracted with VA/military organizations throughout the United States.

For further information on EMDR training or treatments with veterans or other military, contact Soldier Center by phone: (931) 553-6981; fax: (931) 553-6982; email: emdr@soldier-center.org; or website: www.Soldier-Center.org.

EMDR International Association

The EMDRIA International Association is a professional organization of EMDR-trained therapists and researchers devoted to promoting the highest possible standards of excellence and integrity in EMDR practice, research, and education for the public good throughout the United States.

To identify a clinician near you who has been trained by an EMDRIA-approved basic training provider, visit the EMDRIA website and click on "Find an EMDR Therapist." If you are looking for a specific name but cannot find it, contact the organization by telephone or email. Remember that many clinicians may not be aware that they have received substandard EMDR training.

For more information about EMDRIA, contact the association by phone: (866) 451–5200; fax: (512) 451–5256; email: info@emdria.org; mail: 5806 Mesa Drive, Suite 360 Austin, TX 78731–3785; or website: www.emdria.org.

EMDR Canada

EMDR Canada maintains a list of trained therapists in Canada. For more information, contact this organization by website, www.emdcanada.org or email: info@emdrcanada.org.

EMDR Therapy and Training Resources, Beyond North America

As the overseeing professional organizations of their respective regions, all the multinational regional associations below perform a similar function to that of EMDRIA. They are devoted to promoting the highest possible standard of excellence and integrity in EMDR practice, research, and education.

EMDR Asia Association

The EMDR Asia Association is the governing body for all the national EMDR associations throughout Asia, Australia, and New Zealand. Links to the individual national associations can be found on EMDR Asia's website, below. The various national associations help coordinate pro bono training and treatment after disasters.

Further details can be found on its website: www.emdrasia-assoc.org. or by email: emdrasia @gmail.com.

EMDR Europe Association

The EMDR Europe Association is the governing body for all the national European EMDR associations, including Turkey and Israel. Links to the individual national associations can be found on the website, below. Each national association maintains a list of members who have gone through the accredited training.

National European associations also provide pro bono training and treatment after domestic disasters. The EMDR Europe Humanitarian Assistance Programmes provide similar support (pro bono training and treatment) after international disasters.

Further details can be found on its website: www.emdr-europe.org or by email: info@emdr-europe.org.

EMDR Iberoamérica Association

The EMDR Iberoamérica Association is the governing body for all the national EMDR associations throughout Latin America. Each national association maintains a list of members who have gone through the accredited training. Links to the individual national associations can be found on the website below.

The Mexican Association for Mental Health Support in Crisis also coordinates pro bono EMDR training and treatment after disasters throughout Iberoamerica.

Further details can be found on its website: www.emdriberoamerica.org or by email: info@ emdriberoamerica.org

EMDRIA Latinoamérica

EMDRIA Latinoamérica lists additional therapists on its website, www.emdr.org.ar.

Trauma Recovery/EMDR Humanitarian Assistance Programs

Trauma Recovery/EMDR Humanitarian Assistance Programs (HAP), a 501(c)(3) nonprofit organization based in the United States, provides low-cost trainings for domestic nonprofit organizations and pro bono training and treatment after natural and human-made disasters domestically and internationally.

HAP's services include the Trauma Recovery Network, which supports ongoing local groups of clinicians who volunteer their time and expertise to stop emotional suffering and prevent the psychological aftereffects of trauma and violence in their areas. HAP's goal is to help break the cycle of suffering that ruins lives and devastates families.

The HAP model emphasizes training and other professional support for local clinicians to continue the healing process. This training-focused model has several advantages. By teaching EMDR therapy to local clinicians, the program equips them with an efficient and effective tool with which to treat the emotional effects of trauma. The professionals who are already part of the affected community are not being replaced by outsiders; rather, they are given an important resource to be used when and how they think is best. Because reactions to traumatic events are sometimes delayed and individuals often try to resolve problems on their own before they seek professional intervention, training local clinicians helps ensure that when people do come for help, their needs can be met. In this way, effective psychological treatment of trauma extends far beyond the parameters of a single event.

Over the past years, more than 10,000 clinicians have enrolled in Trauma Recovery/HAP training workshops to learn basic EMDR therapy. All the training sessions have been provided by volunteers who are licensed mental health professionals. Trauma Recovery/HAP provides very low-cost EMDR training, in their own community, to therapists working in public and nonprofit agencies. U.S. or international agencies that wish to sponsor such training should contact Trauma Recovery/HAP directly (see below).

In addition to training, HAP's Trauma Recovery Network coordinates clinicians to treat victims and emergency service workers after crises such as the Oklahoma City bombing and the 9/11 terrorist attacks.

Since the Oklahoma City bombing in 1995, a growing network of Trauma Recovery/HAP volunteers have responded to the calls for healing that come from all over the world, be it after Hurricanes Sandy and Katrina or tornadoes in Tuscaloosa, Alabama, and Moore, Oklahoma; bombings in Boston; earthquakes in Turkey, India, China, Haiti, and Nepal; flooding in Kashmir; hurricanes in Haiti and Mexico; or tsunamis in the Philippines. We have reached out to communities traumatized by war and terror in Palestine and Israel, Croatia and Bosnia, Northern Ireland, and Kenya and weakened by epidemics in Ethiopia. We have helped to fill the void in mental health services for inner-city communities from Bedford Stuyvesant to Oakland and underserved populations in rural and suburban communities, Native American reservations, Sri Lanka, Uganda, Hungary, Poland, China, South Africa, Ukraine, Mexico, Nicaragua, El Salvador, and beyond. We have treated and trained and sowed the seeds for healing in the aftermaths of the school shootings at Columbine High School, Sandy Hook Elementary, and Dunblane, Scotland, and after the 9/11 terrorist attacks in New York City and Washington, D.C.

Trauma Recovery/HAP volunteers donate a significant amount of time per year of therapy or training time to make healing available to those who are suffering but who can least afford to pay for treatment. However, funding is needed to get the clinicians to where they are most needed allowing them to provide pro bono clinical services while training local clinicians to develop a trauma-informed community. While individual trainings in Bangladesh, the Balkans,

Africa, and the Middle East have been co-sponsored by organizations like UNICEF, Catholic Relief Services, the World Health Organization, and Save the Children, most sessions are funded exclusively by individual contributions.

To learn more about Trauma Recovery/EMDR Humanitarian Assistance Programs and what we have accomplished, go to our website: www.emdrhap.org

Tax-deductible gifts can be made online or sent to:

Trauma Recovery, EMDR Humanitarian Assistance Programs

2911 Dixwell Avenue, Ste. 201

Hamden, CT 06518

Phone: (203) 288-4450

Fax: (203) 288-4060

TRAUMA RESEARCH AND FURTHER READING

International Treatment Guidelines

- **American Psychiatric Association (2004).** *Practice Guideline for the Treatment of Patients with Acute Stress Disorder and Posttraumatic Stress Disorder.* Arlington, VA: American Psychiatric Association Practice Guidelines.

  EMDR is recommended as an effective treatment for trauma.

- **Bleich, A., Kotler, M., Kutz, I., and Shalev, A. (2002).** A position paper of the (Israeli) National Council for Mental Health: Guidelines for the assessment and professional intervention with terror victims in the hospital and in the community. Jerusalem, Israel.

  EMDR is one of three methods recommended for treatment of terror victims.

- **California Evidence-Based Clearinghouse for Child Welfare (2010).** Trauma Treatment for Children. www.cebc4cw.org.

  EMDR and Trauma-focused CBT are considered "Well-supported by research evidence."

- **Chambless, D. L., et al. (1998).** Update of empirically validated therapies, II. *Clinical Psychologist, 51,* 3–16.

  According to a taskforce of the Clinical Division of the American Psychological Association, the only methods empirically supported ("probably efficacious") for the treatment of any post-traumatic stress disorder population were EMDR, exposure therapy, and stress inoculation therapy. Note that this evaluation does not cover the last decade of research.

- **CREST (Clinical Resource Efficiency Support Team) (2003).** *The Management of Post Traumatic Stress Disorder in Adults.* A publication of the Clinical Resource Efficiency Support Team of the Northern Ireland Department of Health, Social Services and Public Safety, Belfast.

  EMDR and CBT were stated to be the treatments of choice.

- **Department of Veterans Affairs and Department of Defense (2010).** *VA/DoD Clinical Practice Guideline for the Management of Post-Traumatic Stress.* Washington, D.C.: Veterans Health Administration, Department of Veterans Affairs and Health Affairs, Department of Defense.

  EMDR was placed in the category of the most effective PTSD psychotherapies. This "A" category is described as "A strong recommendation that clinicians provide the intervention to eligible patients. Good evidence was found that the intervention improves important health outcomes and concludes that benefits substantially outweigh harm."

- **Dutch National Steering Committee Guidelines Mental Health Care (2003).** Multidisciplinary Guideline Anxiety Disorders. Quality Institute Heath Care CBO/Trimbos Institute. Utrecht, Netherlands.

  EMDR and CBT are both designated as treatments of choice for PTSD.

- **Foa, E. B., Keane, T. M., Friedman, M. J., and Cohen, J. A. (2009).** Effective Treatments for PTSD: Practice Guidelines of the International Society for Traumatic Stress Studies. New York: Guilford Press.

  EMDR was listed as an effective and empirically supported treatment for PTSD, and was given an A rating for adult PTSD by the Agency for Health Care Policy and Research (AHCPR). This guideline specifically rejected the findings of the previous Institute of Medicine report, which stated that more research was needed to judge EMDR effective for adult PTSD. With regard to the application of EMDR to children, an AHCPR rating of Level B was assigned. Since the time of this publication, three additional randomized studies on EMDR have been completed (see Randomized Clinical Trials).

- **INSERM (2004).** *Psychotherapy: An Evaluation of Three Approaches.* French National Institute of Health and Medical Research, Paris, France.

  EMDR and CBT were stated to be the treatments of choice for trauma victims.

- **National Collaborating Centre for Mental Health (2005).** *Post Traumatic Stress Disorder (PTSD): The Management of Adults and Children in Primary and Secondary Care.* London: National Institute for Clinical Excellence.

  Trauma-focused CBT and EMDR were stated to be empirically supported treatments of choice for adult PTSD.

- **SAMHSA's National Registry of Evidence-Based Programs and Practices (2011).** http://legacy.nreppadmin.net/ViewIntervention.aspx?id=199.

  The Substance Abuse and Mental Health Services Administration (SAMHSA) is an agency of the U.S. Department of Health and Human Services (HHS). This national registry (NREPP) cites EMDR as evidence-based practice for treatment of PTSD, anxiety, and depression symptoms. Their review of the evidence also indicated that EMDR leads to an improvement in mental health functioning.

- **Therapy Advisor (2004–2011). www.therapyadvisor.com.** An NIMH-sponsored website listing empirically supported methods for a variety of disorders. EMDR is one of three treatments listed for PTSD.

- **United Kingdom Department of Health (2001).** Treatment choice in psychological therapies and counselling evidence based clinical practice guideline. London.

  Best evidence of efficacy was reported for EMDR, exposure, and stress inoculation.

- **World Health Organization (2013).** Guidelines for the Management of Conditions That Are Specifically Related to Stress. Geneva: WHO.

  Trauma-focused CBT and EMDR are the only psychotherapies recommended for children, adolescents, and adults with PTSD. "Like CBT with a trauma focus, EMDR aims to reduce subjective distress and strengthen adaptive cognitions related to the traumatic event. Unlike CBT with a trauma focus, EMDR does not involve (a) detailed descriptions of the event, (b) direct challenging of beliefs, (c) extended exposure, or (d) homework." (p. 1)

Meta-analyses

EMDR therapy has been compared to numerous exposure therapy protocols, with and without CBT techniques. It should be noted that exposure therapy uses one to two hours of daily homework and EMDR uses none. The most recent meta-analyses are listed here.

- **Bisson, J., Roberts, N. P., Andrew, M., Cooper, R., and Lewis, C. (2013).** Psychological therapies for chronic post-traumatic stress disorder (PTSD) in adults. Cochrane Database of Systematic Reviews 2013, doi: 10.1002/14651858.CD003388.pub4

  Research indicates that CBT and EMDR therapy are superior to all other treatments.

- **Bradley, R., Greene, J., Russ, E., Dutra, L., and Westen, D. (2005).** A multidimensional meta-analysis of psychotherapy for PTSD. *American Journal of Psychiatry, 162,* 214–227.

  EMDR therapy is equivalent to exposure and other cognitive behavioral treatments and all "are highly efficacious in reducing PTSD symptoms."

- **Davidson, P. R., and Parker, K. C. H. (2001).** Eye movement desensitization and reprocessing (EMDR): A meta-analysis. *Journal of Consulting and Clinical Psychology, 69,* 305–316.

  EMDR therapy is equivalent to exposure and other cognitive behavioral treatments.

- **Lee, C. W., and Cuijpers, P. (2013).** A meta-analysis of the contribution of eye movements in processing emotional memories. *Journal of Behavior Therapy and Experimental Psychiatry, 44,* 231–239.

  "The effect size for the additive effect of eye movements in EMDR treatment studies was moderate and significant (Cohen's $d = 0.41$). For the second group of laboratory studies the effect size was large and significant ($d = 0.74$)."

- **Maxfield, L., and Hyer, L. A. (2002).** The relationship between efficacy and methodology in studies investigating EMDR treatment of PTSD. *Journal of Clinical Psychology, 58,* 23–41.

  A comprehensive meta-analysis reported the more rigorous the study, the larger the effect.

- **Rodenburg, R., Benjamin, A., de Roos, C., Meijer, A. M., and Stams, G. J. (2009).** Efficacy of EMDR in children: A meta-analysis. *Clinical Psychology Review, 29,* 599–606.

"Results indicate efficacy of EMDR when effect sizes are based on comparisons between EMDR and non-established trauma treatment or no-treatment control groups, and incremental efficacy when effect sizes are based on comparisons between EMDR and established (CBT) trauma treatment."

- **Seidler, G. H., and Wagner, F. E. (2006).** Comparing the efficacy of EMDR and trauma-focused cognitive-behavioral therapy in the treatment of PTSD: A meta-analytic study. *Psychological Medicine, 36*, 1515–1522.

  "Results suggest that in the treatment of PTSD, both therapy methods tend to be equally efficacious."

- **Watts, B. V. et al. (2013).** Meta-analysis of the efficacy of treatments for posttraumatic stress disorder. *Journal of Clinical Psychiatry, 74*, e541–550. doi: 10.4088/JCP.12r08225.

  "CBT and eye movement desensitization and reprocessing were the most often-studied types of psychotherapy. Both were effective."

Randomized Clinical Trials

- **Abbasnejad, M., Mahani, K. N., and Zamyad, A. (2007).** Efficacy of "eye movement desensitization and reprocessing" in reducing anxiety and unpleasant feelings due to earthquake experience. *Psychological Research, 9*, 104–117.

  "EMDR is effective in reducing earthquake anxiety and negative emotions (e.g. PTSD, grief, fear, intrusive thoughts, depression, etc.) resulting from earthquake experience. Furthermore, results show that improvement due to EMDR was maintained at a one month follow up."

- **Ahmad, A., Larsson, B., and Sundelin-Wahlsten, V. (2007).** EMDR treatment for children with PTSD: Results of a randomized controlled trial. *Nordic Journal of Psychiatry, 61*, 349–354.

  "Post-treatment scores of the EMDR group were significantly lower than the WLC indicating improvement in total PTSS-C scores, PTSD-related symptom scale, and the subscales re-experiencing and avoidance among subjects in the EMDR group, while untreated children improved in PTSD-non-related symptom scale."

- **Arabia, E., Manca, M. L., and Solomon, R. M. (2011).** EMDR for survivors of life-threatening cardiac events: Results of a pilot study. *Journal of EMDR Practice and Research, 5*, 2–13.

  "Forty-two patients undergoing cardiac rehabilitation . . . were randomized to a 4-week treatment of EMDR or imaginal exposure (IE). . . . EMDR was effective in reducing PTSD, depressive, and anxiety symptoms and performed significantly better than IE for all variables. . . . Because the standardized IE procedures used were those employed in-session during [prolonged exposure] the results are also instructive regarding the relative efficacy of both treatments without the addition of homework."

- **Capezzani et al. (2013).** EMDR and CBT for cancer patients: Comparative study of effects on PTSD, anxiety, and depression. *Journal of EMDR Practice and Research, 5*, 2–13.

This randomized pilot study reported that after eight sessions of treatment, EMDR therapy was superior to a variety of CBT techniques. "Almost all the patients (20 out of 21, 95.2%) did not have PTSD after the EMDR treatment."

- **Carlson, J., Chemtob, C. M., Rusnak, K., Hedlund, N. L., and Muraoka, M. Y. (1998).** Eye movement desensitization and reprocessing (EMDR): Treatment for combat-related post-traumatic stress disorder. *Journal of Traumatic Stress, 11,* 3–24.

Twelve sessions of EMDR eliminated posttraumatic stress disorder in 77.7 percent of the multiply traumatized combat veterans studied. There was 100 percent retention in the EMDR condition. Effects were maintained at follow-up. This is the only randomized study to provide a full course of treatment with combat veterans. Other studies (e.g., Boudewyns; Devilly and Spence, 1999; Jensen; Pitman et al.; Macklin et al.) evaluated treatment of only one or two memories, which, according to the International Society for Traumatic Stress Studies Practice Guidelines *(2000), is inappropriate for multiple-trauma survivors. The VA/DoD* Clinical Practice Guideline for the Management of Post-Traumatic Stress *(VA/DoD, 2004) also indicates these studies (often with only two sessions) offered insufficient treatment doses for veterans. EMDR therapy is listed as an "A"-level treatment in the VA/DoD (2004, 2010).*

- **Carletto, S., Borghi, M., Bertino, G., Oliva, F., Cavallo, M., Hoffmann, A., and Ostacoli, L., (2016).** Treating posttraumatic stress disorder in patients with multiple sclerosis: A randomized controlled trial comparing the efficacy of eye movement desensitization and reprocessing and relaxation therapy. *Frontiers in Psychology, 7.*

In the EMDR condition, measurements at posttest and follow-up revealed 85 percent and 100 percent PTSD remission, respectively.

- **Chemtob, C. M., Nakashima, J., and Carlson, J. G. (2002).** Brief-treatment for elementary school children with disaster-related PTSD: A field study. *Journal of Clinical Psychology, 58,* 99–112.

EMDR was found to be an effective treatment for children with disaster-related PTSD who had not responded to another intervention.

- **Cvetek, R. (2008).** EMDR treatment of distressful experiences that fail to meet the criteria for PTSD. *Journal of EMDR Practice and Research, 2,* 2–14.

EMDR treatment of disturbing life events (small "t" trauma) was compared to active listening, and waitlist. EMDR produced significantly lower scores on the Impact of Event Scale (mean reduced from "moderate" to "subclinical") and a significantly smaller increase on the STAI after memory recall.

- **de Bont, P. A., van den Berg, D. P., van der Vleugel, B. M., de Roos, C., de Jongh, A., van der Gaag, M., and van Minnen, A. M. (2016).** Prolonged exposure and EMDR for PTSD v. a PTSD waiting-list condition: Effects on symptoms of psychosis, depression and social functioning in patients with chronic psychotic disorders. *Psychological Medicine,* 1–11.

"In patients with chronic psychotic disorders PE and EMDR not only reduced PTSD symptoms, but also paranoid thoughts. Importantly, in PE and EMDR more patients accomplished the status of their psychotic disorder in remission."

- **de Roos, C., Greenwald, R., den Hollander-Gijsman, M., Noorthoorn, E., van Buuren, S., and de Jongh, A. (2011).** A randomised comparison of cognitive behavioural therapy (CBT) and eye movement desensitisation and reprocessing (EMDR) in disaster exposed children. *European Journal of Psychotraumatology, 2,* 5694. doi: 10.3402/ejpt.v2i0.5694.

    "Children (n = 52, aged 4–18) were randomly allocated to either CBT (n = 26) or EMDR (n = 26) in a disaster mental health after-care setting after an explosion of a fireworks factory. . . . Both treatment approaches produced significant reductions on all measures and results were maintained at follow-up. Treatment gains of EMDR were reached in fewer sessions."

- **Diehle, J., Opmeer, B. C., Boer, F., Mannarino, A. P., and Lindauer, R. J. (2014).** Trauma-focused cognitive behavioral therapy or eye movement desensitization and reprocessing: What works in children with posttraumatic stress symptoms? A randomized controlled trial. *European Child and Adolescent Psychiatry, 226,* 227–236.

    A mixed sample of full and partial PTSD was evaluated. "[B]oth treatments are effective in children with PTSS in an outpatient setting. Results on both child and parent measures support this conclusion."

- **Edmond, T., Rubin, A., and Wambach, K. (1999).** The effectiveness of EMDR with adult female survivors of childhood sexual abuse. *Social Work Research, 23,* 103–116.

    EMDR treatment resulted in lower scores (fewer clinical symptoms) on all four of the outcome measures at the three-month follow-up, compared to those in the routine treatment condition. The EMDR group also improved on all standardized measures at eighteen months follow-up.

- **Edmond, T., and Rubin, A. (2004). Assessing the long-term effects of EMDR: Results from an 18-month follow up study with adult female survivors of CSA.** *Journal of Childhood Sexual Abuse, 13,* **69–86.**

- **Edmond, T., Sloan, L., and McCarty, D. (2004).** Sexual abuse survivors' perceptions of the effectiveness of EMDR and eclectic therapy: A mixed-methods study. *Research on Social Work Practice, 14,* 259–272.

    Combination of qualitative and quantitative analyses of treatment outcomes with important implications for future rigorous research. Survivors' narratives indicate that EMDR produces greater trauma resolution, while within eclectic therapy, survivors more highly value their relationship with their therapist, through whom they learn effective coping strategies.

- **Högberg, G., Pagani, M., Sundin, O., Soares, J., Åberg-Wisted, A., Tärnell, B., and Hällström, T. (2007).** On treatment with eye movement desensitization and reprocessing of chronic post-traumatic stress disorder in public transportation workers: A randomized controlled study. *Nordic Journal of Psychiatry, 61,* 54–61.

    Employees who had experienced "person-under-train accident or had been assaulted at work were recruited." Six sessions of EMDR resulted in remission of PTSD in 67 percent compared to 11 percent in the wait-list control. Significant effects were documented in Global Assessment of Function (GAF) and Hamilton Depression (HAM-D) score. Follow-up: Högberg, G. et al.

(2008). Treatment of post-traumatic stress disorder with eye movement desensitization and reprocessing: Outcome is stable in 35-month follow-up. Psychiatry Research, *159, 101–108.*

- **Ironson, G. I., Freund, B., Strauss, J. L., and Williams, J. (2002).** Comparison of two treatments for traumatic stress: A community-based study of EMDR and prolonged exposure. *Journal of Clinical Psychology, 58,* 113–128.

  Both EMDR and prolonged exposure produced a significant reduction in PTSD and depression symptoms. This is the only research comparing EMDR and exposure therapy that added in vivo homework to the EMDR condition. The study found that 70 percent of EMDR participants achieved a good outcome in three active treatment sessions, compared to 17 percent of persons in the prolonged-exposure condition. EMDR also had fewer dropouts (0 versus 30 percent).

- **Jaberghaderi, N., Greenwald, R., Rubin, A., Dolatabadim S., and Zand, S. O. (2004).** A comparison of CBT and EMDR for sexually abused Iranian girls. *Clinical Psychology and Psychotherapy, 11,* 358–368.

  Both EMDR and CBT produced significant reduction in PTSD and behavior problems. EMDR was significantly more efficient, using approximately half the number of sessions to achieve results.

- **Jarero, I., Artigas, L., and Luber, M. (2011).** The EMDR protocol for recent critical incidents: Application in a disaster mental health continuum of care context. *Journal of EMDR Practice and Research, 5,* 82–94.

  Participants were treated two weeks following a 7.2 earthquake in Mexico. "One session of EMDR-PRECI produced significant improvement on symptoms of posttraumatic stress for both the immediate-treatment and waitlist/delayed treatment groups, with results maintained at 12-week follow-up, even though frightening aftershocks continued to occur frequently."

- **Jarero, I., Uribe, S., Artigas, L., and Givaudan, M. (2015).** EMDR protocol for recent critical incidents: A randomized controlled trial in a technological disaster context. *Journal of EMDR Practice and Research, 9,* 166–173.

  Evaluation of co-workers ten days after they witnessed seven people killed in an explosion revealed a mean score of 22 on the SPRINT, indicating severe PTSD symptoms. After two consecutive-day sixty-minute EMDR sessions, the mean SPRINT scores for immediate- and delayed-treatment groups declined to equally low levels on both posttest and follow-up.

- **Kemp M., Drummond P., and McDermott, B. (2010).** A wait-list controlled pilot study of eye movement desensitization and reprocessing (EMDR) for children with post-traumatic stress disorder (PTSD) symptoms from motor vehicle accidents. *Clinical Child Psychology and Psychiatry, 15,* 5–25.

  "An effect for EMDR was identified on primary outcome and process measures including the Child Post-Traumatic Stress–Reaction Index, clinician rated diagnostic criteria for PTSD, Subjective Units of Disturbance and Validity of Cognition scales. All participants initially met

two or more PTSD criteria. After EMDR treatment, this decreased to 25% in the EMDR group but remained at 100% in the wait-list group."

- **Lee, C., Gavriel, H., Drummond, P., Richards, J., and Greenwald, R. (2002).** Treatment of post-traumatic stress disorder: A comparison of stress inoculation training with prolonged exposure and eye movement desensitization and reprocessing. *Journal of Clinical Psychology, 58,* 1071–1089.

  Both EMDR and stress inoculation therapy plus prolonged exposure (SITPE) produced significant improvement, with EMDR achieving greater improvement on PTSD intrusive symptoms. Participants in the EMDR condition showed greater gains at three-month follow-up. EMDR condition used three hours of homework compared to twenty-eight hours for SITPE.

- **Marcus, S., Marquis, P., and Sakai, C. (1997).** Controlled study of treatment of PTSD using EMDR in an HMO setting. *Psychotherapy, 34,* 307–315.

  Funded by Kaiser Permanente. Results show that 100 percent of single-trauma and 77 percent of multiple-trauma survivors were no longer diagnosed with posttraumatic stress disorder after six 50-minute sessions.

- **Marcus, S., Marquis, P., and Sakai, C. (2004).** Three- and 6-month follow-up of EMDR treatment of PTSD in an HMO setting. *International Journal of Stress Management, 11,* 195–208.

  Funded by Kaiser Permanente, follow-up evaluation indicates that a relatively small number of EMDR sessions result in substantial benefits that are maintained over time.

- **Nijdam, M. J., Gersons, B. P. R, Reitsma, J. B., de Jongh, A., and Olff, M. (2012).** Brief eclectic psychotherapy v. eye movement desensitisation and reprocessing therapy in the treatment of post-traumatic stress disorder: Randomised controlled trial. *British Journal of Psychiatry, 200,* 224–231.

  A comparison of "the efficacy and response pattern of a trauma-focused CBT modality, brief eclectic psychotherapy for PTSD, with EMDR. . . . Although both treatments are effective, EMDR results in a faster recovery compared with the more gradual improvement with brief eclectic psychotherapy."

- **Novo, P. et al. (2014).** Eye movement desensitization and reprocessing therapy in subsyndromal bipolar patients with a history of traumatic events: A randomized, controlled pilot-study. *Psychiatry Research, 219,* 122–128.

  "Although preliminary, our findings support the utility of this treatment approach and suggest that eye movement desensitization and reprocessing therapy could be a promising and safe therapeutic strategy to reduce trauma symptoms and stabilize mood in traumatized bipolar patients with subsyndromal symptoms."

- **Power, K. G., McGoldrick, T., Brown, K., et al. (2002).** A controlled comparison of eye movement desensitization and reprocessing versus exposure plus cognitive restructuring, versus waiting list in the treatment of post-traumatic stress disorder. *Journal of Clinical Psychology and Psychotherapy, 9,* 299–318.

Both EMDR and exposure therapy plus cognitive restructuring (with daily homework) produced significant improvement. EMDR was more beneficial for depression and social functioning and required fewer treatment sessions. Subsequent reevaluation of the data indicated that "For pre-to post-treatment IES mean change score, EMDR patients also appeared to have had better treatment outcome than E+CR patients" and that EMDR therapy was a predictor of positive outcome: Karatzias, A., Power, K., McGoldrick, T., Brown, K., Buchanan, R., Sharp, D. and Swanson, V. (2006). Predicting treatment outcome on three measures for post-traumatic stress disorder. European Archives of Psychiatry and Clinical Neuroscience, 20, 1–7.

- **Rothbaum, B. O. (1997).** A controlled study of eye movement desensitization and reprocessing in the treatment of post-traumatic stress disordered sexual assault victims. *Bulletin of the Menninger Clinic, 61,* 317–334.

  Three 90-minute sessions of EMDR eliminated posttraumatic stress disorder in 90 percent of rape victims.

- **Rothbaum, B. O., Astin, M. C., and Marsteller, F. (2005).** Prolonged exposure versus eye movement desensitization (EMDR) for PTSD rape victims. *Journal of Traumatic Stress, 18,* 607–616.

  In this NIMH-funded study, both treatments were effective: "An interesting potential clinical implication is that EMDR seemed to do equally well in the main despite less exposure and no homework. It will be important for future research to explore these issues." (p. 614)

- **Scheck, M., Schaeffer, J. A., and Gillette, C. (1998).** Brief psychological intervention with traumatized young women: The efficacy of eye movement desensitization and reprocessing. *Journal of Traumatic Stress, 11,* 25–44.

  Two sessions of EMDR reduced psychological distress in traumatized adolescents and young women and brought scores within one standard deviation of the norm.

- **Shapiro, E., and Laub, B. (2015).** Early EMDR intervention following a community critical incident: A randomized clinical trial. *Journal of EMDR Practice and Research, 9,* 17–27.

  "At 1 week posttreatment, the scores of the immediate treatment group were significantly improved on the IES-R compared to the waitlist/delayed treatment group, who showed no improvement prior to their treatment. At 3 months follow-up, results on the IES-R were maintained and there was a significant improvement on PHQ-9 scores."

- **Shapiro, F. (1989).** Efficacy of the eye movement desensitization procedure in the treatment of traumatic memories. *Journal of Traumatic Stress, 2,* 199–223.

  Seminal study appeared the same year as first controlled studies of CBT treatments. Three-month follow-up indicated substantial effects on distress and behavioral reports. Marred by lack of standardized measures and the originator's serving as sole therapist.

- **Soberman, G. B., Greenwald, R., and Rule, D. L. (2002).** A controlled study of eye movement desensitization and reprocessing (EMDR) for boys with conduct problems. *Journal of Aggression, Maltreatment, and Trauma, 6,* 217–236.

  The addition of three sessions of EMDR resulted in large and significant reductions of memory-related distress and problem behaviors at two-month follow-up.

- **Taylor, S. et al. (2003).** Comparative efficacy, speed, and adverse effects of three PTSD treatments: Exposure therapy, EMDR, and relaxation training. *Journal of Consulting and Clinical Psychology, 71,* 330–338.

  The only randomized study to show exposure statistically superior to EMDR on some measures. This study used therapist-assisted in vivo exposure, where the therapist takes the person to previously avoided areas, in addition to imaginal exposure and one hour of daily homework (@ 50 hours). The EMDR group used only standard sessions and no homework.

- **van den Berg, D. P. G. et al. (2015).** Prolonged exposure versus eye movement desensitization and reprocessing versus waiting list for posttraumatic stress disorder in patients with a psychotic disorder: A randomized clinical trial. *JAMA Psychiatry, 72,* 259–267.

  Standard PE (prolonged exposure) and EMDR therapy protocols are effective, safe, and feasible in patients with PTSD and severe psychotic disorders, including current symptoms. Additional evaluation indicated trauma-focused treatment was associated with significantly less exacerbation, fewer adverse events, and reduced revictimization compared with the WL condition: van den Berg D. P. G. et al. (2015). Trauma-focused treatment in PTSD-patients with psychosis: Symptom exacerbation, adverse events, and revictimization. Schizophrenia Bulletin. doi: 10.1093/schbul/sbv172.

- **Van der Kolk, B., Spinazzola, J., Blaustein, M., Hooper, J., Hooper, E., Korn, D., and Simpson, W. (2007).** A randomized clinical trial of EMDR, fluoxetine and pill placebo in the treatment of PTSD: Treatment effects and long-term maintenance. *Journal of Clinical Psychiatry, 68,* 37–46.

  EMDR was superior to both control conditions in the amelioration of both PTSD symptoms and depression. Upon termination of therapy, the EMDR group continued to improve while fluoxetine participants again became symptomatic.

- **Vaughan, K., Armstrong, M. F., Gold, R., O'Connor, N., Jenneke, W., and Tarrier, N. (1994).** A trial of eye movement desensitization compared to image habituation training and applied muscle relaxation in post-traumatic stress disorder. *Journal of Behavior Therapy and Experimental Psychiatry, 25,* 283–291.

  All treatments led to significant decreases in PTSD symptoms for subjects in the treatment groups as compared to those on a waiting list, with a greater (albeit nonsignificant) reduction in the EMDR group, particularly with respect to intrusive symptoms. In the two to three weeks of the study, forty to sixty additional minutes of daily homework were part of the treatment in the other two conditions.

- **Wanders, F., Serra, M., and de Jongh, A. (2008).** EMDR versus CBT for children with self-esteem and behavioral problems: A randomized controlled trial. *Journal of EMDR Practice and Research, 2,* 180–189.

  Twenty-six children (average age 10.4 years) with behavioral problems were randomly assigned to receive either four sessions of EMDR or CBT. Both were found to have significant positive effects on behavioral and self-esteem problems, with the EMDR group showing significantly larger changes in target behaviors.

- **Wilson, S., Becker, L. A., and Tinker, R. H. (1995).** Eye movement desensitization and reprocessing (EMDR): Treatment for psychologically traumatized individuals. *Journal of Consulting and Clinical Psychology, 63,* 928–937.

  Three sessions of EMDR produced clinically significant change in traumatized civilians on multiple measures.

- **Wilson, S., Becker, L. A., and Tinker, R. H. (1997).** Fifteen-month follow-up of eye movement desensitization and reprocessing (EMDR) treatment of post-traumatic stress disorder and psychological trauma. *Journal of Consulting and Clinical Psychology, 65,* 1047–1056.

  Follow-up at fifteen months showed maintenance of positive treatment effects, with 84 percent remission of PTSD diagnosis.

Nonrandomized Studies

- **Aduriz, M. E., Bluthgen, C., and Knopfler, C. (2009).** Helping child flood victims using group EMDR intervention in Argentina: Treatment outcome and gender differences. *International Journal of Stress Management, 16,* 138–153.

  A comprehensive group intervention with 124 children who experienced disaster-related trauma during a massive flood, utilizing a one-session group protocol. Significant differences were obtained and maintained at three-month follow-up.

- **Devilly, G. J., and Spence, S. H. (1999).** The relative efficacy and treatment distress of EMDR and a cognitive behavioral trauma treatment protocol in the amelioration of post-traumatic stress disorder. *Journal of Anxiety Disorders, 13,* 131–157.

  This study found CBT superior to EMDR. The research is marred by higher expectations in the CBT condition. Treatment was delivered in both conditions by the developer of the CBT protocol.

- **Fernandez, I. (2007).** EMDR as treatment of post-traumatic reactions: A field study on child victims of an earthquake. *Educational and Child Psychology. Special Issue: Therapy, 24,* 65–72.

  This field study explores the effectiveness of EMDR and the level of post-traumatic reactions in a post-emergency context on twenty-two children, victims of an earthquake. The results show that EMDR contributed to the reduction or remission of PTSD symptoms and facilitated the processing of the traumatic experience.

- **Fernandez, I., Gallinari, E., and Lorenzetti, A. (2004).** A school-based EMDR intervention for children who witnessed the Pirelli building airplane crash in Milan, Italy. *Journal of Brief Therapy, 2,* 129–136.

  A group intervention of EMDR was provided to 236 schoolchildren exhibiting PTSD symptoms thirty days post-incident. At four-month follow-up, teachers reported that all but two children evinced a return to normal functioning after treatment.

- **Grainger, R. D., Levin, C., Allen-Byrd, L., Doctor, R. M., and Lee, H. (1997).** An empirical evaluation of eye movement desensitization and reprocessing (EMDR) with survivors of a natural catastrophe. *Journal of Traumatic Stress, 10,* 665–671.

  A study of Hurricane Andrew survivors found significant differences on the Impact of Event Scale and subjective distress in a comparison of EMDR and nontreatment condition.

- **Hensel, T. (2009).** EMDR with children and adolescents after single-incident trauma: An intervention study. *Journal of EMDR Practice and Research, 3,* 2–9.

  Thirty-six children and adolescents ranging in age from 1 year 9 months to 18 years 1 month were assessed at intake, post-waitlist/pretreatment, and at follow-up. EMDR treatment resulted in significant improvement, demonstrating that children younger than 4 years of age showed the same benefit as the school-aged children.

- **Jarero, I., and Artigas, L. (2010).** The EMDR integrative group treatment protocol: Application with adults during ongoing geopolitical crisis. *Journal of EMDR Practice and Research, 4,* 148–155.

  "In this study, the EMDR-IGTP was applied during three consecutive days to a group of 20 adults during ongoing geopolitical crisis in a Central American country in 2009. . . . Changes on the IES were maintained at 14 weeks follow-up even though participants were still exposed to ongoing crisis."

- **Jarero, I., Artigas, L., and Hartung, J. (2006).** EMDR integrative group treatment protocol: A post-disaster trauma intervention for children and adults. Traumatology, *12,* 121–129.

  A study of two hundred children treated with a group protocol after a flood in Mexico indicates that one session of treatment reduced trauma symptoms from the severe range to low (subclinical) levels of distress. Data from successful treatment at other disaster sites are also reported.

- **Jarero, I., Artigas, L., and Lopez-Lena, M. (2008).** The EMDR integrative group treatment protocol: Application with child victims of mass disaster. *Journal of EMDR Practice and Research, 2,* 97–105.

  "In this study the EMDR-IGTP was used with 16 bereaved children after a human provoked disaster in the Mexican State of Coahuila in 2006. Results showed a significant decrease in scores on the Child's Reaction to Traumatic Events Scale that was maintained at 3-month follow-up."

- **Jarero, I., and Uribe, S. (2011).** The EMDR protocol for recent critical incidents: Brief report of an application in a human massacre situation. *Journal of EMDR Practice and Research, 5,* 156–165.

  "Each individual client session lasted between 90 and 120 minutes. Results showed that one session of EMDR-PRECI produced significant improvement on self-report measures of post-traumatic stress and PTSD symptoms for both the immediate treatment and waitlist/delayed treatment groups." There were no dropouts during treatment.

- **Jarero, I., and Uribe, S. (2012).** The EMDR protocol for recent critical incidents: Follow-up report of an application in a human massacre situation. *Journal of EMDR Practice and Research, 6,* 50–61.

  "Follow-up scores showed that the original treatment results were maintained, with a further significant reduction of self-reported symptoms of posttraumatic stress and PTSD between posttreatment and follow-up. . . . [S]cores of all participants were far below PTSD cutoff levels."

- **Konuk, E., Knipe, J., Eke, I., Yuksek, H., Yurtsever, A., and Ostep, S. (2006).** The effects of EMDR therapy on post-traumatic stress disorder in survivors of the 1999 Marmara, Turkey, earthquake. *International Journal of Stress Management, 13,* 291–308.

  Data reported on a representative sample of fifteen hundred earthquake victims indicated that five sessions of EMDR successfully eliminated PTSD in 92.7 percent of those treated, with a reduction of symptoms in the remaining participants. Gains were maintained at six-month follow-up.

- **McLay, R. N., Webb-Murphy, J. A., Fesperman, S. F., Delaney, E. M., Gerard, S. K., Roesch, S. C., Nebeker, B. J., Pandzic, I., Vishnyak, E. A., and Johnston, S. L. (2016).** Outcomes from eye movement desensitization and reprocessing in active-duty service members with posttraumatic stress disorder. *Psychological Trauma: Theory, Research, Practice, and Policy.* Advance online publication. http://dx.doi.org/10.1037/tra0000120.

  "Results indicated that patients receiving EMDR had significantly fewer therapy sessions over ten weeks but had significantly greater gains in their PCL-M scores than did individuals not receiving EMDR."

- **Puffer, M., Greenwald, R., and Elrod, D. (1997).** A single session EMDR study with twenty traumatized children and adolescents. *Traumatology, 32,* art. 6.

  In this delayed-treatment comparison, over half of the participants moved from clinical to normal levels on the Impact of Events Scale, and all but three showed at least partial symptom relief on several measures at 1–3 months following a single EMDR session.

- **Ribchester, T., Yule, W., and Duncan, A. (2010).** EMDR for childhood PTSD after road traffic accidents: Attentional, memory, and attributional processes. *Journal of EMDR Practice and Research, 4,* 138–147.

  "EMDR was used with 11 children who developed posttraumatic stress disorder (PTSD) after road traffic accidents. All improved such that none met criteria for PTSD on standardized assessments after an average of only 2.4 sessions. . . . Treatment was associated with a significant trauma-specific reduction in attentional bias on the modified Stroop task, with results apparent both immediately after therapy and at follow-up."

- **Russell, M. C., Silver, S. M., Rogers, S., and Darnell, J. (2007).** Responding to an identified need: A joint Department of Defense–Department of Veterans Affairs training program in eye movement desensitization and reprocessing (EMDR) for clinicians providing trauma services. *International Journal of Stress Management, 14,* 61–71.

Seventy-two active-duty military personnel were treated with EMDR therapy by nine different therapists in actual clinic settings. Results indicated that "the disturbance associated with the targeted traumatic memories had been largely eliminated and a new more positive perspective had developed. These changes were corroborated with the IES-R and BDI scores falling from the severe range to the mild or subclinical range." Average treatment time: 8.50 sessions if wounded and 3.82 sessions if nonwounded.

- **Schubert, S. J., Lee, C. W., de Araujo, G., Butler, S. R., Taylor, G., and Drummond, P. (2016).** The effectiveness of eye movement desensitization and reprocessing (EMDR) therapy to treat symptoms following trauma in Timor Leste. *Journal of Traumatic Stress, 29(2),* 141–148.

  "These findings suggest that benefits can be achieved with EMDR therapy for decreasing PTSD symptoms in a post-war, cross-cultural setting in a relatively short period (on average 4 treatment sessions over 13 days)."

- **Silver, S. M., Brooks, A., and Obenchain, J. (1995).** Eye movement desensitization and reprocessing treatment of Vietnam war veterans with PTSD: Comparative effects with biofeedback and relaxation training. *Journal of Traumatic Stress, 8,* 337–342.

  The analysis of an inpatient veterans' PTSD program (n = 100) found EMDR to be superior to biofeedback and relaxation training.

- **Silver, S. M., Rogers, S., Knipe, J., and Colelli, G. (2005).** EMDR therapy following the 9/11 terrorist attacks: A community-based intervention project in New York City. *International Journal of Stress Management, 12,* 29–42.

  Clients made highly significant positive gains on a range of outcome variables, including validated psychometrics and self-report scales. Analyses of the data indicate that EMDR is a useful treatment intervention both in the immediate aftermath of disaster as well as later.

- **Solomon, R. M., and Kaufman, T. E. (2002).** A peer support workshop for the treatment of traumatic stress of railroad personnel: Contributions of eye movement desensitization and reprocessing (EMDR). *Journal of Brief Therapy, 2,* 27–33.

  Sixty railroad employees who had experienced fatal-grade crossing accidents were evaluated for workshop outcomes and for the additive effects of EMDR treatment. Although the workshop was successful, in this setting, the addition of a short session of EMDR (5–40 minutes) led to significantly lower, subclinical scores, which further decreased at follow-up.

- **Sprang, G. (2001).** The use of eye movement desensitization and reprocessing (EMDR) in the treatment of traumatic stress and complicated mourning: Psychological and behavioral outcomes. *Research on Social Work Practice, 11,* 300–320.

  In a multisite study, EMDR significantly reduced symptoms more often than the CBT treatment on behavioral measures and on four of five psychosocial measures. EMDR was more efficient, inducing change at an earlier stage and requiring fewer sessions. Positive recall of the deceased was significantly greater posttreatment in the EMDR condition.

- **Wadaa, N. N., Zaharim, N. M., and Alqashan, H. F. (2010).** The use of EMDR in treatment of traumatized Iraqi children. *Digest of Middle East Studies, 19,* 26–36.

"Our findings are consistent with the conclusion . . . that EMDR is effective for civilian PTSD, and it applies its treatment in a user-friendly manner. . . . The results of the study demonstrated the effectiveness of EMDR in the treatment of PTSD in the experimental group compared to the control group."

- **Zaghrout-Hodali, M., Alissa, F., and Dodgson, P. W. (2008).** Building resilience and dismantling fear: EMDR group protocol with children in an area of ongoing trauma. *Journal of EMDR Practice and Research, 2,* 106–113.

  Results indicate that the EMDR approach can be effective in a group setting and in an acute situation both in reducing symptoms of posttraumatic and peritraumatic stress and in "inoculation" or building resilience in a setting of ongoing conflict and trauma.

Adaptive Information Processing and EMDR Therapy Procedures

The Adaptive Information Processing model (Shapiro, 2001, 2002, 2007, 2014) is used to explain EMDR's clinical effects and guide clinical practice. This section includes literature to provide an overview of the model and procedures, as well as selected research and case reports that demonstrate the predictive value of the model in the treatment of life experiences that appear to underlie a variety of clinical complaints.

- **Afifi, T. O., Mota, N. P., Dasiewicz, P., MacMillan, H. L., and Sareen, J. (2012).** Physical punishment and mental disorders: Results from a nationally representative US sample. *Pediatrics, 130,* 184–192.

  "Harsh physical punishment [i.e., pushing, grabbing, shoving, slapping, hitting] in the absence of [more severe] child maltreatment is associated with mood disorders, anxiety disorders, substance abuse/dependence, and personality disorders in a general population sample."

- **Allon, M. (2015).** EMDR group therapy with women who were sexually assaulted in the Congo. *Journal of EMDR Practice and Research, 9,* 28–34.

  Rape victims were successfully treated within three sessions using both individual and group protocols. They reported the simultaneous remission of back and abdominal pain. These processing results are consistent with the reported remission of PLP with EMDR therapy.

- **Arseneault, L., Cannon, M., Fisher, H. L., Polanczyk, G., Moffitt, T. E., and Caspi, A. (2011).** Childhood trauma and children's emerging psychotic symptoms: A genetically sensitive longitudinal cohort study. *American Journal of Psychiatry, 168,* 65–72.

  "Trauma characterized by intention to harm is associated with children's reports of psychotic symptoms. Clinicians working with children who report early symptoms of psychosis should inquire about traumatic events such as maltreatment and bullying."

- **Bae, H., Kim, D., and Park, Y. C. (2008).** Eye movement desensitization and reprocessing for adolescent depression. *Psychiatry Investigation, 5,* 60–65.

  Processing of etiological disturbing memories, triggers, and templates resulted in complete remission of Major Depressive Disorder in two teenagers. Treatment duration was three to seven sessions, and effects were maintained at follow-up.

- **Behnam Moghadam, M., Alamdari, A. K., Behnam Moghadam, A., and Darban, F.
  (2015).** Effect of EMDR on depression in patients with myocardial infarction. *Global Journal of Health Science, 7,* 258–262.

  In this randomized study, the mean depression level in experimental group significantly decreased following the intervention. These changes were significantly greater compared to the control group. Conclusion: "EMDR is an effective, useful, efficient, and non-invasive method for treatment and reducing depression in patients with MI." A twelve-month follow-up reported maintenance of treatment effects: Behnam, M. M., Behnam, M. A., and Salehian, T. (2015). Efficacy of eye movement desensitization and reprocessing (EMDR) on depression in patients with myocardial infarction (MI) in a 12-month follow up. Iranian Journal of Critical Care Nursing, 7, *221–226.*

- **Brown, K. W., McGoldrick, T., and Buchanan, R. (1997).** Body dysmorphic disorder: Seven cases treated with eye movement desensitization and reprocessing. *Behavioural and Cognitive Psychotherapy, 25,* 203–207.

  Seven consecutive cases were treated with up to three sessions of EMDR. Complete remission of body dysmorphic disorder symptoms were reported in five cases, with effects maintained at one-year follow-up.

- **Brown, S., and Shapiro, F. (2006).** EMDR in the treatment of borderline personality disorder. *Clinical Case Studies, 5,* 403–420.

  Twenty EMDR sessions that focused on reprocessing the memories seemingly at the foundation of the pathology, along with triggers and future templates, resulted in a complete remission of borderline personality disorder, including symptoms of affect dysregulation, as measured on the Inventory of Altered Self Capacities.

- **de Roos, C. et al. (2010).** Treatment of chronic phantom limb pain (PLP) using a trauma-focused psychological approach. *Pain Research and Management, 15,* 65–71.

  Ten consecutive cases of phantom limb pain were treated with EMDR resulting in the reduction or elimination of pain in all but two cases. Results were maintained at 2.8-year follow-up.

- **Doering, S., Ohlmeier, M., de Jongh, A., Hofmann, A., and Bisping, V. (2013).** Efficacy of a trauma-focused treatment approach for dental phobia: A randomized clinical trial. *European Journal of Oral Sciences, 121,* 584–593.

  Three sessions of EMDR therapy memory processing resulted in remission of dental phobia. "After 1 yr, 83.3% of the patients were in regular dental treatment (d = 3.20). The findings suggest that therapy aimed at processing memories of past dental events can be helpful for patients with dental phobia."

- **Faretta, E. (2013).** EMDR and cognitive behavioral therapy in the treatment of panic disorder: A comparison. *Journal of EMDR Practice and Research, 7,* 121–133.

  As predicted by Adaptive Information Processing, the processing of etiological events, triggers, and memory templates was sufficient to alleviate the diagnosis without the use of treatment-specific homework, in contrast to the CBT group. In this study, there was "a continuing decrease in frequency of panic attacks for participants with PD or PDA in the EMDR condition at follow-up that was significantly greater than that found in the CBT treatment group."

- **Felitti, V. J. et al. (1998).** Relationship of childhood abuse and household dysfunction to many of the leading causes of death in adults: The adverse childhood experiences (ACE) study. *American Journal of Preventive Medicine, 14*, 245–258.

  "We found a strong dose-response relationship between the breadth of exposure to abuse or household dysfunction during childhood and multiple risk factors for several of the leading causes of death in adults."

- **Fernandez, I., and Faretta, E. (2007).** EMDR in the treatment of panic disorder with agoraphobia. *Clinical Case Studies, 6*, 44–63.

  As predicted by Adaptive Information Processing, the processing of etiological events, triggers, and memory templates was sufficient to alleviate the diagnosis without the use of therapist-assisted in vivo exposure.

- **Gauvreau, P., and Bouchard, S. (2008).** Preliminary evidence for the efficacy of EMDR in treating generalized anxiety disorder. *Journal of EMDR Practice and Research, 2*, 26–40.

  Four subjects were evaluated using a single case design with multiple baselines. Results indicate that subsequent to targeting the experiential contributors, at posttreatment and at two months follow-up, all four participants no longer presented with generalized anxiety disorder diagnosis.

- **Gold, S. D., Marx, B. P., Soler-Baillo, J. M., and Sloan, D. M. (2005).** Is life stress more traumatic than traumatic stress? *Journal of Anxiety Disorders, 19*, 687–698.

  "[The non-Criterion A] group reported significantly greater severity of PTSD symptomatology than those who reported a Criterion A1 PTSD event. In addition, significantly more people in the DSM trauma-incongruent group met criteria for PTSD than those in the DSM trauma-congruent group."

- **Heim, C., Plotsky, P. M., and Nemeroff, C. B. (2004).** Importance of studying the contributions of early adverse experience to neurobiological findings in depression. *Neuropsychopharmacology, 29*, 641–648.

  "The available data suggest that (1) early adverse experience contributes to the pathophysiology of depression, (2) there are neurobiologically different subtypes of depression depending on the presence or absence of early adverse experience, likely having confounded previous research on the neurobiology of depression, and (3) early adverse experience likely influences treatment response in depression."

- **Heins, M. et al. (2011).** Childhood trauma and psychosis: A case-control and case-sibling comparison across different levels of genetic liability, psychopathology, and type of trauma. *American Journal of Psychiatry, 168*, 1286–1294.

  "Discordance in psychotic illness across related individuals can be traced to differential exposure to trauma. The association between trauma and psychosis is apparent across different levels of illness and vulnerability to psychotic disorder, suggesting true association rather than reporting bias, reverse causality, or passive gene-environment correlation."

- **Madrid, A., Skolek, S., and Shapiro, F. (2006).** Repairing failures in bonding through EMDR. *Clinical Case Studies, 5*, 271–286.

EMDR processing of experiential contributors to bonding disruption, in addition to current triggers, and a memory template of an alternative/problem-free pregnancy and birth resulted in the repair of maternal bonding, analogous to the positive findings with the repair of disrupted attachment.

- **McGoldrick, T., Begum, M., and Brown, K. W. (2008).** EMDR and olfactory reference syndrome: A case series. *Journal of EMDR Practice and Research 2*, 63–68.

EMDR treatment of four consecutive cases of olfactory reference syndrome whose pathological symptoms had endured for eight to forty-eight years resulted in a complete resolution of symptoms in all four cases, which was maintained at follow-up.

- **Mol, S. S. L., Arntz, A., Metsemakers, J. F. M., Dinant, G., Vilters-Van Montfort, P. A. P., and Knottnerus, A. (2005).** Symptoms of post-traumatic stress disorder after non-traumatic events: Evidence from an open population study. *British Journal of Psychiatry, 186,* 494–499.

Supports a basic tenet of the Adaptive Information Processing model that "Life events can generate at least as many PTSD symptoms as traumatic events." In a survey of 832 people, "For events from the past 30 years the PTSD scores were higher after life events than after traumatic events."

- **Nazari, H., Momeni, N., Jariani, M., and Tarrahi, M. J. (2011).** Comparison of eye movement desensitization and reprocessing with citalopram in treatment of obsessive-compulsive disorder. *International Journal of Psychiatry in Clinical Practice, 15,* 270–274.

"There was significant difference between the mean Yale–Brown scores of the two groups after treatment and EMDR was more effective than citalopram in improvement of OCD signs."

- **Obradović, J., Bush, N. R., Stamperdahl, J., Adler, N. E., and Boyce, W. T. (2010).** Biological sensitivity to context: The interactive effects of stress reactivity and family adversity on socioemotional behavior and school readiness. *Child Development, 1,* 270–289.

"A substantive body of work has established that environmental adversity can have a deleterious effect on children's functioning. . . . Exposure to adverse, stressful events . . . has been linked to socioemotional behavior problems and cognitive deficits."

- **Perkins, B. R., and Rouanzoin, C. C. (2002).** A critical evaluation of current views regarding eye movement desensitization and reprocessing (EMDR): Clarifying points of confusion. *Journal of Clinical Psychology, 58,* 77–97.

Reviews common errors and misperceptions of the procedures, research, and theory.

- **Raboni, M. R., Tufik, S., and Suchecki, D. (2006).** Treatment of PTSD by eye movement desensitizatio..n and reprocessing improves sleep quality, quality of life and perception of stress. *Annals of the New York Academy of Science, 1071,* 508–513.

Specifically citing the hypothesis that EMDR induces processing effects similar to REM sleep (see also Stickgold, 2002, 2008), polysomnograms indicated a change in sleep patterns post treatment, and improvement on all measures, including anxiety, depression, and quality of life after a mean of five sessions.

- **Ray, A. L., and Zbik, A. (2001).** Cognitive behavioral therapies and beyond. In *Practical Pain Management*, 3rd ed., edited by C. D. Tollison, J. R. Satterthwaite, and J. W. Tollison, 189–208. Philadelphia: Lippincott.

  The authors note that the application of EMDR guided by the Adaptive Information Processing model appears to afford benefits to chronic pain patients not found in other treatments.

- **Read, J., Fosse, R., Moskowitz, A., and Perry, B. (2014).** The traumagenic neurodevelopmental model of psychosis revisited. *Neuropsychiatry, 4*, 65–79.

  "[C]ontrary to long-held beliefs among biologically oriented researchers and clinicians, the etiology of psychosis and schizophrenia are just as socially based [e.g., early-life adversity] as are nonpsychotic mental health problems, such as anxiety and depression."

- **Ricci, R. J., Clayton, C. A., and Shapiro, F. (2006).** Some effects of EMDR treatment with previously abused child molesters: Theoretical reviews and preliminary findings. *Journal of Forensic Psychiatry and Psychology, 17*, 538–562.

  As predicted by the Adaptive Information Processing model, the EMDR treatment of the molesters' own childhood victimization resulted in a decrease in deviant arousal as measured by the plethysmograph, a decrease in sexual thoughts, and increased victim empathy. Effects were maintained at one-year follow-up.

- **Robinson, J. S. and Larson, C. (2010).** Are traumatic events necessary to elicit symptoms of posttraumatic stress? *Psychological Trauma: Theory, Research, Practice, and Policy, 2*, 71–76.

  Research data "indicated similar levels of posttrauma syndrome severity for all three symptom clusters among people who had endorsed the experience of only a traumatic type even and people who had reported the experience of only stressful negative life events (e.g., loss of job, problems with school or work, or change in financial status)."

- **Russell, M. (2008).** Treating traumatic amputation-related phantom limb pain: a case study utilizing eye movement desensitization and reprocessing (EMDR) within the armed services. *Clinical Case Studies, 7*, 136–153.

  "Since September 2006, over 725 service-members from the global war on terrorism have survived combat-related traumatic amputations that often result in phantom limb pain (PLP) syndrome. . . . Four sessions of eye movement desensitization and reprocessing (EMDR) led to elimination of PLP, and a significant reduction in PTSD, depression, and phantom limb tingling sensations."

- **Schneider, J., Hofmann, A., Rost, C., and Shapiro, F. (2007).** EMDR and phantom limb pain: Case study, theoretical implications, and treatment guidelines. *Journal of EMDR Science and Practice, 1*, 31–45.

  Detailed presentation of case treated by EMDR that resulted in complete elimination of PTSD, depression, and phantom limb pain, with effects maintained at eighteen-month follow-up.

- **Schneider, J., Hofmann, A., Rost, C., and Shapiro, F. (2008).** EMDR in the treatment of chronic phantom limb pain. *Pain Medicine, 9*, 76–82.

As predicted by the Adaptive Information Processing model, the EMDR treatment of the event involving the limb loss, and the stored memories of the pain sensations, resulted in a decrease or elimination of the phantom limb pain, which was maintained at one-year follow-up.

- **Shapiro, F. (2001).** *Eye Movement Desensitization and Reprocessing: Basic Principles, Protocols and Procedures.* 2nd ed. New York: Guilford Press.

  EMDR is an eight-phase psychotherapy with standardized procedures and protocols that are all believed to contribute to therapeutic effect. This text provides description and clinical transcripts and an elucidation of the guiding Adaptive Information Processing model.

- **Shapiro, F., ed. (2002).** EMDR as an Integrative Psychotherapy Approach: Experts of Diverse Orientations Explore the Paradigm Prism. Washington, D.C.: American Psychological Association Books.

  EMDR is an integrative approach distinct from other forms of psychotherapy. Experts of the major psychotherapy orientations identify and highlight various procedural elements.

- **Shapiro, F. (2006).** EMDR and new notes on Adaptive Information Processing: Case formulation principles, scripts and worksheets. Camden, Conn.: EMDR Humanitarian Assistance Programs (www.emdrhap.org).

  Overview of Adaptive Information Processing model, including how the principles are reflected in the procedures, phases, and clinical applications of EMDR. Comprehensive worksheets for client assessment, case formulation, and treatment, as well as scripts for various procedures.

- **Shapiro, F. (2007).** EMDR, Adaptive Information Processing, and case conceptualization. *Journal of EMDR Practice and Research, 1,* 68–87.

  Overview of EMDR treatment based upon an Adaptive Information Processing case conceptualization. Early life experiences are viewed as the basis of pathology and used as targets for processing. The three-pronged protocol includes processing of past events that have set the foundation for the pathology, the current triggers, and templates for appropriate future functioning to address skill and developmental deficits.

- **Shapiro, F. (2012).** EMDR therapy: An overview of current and future research. *European Review of Applied Psychology, 62,* 193–195.

  "Research findings indicate that EMDR therapy and TF-CBT are based on different mechanisms of action in that EMDR therapy does not necessitate daily homework, sustained arousal or detailed descriptions of the event, and appears to take fewer sessions. EMDR is guided by the Adaptive Information Processing model, which posits a wide range of adverse life experiences as the basis of pathology."

- **Shapiro, F. (2014).** The role of eye movement desensitization and reprocessing (EMDR) therapy in medicine: Addressing the psychological and physical symptoms stemming from adverse life experiences. *Permanente Journal, 18,* 71–77.

  An overview of the substantial body of research demonstrating that adverse life experiences contribute to both psychological and biomedical pathology, as well as the research demonstrating the clinical effects of EMDR therapy as guided by the Adaptive Information Processing model.

- **Shapiro, F., Kaslow, F., and Maxfield, L., eds. (2007).** *Handbook of EMDR and Family Therapy Processes.* Hoboken, N.J.: Wiley.

  Using an Adaptive Information Processing conceptualization a wide range of family problems and impasses can be addressed through the integration of EMDR and family therapy techniques. Family therapy models are also useful for identifying the targets in need of processing for those engaged in individual therapy.

- **Simhandl, C., Radua, J., König, B., and Amann, B. L. (2014).** The prevalence and effect of life events in 222 bipolar I and II patients: A prospective, naturalistic 4 year follow-up study. *Journal of Affective Disorders.* doi: 10.1016/j.jad.2014.08.043.

  "Our data suggest a high and continuous number of life events prior to affective episodes. Life events after the index episode worsened the course of bipolar I patients with more depressive episodes. This underlines the importance of detection and treatment of emerging life events."

- **Solomon, R. M., and Shapiro, F. (2008).** EMDR and the Adaptive Information Processing model: Potential mechanisms of change. *Journal of EMDR Practice and Research, 2,* 315–325.

  This article provides a brief overview of some of the major precepts of the Adaptive Information Processing model, a comparison and contrast to extinction-based information processing models and treatment, and a discussion of a variety of mechanisms of action.

- **Teicher, M. H., Samson, J. A., Sheu, Y. S., Polcari, A., and McGreenery, C. E. (2010).** Hurtful words: Association of exposure to peer verbal abuse with elevated psychiatric symptom scores and corpus callosum abnormalities. *American Journal of Psychiatry, 167,* 1464–1471.

  "These findings parallel results of previous reports of psychopathology associated with childhood exposure to parental verbal abuse and support the hypothesis that exposure to peer verbal abuse is an aversive stimulus associated with greater symptom ratings and meaningful alterations in brain structure."

- **Uribe, M. E. R., and Ramirez, E. O. L. (2006).** The effect of EMDR therapy on the negative information processing on patients who suffer depression. *Revista Electrónica de Motivación y Emoción (REME), 9,* 23–24.

  The study evaluated the impact of EMDR treatment on bias mechanisms in depressed subjects in regard to negative emotional valence evaluation. "The results indicated that it generated important cognitive emotional changes in such mechanisms. Priming tests indicated changes in the negative valence evaluation of emotional information indicative of recovery with decreased reaction times in the neutral and positive stimuli processing."

- **van den Berg, D. P. G., and van den Gaag, M. (2012).** Treating trauma in psychosis with EMDR: A pilot study. *Journal of Behavior Therapy and Experimental Psychiatry, 43,* 664–671.

  "This pilot study shows that a short EMDR therapy is effective and safe in the treatment of PTSD in subjects with a psychotic disorder. Treatment of PTSD has a positive effect on auditory verbal hallucinations, delusions, anxiety symptoms, depression symptoms, and self-esteem."

- **Varese, F., Smeets, F., Drukker, M., Lieverse, R., Lataster, T., Vichetbauer, W. (2012).** Childhood adversities increase the risk of psychosis: a meta-analysis of patient-control, prospective- and cross-sectional cohort studies. *Schizophrenia Bulletin, 38*, 661–671.

  "These findings indicate that childhood adversity is strongly associated with increased risk for psychosis."

- **Wesselmann, D., and Potter, A. E. (2009).** Change in adult attachment status following treatment with EMDR: Three case studies. *Journal of EMDR Practice and Research, 3*, 178–191.

  Subsequent to EMDR treatment, "all three patients made positive changes in attachment status as measured by the [Adult Attachment Inventory], and all three reported positive changes in emotions and relationships."

- **Wilensky, M. (2006).** Eye movement desensitization and reprocessing (EMDR) as a treatment for phantom limb pain. *Journal of Brief Therapy, 5*, 31–44.

  "Five consecutive cases of phantom limb pain were treated with EMDR. Four of the five clients completed the prescribed treatment and reported that pain was completely eliminated, or reduced to a negligible level. . . . The standard EMDR treatment protocol was used to target the accident that caused the amputation, and other related events."

Mechanism of Action

EMDR contains many procedures and elements that contribute to treatment effects. While the methodology used in EMDR has been extensively validated (see above), questions still remain regarding mechanism of action. However, since EMDR achieves clinical effects without the need for homework or the prolonged focus used in exposure therapies, attention has been paid to the possible neurobiological processes that might be evoked. Although the eye movements (and other dual-attention stimulation) constitute only one procedural element, this element has come under greatest scrutiny. Randomized controlled studies evaluating the mechanism of action of the eye movement component follow this section.

- **De Jongh, A., Ernst, R., Marques, L., and Hornsveld, H. (2013).** The impact of eye movements and tones on disturbing memories of patients with PTSD and other mental disorders. *Journal of Behavior Therapy and Experimental Psychiatry, 44*, 447–483.

  "The findings provide further evidence for the value of employing eye movements in EMDR treatments. The results also support the notion that EMDR is a suitable option for resolving disturbing memories underlying a broader range of mental health problems than PTSD alone."

- **El Khoury-Malhame, M. et al. (2011).** Attentional bias in post-traumatic stress disorder diminishes after symptom amelioration. *Behaviour Research and Therapy, 49*, 796–801.

  "Attentional bias toward aversive cues in PTSD has been hypothesized as being part of the dysfunction causing etiology and maintenance of PTSD. The aim of the present study was to investigate the cognitive strategy underlying attentional bias in PTSD and whether normal cognitive processing is restored after a treatment suppressing core PTSD symptoms." An average of 4.1 EMDR sessions resulted in remission of PTSD. Post treatment, *"similarly to controls, EMDR treated patients who were symptom free had null e-Stroop and disengagement indices."*

- **Elofsson, U. O. E., von Scheele, B., Theorell, T., and Sondergaard, H. P. (2008).** Physiological correlates of eye movement desensitization and reprocessing. *Journal of Anxiety Disorders, 22,* 622–634.

  Changes in heart rate, skin conductance and LF/HF ratio, finger temperature, breathing frequency, carbon dioxide and oxygen levels were documented during the eye-movement condition. It was concluded the "eye movements during EMDR activate cholinergic and inhibit sympathetic systems. The reactivity has similarities with the pattern during REM sleep."

- **Hornsveld, H. K., Landwehr, F., Stein, W., Stomp, M., Smeets, S., and van den Hout, M. A. (2010).** Emotionality of loss-related memories is reduced after recall plus eye movements but not after recall plus music or recall only. *Journal of EMDR Practice and Research,* 4, 106–112.

  "Recall-plus-music was added to investigate whether reductions in emotionality are associated with relaxation. . . . Participants reported a greater decline in emotionality and concentration after eye movements in comparison to recall-only and recall-with-music. It is concluded that eye movements are effective when negative memories pertain to loss and grief."

- **Kapoula, Z., Yang, Q., Bonnet, A., Bourtoire, P., and Sandretto, J. (2010).** EMDR effects on pursuit eye movements. *PLoS ONE, 5(5): e10762.* doi:10.1371/journal.pone.0010762.

  EMDR treatment of autobiographic worries causing moderate distress resulted in an "increase in the smoothness of pursuit [which] presumably reflects an improvement in the use of visual attention needed to follow the target accurately. Perhaps EMDR reduces distress thereby activating a cholinergic effect known to improve ocular pursuit."

- **Kristjánsdóttir, K., and Lee, C. M. (2011).** A comparison of visual versus auditory concurrent tasks on reducing the distress and vividness of aversive autobiographical memories. *Journal of EMDR Practice and Research, 5,* 34–41.

  "Results showed that vividness and emotionality ratings of the memory decreased significantly after eye movement and counting, and that eye movement produced the greatest benefit. Furthermore, eye movement facilitated greater decrease in vividness irrespective of the modality of the memory. Although this is not consistent with the hypothesis from a working memory model of mode-specific effects, it is consistent with a central executive explanation."

- **Lee, C. W., Taylor, G., and Drummond, P. D. (2006).** The active ingredient in EMDR: Is it traditional exposure or dual focus of attention? *Clinical Psychology and Psychotherapy, 13,* 97–107.

  This study tested whether the content of participants' responses during EMDR is similar to that thought to be effective for traditional exposure treatments (reliving) or is more consistent with distancing, which would be expected, given Shapiro's proposal of dual focus of attention. Greatest improvement on a measure of PTSD symptoms occurred when the participant processed the trauma in a more detached manner, which indicates the underlying mechanisms of EMDR and exposure therapy are different.

- **Leer, A., Engelhard, I. M., and van den Hout, M. A. (2014).** How eye movements in EMDR work: Changes in memory vividness and emotionality. *Journal of Behavior Therapy and Experimental Psychiatry, 45,* 396–401.

"[T]his study provides corroborating evidence that EM during recall causes reductions in memory vividness and emotionality at a delayed post-test and that the magnitude of these effects is related to intervention duration."

- **Lilley, S. A., Andrade, J., Graham Turpin, G., Sabin-Farrell, R., and Holmes, E. A. (2009).** Visuospatial working memory interference with recollections of trauma. *British Journal of Clinical Psychology, 48,* 309–321.

  Tested patients awaiting PTSD treatment and demonstrated that the eye-movement condition had a significant effect on vividness of trauma memory and emotionality compared to counting and exposure only. In addition, "the counting task had no effect on vividness compared to exposure only, suggesting that the eye-movement task had a specific effect rather than serving as a general distractor." (p. 317)

- **MacCulloch, M. J., and Feldman, P. (1996).** Eye movement desensitization treatment utilizes the positive visceral element of the investigatory reflex to inhibit the memories of post-traumatic stress disorder: A theoretical analysis. *British Journal of Psychiatry, 169,* 571–579.

  One of a variety of articles positing an orienting response as a contributing element (see Shapiro, 2001, for comprehensive examination of theories and suggested research parameters). This theory has received controlled research support (see Barrowcliff et al., 2003, 2004).

- **Propper, R., Pierce, J. P., Geisler, M. W., Christman, S. D., and Bellorado, N. (2007).** Effect of bilateral eye movements on frontal interhemispheric gamma EEG coherence: Implications for EMDR therapy. *Journal of Nervous and Mental Disease, 195,* 785–788.

  "Specifically, the EM manipulation used in the present study, reported previously to facilitate episodic memory, resulted in decreased interhemispheric EEG coherence in anterior prefrontal cortex. Because the gamma band includes the 40 Hz wave that may indicate the active binding of information during the consolidation of long-term memory storage (e.g., Cahn and Polich, 2006), it is particularly notable that the changes in coherence we found are in this band. With regard to PTSD symptoms, it may be that by changing interhemispheric coherence in frontal areas, the EMs used in EMDR foster consolidation of traumatic memories, thereby decreasing the memory intrusions found in this disorder."

- **Rogers, S., and Silver, S. M. (2002).** Is EMDR an exposure therapy? A review of trauma protocols. *Journal of Clinical Psychology, 58,* 43–59.

  Theoretical, clinical, and procedural differences referencing two decades of CBT and EMDR research.

- **Rogers, S., Silver, S., Goss, J., Obenchain, J., Willis, A., and Whitney, R. (1999).** A single session, controlled group study of flooding and eye movement desensitization and reprocessing in treating posttraumatic stress disorder among Vietnam war veterans: Preliminary data. *Journal of Anxiety Disorders, 13,* 119–130.

  This study was designed as primarily a process report to compare EMDR and exposure therapy. A different recovery pattern was observed with the EMDR group, demonstrating a more rapid decline in self-reported distress.

- **Sack, M., Hofmann, A., Wizelman, L., and Lempa, W. (2008).** Psychophysiological changes during EMDR and treatment outcome. *Journal of EMDR Practice and Research, 2,* 239–246.

  During-session changes in autonomic tone were investigated in ten patients suffering from single-trauma PTSD. Results indicate that information processing during EMDR is followed by during-session decreases in psychophysiological activity, reduced subjective disturbance, and reduced stress reactivity to traumatic memory.

- **Sack, M., Lempa, W., Steinmetz, A., Lamprecht, F., and Hofmann, A. (2008).** Alterations in autonomic tone during trauma exposure using eye movement desensitization and reprocessing (EMDR): Results of a preliminary investigation. *Journal of Anxiety Disorders, 22,* 1264–1271.

  The psychophysiological correlates of EMDR were investigated during treatment sessions of trauma patients. The initiation of the eye movements sets resulted in immediate changes that indicated a pronounced de-arousal.

- **Servan-Schreiber, D., Schooler, J., Dew, M. A., Carter, C., and Bartone, P. (2006).** EMDR for PTSD: A pilot blinded, randomized study of stimulation type. *Psychotherapy and Psychosomatics, 75,* 290–297.

  Twenty-one patients with single-event PTSD (average IES: 49.5) received three consecutive sessions of EMDR with three different types of auditory and kinesthetic stimulation. All were clinically useful. However, alternating stimulation appeared to confer an additional benefit to the EMDR procedure.

- **Stickgold, R. (2002).** EMDR: A putative neurobiological mechanism of action. *Journal of Clinical Psychology, 58,* 61–75.

- **Stickgold, R. (2008).** Sleep-dependent memory processing and EMDR action. *Journal of EMDR Practice and Research, 2,* 289–299.

  Comprehensive explanations of mechanisms and the potential links to the processes that occur in REM sleep. Controlled studies have evaluated these theories (see next section; Christman et al., 2003; Kuiken et al., 2001, 2010).

- **Suzuki, A. et al. (2004).** Memory reconsolidation and extinction have distinct temporal and biochemical signatures. *Journal of Neuroscience, 24,* 4787–4795.

  The article explores the differences between memory reconsolidation and extinction. This new area of investigation is worthy of additional attention. Reconsolidation may prove to be the underlying mechanism of EMDR, as opposed to extinction caused by prolonged exposure therapies. "Memory reconsolidation after retrieval may be used to update or integrate new information into long-term memories. . . . Brief exposure . . . seems to trigger a second wave of memory consolidation (reconsolidation), whereas prolonged exposure . . . leads to the formation of a new memory that competes with the original memory (extinction)."

- **van den Hout, M., Engelhard, I. M., Marleen, M., Rijkeboer, M. M., Koekebakker, J., Hornsveld, H., Leer, A., et al. (2012).** EMDR: Tones inferior to eye movements in the EMDR treatment of PTSD. *Behaviour Research and Therapy, 50,* 275–279.

"EMs outperformed tones while it remained unclear if tones add to recall only. . . . EMs were superior to tones in reducing the emotionality and vividness of trauma memories. [I]n contrast to EMs, tones hardly tax working memory and induce a smaller reduction in emotionality and vividness of aversive memories. Interestingly, patients' preferences did not follow this pattern: the perceived effectiveness was higher for tones than for EMs. . . . Clearly, the superior effects of EMs on emotionality and vividness of trauma memories were not due to demand characteristics."

- **Wilson, D., Silver, S. M., Covi, W., and Foster, S. (1996).** Eye movement desensitization and reprocessing: Effectiveness and autonomic correlates. *Journal of Behaviour Therapy and Experimental Psychiatry, 27,* 219–229.

  Study involving biofeedback equipment has supported the hypothesis that the parasympathetic system is activated by finding that eye movements appeared to cause a compelled relaxation response. More rigorous research with trauma populations is needed.

Randomized Studies of Hypotheses Regarding Eye Movements

Numerous memory researchers have evaluated the eye movements used in EMDR therapy. A recent meta-analysis of the eye movement research has reported positive effects (Lee and Cuijpers, 2013) in both clinical and laboratory trials (see above). It is hypothesized that a number of mechanisms interact synergistically. The following studies have tested specific hypotheses regarding mechanism of action and found a direct effect on emotional arousal, imagery vividness, attentional flexibility, retrieval, distancing, and memory association.

- **Andrade, J., Kavanagh, D., and Baddeley, A. (1997).** Eye-movements and visual imagery: A working memory approach to the treatment of post-traumatic stress disorder. *British Journal of Clinical Psychology, 36,* 209–223.

  Tested the working-memory theory. Eye movements were superior to control conditions in reducing image vividness and emotionality.

- **Barrowcliff, A. L., Gray, N. S., Freeman, T. C. A., and MacCulloch, M. J. (2004).** Eye-movements reduce the vividness, emotional valence and electrodermal arousal associated with negative autobiographical memories. *Journal of Forensic Psychiatry and Psychology, 15,* 325–345.

  Tested the reassurance reflex model. Eye movements were superior to control conditions in reducing image vividness and emotionality.

- **Barrowcliff, A. L., Gray, N. S., MacCulloch, S., Freeman, T. C. A., and MacCulloch, M. J. (2003).** Horizontal rhythmical eye-movements consistently diminish the arousal provoked by auditory stimuli. *British Journal of Clinical Psychology, 42,* 289–302.

  Tested the reassurance reflex model. Eye movements were superior to control conditions in reducing arousal provoked by auditory stimuli.

- **Christman, S. D., Garvey, K. J., Propper, R. E., and Phaneuf, K. A. (2003).** Bilateral eye movements enhance the retrieval of episodic memories. *Neuropsychology. 17,* 221–229.

Tested cortical activation theories. Results provide indirect support for the orienting response/ REM theories suggested by Stickgold (2002, 2008). Saccadic eye movements, but not tracking eye movements, were superior to control conditions in episodic retrieval.

- **Christman, S. D., Propper, R. E., and Brown, T. J. (2006).** Increased interhemispheric interaction is associated with earlier offset of childhood amnesia. *Neuropsychology, 20,* 336.

  "The results of the current Experiment 2 suggest that the eye movements employed in EMDR may induce a neurobiological change in interhemispheric interaction and an attendant psychological change in episodic retrieval."

- **Engelhard, I. M., van den Hout, M. A., Janssen, W. C., and van der Beek, J. (2010).** Eye movements reduce vividness and emotionality of "flashforwards." *Behaviour Research and Therapy, 48,* 442–447.

  Distressing images were randomly assigned to two conditions. "This study examined whether eye movements reduce vividness and emotionality of visual distressing images about feared future events. . . . Relative to the no-dual task condition, eye movements while thinking of future-oriented images resulted in decreased ratings of image vividness and emotional intensity."

- **Engelhard, I. M., van Uijen, S., and van den Hout, M. A. (2010).** The impact of taxing working memory on negative and positive memories. *European Journal of Psychotraumatology, 5623,* doi: 10.3402/ejpt.v1i0.5623.

  "The effects of EM and Tetris on negative and positive memories did not differ, even though Tetris taxed to a greater extent than EM."

- **Engelhard, I. M. et al. (2011).** Reducing vividness and emotional intensity of recurrent "flashforwards" by taxing working memory: An analogue study. *Journal of Anxiety Disorders 25,* 599–603.

  "Results showed that vividness of intrusive images was lower after recall with eye movement, relative to recall only, and there was a similar trend for emotionality."

- **Gunter, R. W., and Bodner, G. E. (2008).** How eye movements affect unpleasant memories: Support for a working-memory account. *Behaviour Research and Therapy 46,* 913–931.

  Three studies were done that cumulatively support a working-memory account of the eye movement benefits in which the central executive is taxed when a person performs a task while attempting to hold a memory in mind.

- **Kavanagh, D. J., Freese, S., Andrade, J., and May, J. (2001).** Effects of visuospatial tasks on desensitization to emotive memories. *British Journal of Clinical Psychology, 40,* 267–280.

  Tested the working-memory theory. Eye movements were superior to control conditions in reducing within-session image vividness and emotionality. There was no difference one week post-treatment.

- **Kearns, M., and Engelhard, I. M. (2015).** Psychophysiological responsivity to script-driven imagery: An exploratory study of the effects of eye movements on public speaking flashforwards. *Frontiers in Psychiatry, 6,* doi:10.3389/fpsyt.2015.00115.

"Relative to the control condition (imagery only), those who made eye movements whilst hold-ing a mental image of this scenario in-mind demonstrated a significant decrease in heart rate, which acted as a measure of emotionality."

- **Kuiken, D., Bears, M., Miall, D., and Smith, L. (2002).** Eye movement desensitization reprocessing facilitates attentional orienting. *Imagination, Cognition and Personality, 21,* 3–20.

  Tested the orienting response theory related to REM-type mechanisms. Indicated that the eye movement condition was correlated with increased attentional flexibility. Eye movements were superior to control conditions.

- **Kuiken, D., Chudleigh, M., and Racher, D. (2010).** Bilateral eye movements, attentional flexibility and metaphor comprehension: The substrate of REM dreaming? *Dreaming, 20,* 227–247.

  This study adds additional support to the orienting response theory related to REM-type mech-anisms. Evaluations of participants experiencing significant loss or trauma demonstrate differ-ential effects in a comparison of eye-movement and non-eye-movement conditions.

- **Lee, C. W., and Drummond, P. D. (2008).** Effects of eye movement versus therapist in-structions on the processing of distressing memories. *Journal of Anxiety Disorders, 22,* 801–808.

  "There was no significant effect of therapist's instruction on the outcome measures. There was a significant reduction in distress for eye movement at post-treatment and at follow-up. . . . The results were consistent with other evidence that the mechanism of change in EMDR is not the same as traditional exposure."

- **Maxfield, L., Melnyk, W. T., and Hayman, C. A. G. (2008).** A working memory explana-tion for the effects of eye movements in EMDR. *Journal of EMDR Practice and Research, 2,* 247–261.

  In two experiments, participants focused on negative memories while engaging in three dual-attention eye-movement tasks of increasing complexity. Results support a working-memory explanation for the effects of eye-movement dual-attention tasks on autobiographical memory.

- **Nieuwenhuis, S., Elzing, B. M., Ras, P. H., Berends, F., Duijs, P., Samara, Z., and Slagter, H. A. (2013).** Bilateral saccadic eye movements and tactile stimulation, but not auditory stimulation, enhance memory retrieval. *Brain and Cognition, 81,* 52–56.

  Increased memory retrieval in two experiments supports "the possibility that alternating bilat-eral activation of the left and right hemispheres exerts its effects on memory by increasing the functional connectivity between the two hemispheres."

- **Parker, A., Buckley, S., and Dagnall, N. (2009).** Reduced misinformation effects following saccadic bilateral eye movements. *Brain and Cognition, 69,* 89–97.

  Bilateral saccadic eye movements were compared to vertical and no eye movements. "It was found that bilateral eye movements increased true memory for the event, increased recollection, and decreased the magnitude of the misinformation effect." This study supports hypotheses regarding effects of interhemispheric activation and episodic memory.

- **Parker, A., and Dagnall, N. (2007).** Effects of bilateral eye movements on gist based false recognition in the DRM paradigm. *Brain and Cognition, 63,* 221–225.

  Bilateral saccadic eye movements were compared to vertical and no eye movements. Those in the bilateral eye movement condition "were more likely to recognise previously presented words and less likely to falsely recognize critical non-studies associates."

- **Parker, A., Relph, S., and Dagnall, N. (2008).** Effects of bilateral eye movement on retrieval of item, associative and contextual information. *Neuropsychology, 22,* 136–145.

  The effects of saccadic bilateral eye movement were compared to vertical eye movements and no eye movements on the retrieval of item, associative, and contextual information. Saccadic eye movements were superior on all parameters in all conditions.

- **Samara, Z., Bernet M., Elzinga, B. M., Heleen A., Slagter, H. A., and Nieuwenhuis, S. (2011).** Do horizontal saccadic eye movements increase interhemispheric coherence? Investigation of a hypothesized neural mechanism underlying EMDR. *Frontiers in Psychiatry, 2,* 4. doi: 10.3389/fpsyt.2011.00004.

  The study demonstrated that thirty seconds of bilateral saccadic eye movements enhanced the episodic retrieval of nontraumatic emotional stimuli in healthy adults. There was no evidence for an increase in interhemispheric coherence. However, a number of caveats regarding interpretation are noted.

- **Schubert, S. J., Lee, C. W., and Drummond, P. D. (2011).** The efficacy and psychophysiological correlates of dual-attention tasks in eye movement desensitization and reprocessing (EMDR). *Journal of Anxiety Disorders, 25,* 1–11.

  "EMDR-with eye movements led to greater reduction in distress than EMDR-without eye movements. Heart rate decreased significantly when eye movements began; skin conductance decreased during eye movement sets; heart rate variability and respiration rate increased significantly as eye movements continued; and orienting responses were more frequent in the eye movement than no-eye movement condition at the start of exposure."

- **Sharpley, C. F., Montgomery, I. M., and Scalzo, L. A. (1996).** Comparative efficacy of EMDR and alternative procedures in reducing the vividness of mental images. *Scandinavian Journal of Behaviour Therapy, 25,* 37–42.

  Eye movements were superior to control conditions in reducing image vividness.

- **Smeets, M. A., Dijs, M. W., Pervan, I., Engelhard, I. M., and van den Hout, M. A. (2012).** Time-course of eye movement-related decrease in vividness and emotionality of unpleasant autobiographical memories. *Memory, 20,* 346–357.

  "Results revealed a significant drop [in eyes moving condition] compared to the [eyes stationary] group in emotionality after 74 seconds compared to a significant drop in vividness at only 2 seconds into the intervention. These results support that emotionality becomes reduced only after vividness has dropped."

- **van den Hout, M., Muris, P., Salemink, E., and Kindt, M. (2001).** Autobiographical memories become less vivid and emotional after eye movements. *British Journal of Clinical Psychology, 40,* 121–130.

  Tested their theory that eye movements change the somatic perceptions accompanying retrieval, leading to decreased affect, and therefore decreasing vividness. Eye movements were superior to control conditions in reducing image vividness. Unlike control conditions, eye movements also decreased emotionality.

- **van den Hout, M. et al. (2011).** EMDR: Eye movements superior to beeps in taxing working memory and reducing vividness of recollections. *Behaviour Research and Therapy, 49,* 92–98.

  "Vividness of negative memories was reduced after both beeps and eye movements, but effects were larger for eye movements. Findings support a working memory account of EMDR and suggest that effects of beeps on negative memories are inferior to those of eye movements."

Additional Psychophysiological and Neurobiological Evaluations of EMDR Treatment

All psychophysiological studies have indicated significant de-arousal. Neurobiological studies have indicated significant effects, including changes in cortical, and limbic activation patterns, and increase in hippocampal volume.

Aubert-Khalfa, S., Roques, J., and Blin, O. (2008). Evidence of a decrease in heart rate and skin conductance responses in PTSD patients after a single EMDR session. *Journal of EMDR Practice and Research, 2,* 51–56.

Bossini, L., Fagiolini, A., and Castrogiovanni, P. (2007). Neuroanatomical changes after EMDR in posttraumatic stress disorder. *Journal of Neuropsychiatry and Clinical Neuroscience, 19,* 457–458.

Bossini, L., Tavanti, M., Calossi, S., Polizzotto, N. R., Vatti, G., Marino, D., and Castrogiovanni, P. (2011). EMDR treatment for posttraumatic stress disorder, with focus on hippocampal volumes: A pilot study. *Journal of Neuropsychiatry and Clinical Neurosciences, 23,* E1–2, doi:10.1176/appi. neuropsych.23.2.E1

Frustaci, A., Lanza, G. A., Fernandez, I., di Giannantonio, M., and Pozzi, G. (2010). Changes in psychological symptoms and heart rate variability during EMDR treatment: A case series of subthreshold PTSD. *Journal of EMDR Practice and Research, 4,* 3–11.

Grbesa et al. (2010). Electrophysiological changes during EMDR treatment in patients with combat-related PTSD. *Annals of General Psychiatry, 9* (Suppl 1), S209.

Harper, M. L., Rasolkhani-Kalhorn, T., and Drozd, J. F. (2009). On the neural basis of EMDR therapy: Insights from QEEG studies. *Traumatology, 15,* 81–95.

Herkt, D., Tumani, V., Grön, G., Kammer, T., Hofmann, A., and Abler, B. (2014). Facilitating access to emotions: Neural signature of EMDR stimulation. *PLOS ONE, 9*(8), e106350.

Kowal, J. A. (2005). QEEG analysis of treating PTSD and bulimia nervosa using EMDR. *Journal of Neurotherapy, 9 (4),* 114–115.

Lamprecht, F., Kohnke, C., Lempa, W., Sack, M., Matzke, M., and Munte, T. (2004). Event-related potentials and EMDR treatment of post-traumatic stress disorder. *Neuroscience Research, 49,* 267–272.

Landin-Romero, R. et al. (2013). EMDR therapy modulates the default mode network in a subsyndromal, traumatized bipolar patient. *Neuropsychobiology, 67,* 181–184.

Lansing, K., Amen, D. G., Hanks, C., and Rudy, L. (2005). High resolution brain SPECT imaging and EMDR in police officers with PTSD. *Journal of Neuropsychiatry and Clinical Neurosciences, 17,* 526–532.

Levin, P., Lazrove, S., and van der Kolk, B. A. (1999). What psychological testing and neuroimaging tell us about the treatment of posttraumatic stress disorder (PTSD) by eye movement desensitization and reprocessing (EMDR). *Journal of Anxiety Disorders, 13,* 159–172.

Nardo, D. et al. (2010). Gray matter density in limbic and paralimbic cortices is associated with trauma load and EMDR outcome in PTSD patients. *Journal of Psychiatric Research, 44,* 477–485.

Oh, D.-H., and Choi, J. (2004). Changes in the regional cerebral perfusion after eye movement desensitization and reprocessing: A SPECT study of two cases. *Journal of EMDR Practice and Research, 1,* 24–30.

Ohtani, T., Matsuo, K., Kasai, K., Kato, T., and Kato, N. (2009). Hemodynamic responses of eye movement desensitization and reprocessing in posttraumatic stress disorder. *Neuroscience Research, 65,* 375–383.

Pagani, M. et al. (2007). Effects of EMDR psychotherapy on 99mTc-HMPAO distribution in occupation-related post-traumatic stress disorder. *Nuclear Medicine Communications, 28,* 757–765.

Pagani, M. et al. (2011). Pretreatment, intratreatment, and posttreatment EEG imaging of EMDR: Methodology and preliminary results from a single case. *Journal of EMDR Practice and Research, 5,* 42–56.

Pagani, M. et al. (2012). Neurobiological correlates of EMDR monitoring: An EEG study. *PLoS ONE, 7*(9) e45753. doi:10.1371/journal.pone.0045753.

Propper, R., Pierce, J. P., Geisler, M. W., Christman, S. D., and Bellorado, N. (2007). Effect of bilateral eye movements on frontal interhemispheric gamma EEG coherence: Implications for EMDR therapy. *Journal of Nervous and Mental Disease, 195,* 785–788.

Richardson, R., Williams, S. R., Hepenstall, S., Gregory, L., McKie, S., and Corrigan, F. **(2009).** A single-case fMRI study: EMDR treatment of a patient with posttraumatic stress disorder. *Journal of EMDR Practice and Research, 3,* 10–23.

Sack, M., Lempa, W., and Lemprecht, W. (2007). Assessment of psychophysiological stress reactions during a traumatic reminder in patients treated with EMDR. *Journal of EMDR Practice and Research, 1,* 15–23.

Sack, M., Nickel, L., Lempa, W., and Lamprecht, F. (2003). Psychophysiological regulation in patients suffering from PTSD: Changes after EMDR treatment. *Journal of Psychotraumatology and Psychological Medicine, 1,* 47–57. (German)

van der Kolk, B., Burbridge, J., and Suzuki, J. (1997). The psychobiology of traumatic memory: Clinical implications of neuroimaging studies. *Annals of the New York Academy of Sciences, 821,* 99–113.

Treatment of Military Personnel

As noted in the World Health Organization (2013) guidelines and the American Psychiatric Association Practice Guidelines (2004, p. 18), in EMDR therapy, "traumatic material need not be verbalized; instead, patients are directed to think about their traumatic experiences without having to discuss them." Given the reluctance of many combat veterans to divulge the details of their experience, this factor is relevant to willingness to initiate treatment, retention and therapeutic gains. It may be one of the factors responsible for the lower remission and higher dropout rate noted in this population when CBT techniques are used.

As described previously, an RCT by Carlson et al. (1998) reported that after twelve EMDR treatment sessions, 77.7 percent of the combat veterans no longer met criteria for PTSD. There were no dropouts and effects were maintained at three- and nine-month follow-up. In addition, the Silver et al. (1995) analysis of an inpatient veterans' PTSD program ($n = 100$) found EMDR to be superior to biofeedback and relaxation training on seven of eight measures. Russell et al. (2007) evaluated seventy-two active-duty military personnel, forty-eight of them diagnosed with combat PTSD, and reported that pre- and post-treatment changes were significant on all measures. A recent program evaluation of active duty military by McLay et al. (2016) compared various forms of treatment and reported, "Results indicated that patients receiving EMDR had significantly fewer therapy sessions over 10 weeks but had significantly greater gains in their PCL-M scores than did individuals not receiving EMDR."

All other RCT of veterans have used insufficient treatment doses to assess PTSD outcomes (e.g., two sessions; see ISTSS, 2000; DVA/DoD, 2004). Sufficient treatment time must be used for multiply traumatized veterans (e.g., see below: Russell et al., 2007). However, in a process analysis, Rogers et al. (1999) compared one session of EMDR and exposure therapy with inpatient veterans, and a different recovery pattern was observed. The EMDR group demonstrated a more rapid decline in self-reported distress (e.g., SUD levels decreased with EMDR and increased with exposure).

As stated in the *American Psychiatric Practice Guidelines* (2004, p. 36), if viewed as an exposure therapy, "EMDR employs techniques that may give the patient more control over the exposure experience (since EMDR is less reliant on a verbal account) and provides techniques to regulate anxiety in the apprehensive circumstance of exposure treatment. Consequently, it may prove advantageous for patients who cannot tolerate prolonged exposure as well as for patients who have difficulty verbalizing their traumatic experiences. Comparisons of EMDR with other treatments in larger samples are needed to clarify such differences."

Such research is highly recommended. In addition, since EMDR utilizes no homework to achieve its effects, it may be particularly suited for front line alleviation of symptoms (see Russell, 2006; Wesson and Gould, 2009). Further, the prevalent somatic and chronic pain problems experienced by combat veterans indicate the need for additional research based upon the reports of Russell (2008), Schneider et al. (2007, 2008), and Wilensky (2007), which demonstrate EMDR's capacity to successfully treat phantom limb pain (see also Ray and Zbik, 2001). The ability of EMDR to simultaneously address PTSD, depression, and pain can have distinct benefits for DVA/DoD treatment.

The following contains clinically relevant information for the treatment of veterans, including therapy parameters.

Carlson, J., Chemtob, C. M., Rusnak, K., Hedlund, N. L, and Muraoka, M. Y. (1998). Eye movement desensitization and reprocessing (EMDR): Treatment for combat-related posttraumatic stress disorder. *Journal of Traumatic Stress, 11*, 3–24.

Cook, J. M., Biyanova, T., and Coyne, J. C. (2009). Comparative case study of diffusion of eye movement desensitization and reprocessing in two clinical settings: Empirically supported treatment status is not enough. *Professional Psychology: Research and Practice, 40*, 518–524.

Errebo, N., and Sommers-Flanagan, R. (2007). EMDR and emotionally focused couple therapy for war veteran couples. In *Handbook of EMDR and Family Therapy Processes*, edited by F. Shapiro, F. Kaslow, and L. Maxfield. New York: Wiley.

Lipke, H. (2000). *EMDR and Psychotherapy Integration*. Boca Raton, FL: CRC Press.

McLay, R. N., Webb-Murphy, J. A., Fesperman, S. F., Delaney, E. M., Gerard, S. K., Roesch, S. C., Nebeker, B. J., Pandzic, I., Vishnayak, E. A., and Johnston, S. L. (2016). Outcomes from eye movement desensitization and reprocessing in active-duty service members with posttraumatic stress disorder. *Psychological Trauma: Theory, Research, Practice, and Policy*. Advance online publication. http://dx.doi.org/10.1037/tra0000120.

Russell, M. C. (2006). Treating combat-related stress disorders: A multiple case study utilizing eye movement desensitization and reprocessing (EMDR) with battlefield casualties from the Iraqi War. *Military Psychology, 18*, 1–18.

Russell, M. C. (2008a). Treating traumatic amputation-related phantom limb pain: A case study utilizing eye movement desensitization and reprocessing (EMDR) within the armed services. *Clinical Case Studies, 7*, 136–153.

Russell, M. C. (2008b). War-related medically unexplained symptoms, prevalence, and treatment: Utilizing EMDR within the armed services. *Journal of EMDR Practice and Research, 2*, 212–226.

Russell, M. C. (2008c). Scientific resistance to research, training and utilization of eye movement desensitization and reprocessing (EMDR) therapy in treating post-war disorders. *Social Science and Medicine, 67*, 1737–1746.

Russell, M. C., and Figley, C. R. (2013). *Treating Traumatic Stress Injuries in Military Personnel: An EMDR Practitioner's Guide*. New York: Routledge.

Russell, M. C., and Silver, S. M. (2007). Training needs for the treatment of combat-related posttraumatic stress disorder. *Traumatology, 13*, 4–10.

Russell, M. C., Silver, S. M., Rogers, S., and Darnell, J. (2007). Responding to an identified need: A joint Department of Defense–Department of Veterans Affairs training program in eye movement desensitization and reprocessing (EMDR) for clinicians providing trauma services. *International Journal of Stress Management, 14*, 61–71.

Silver, S. M., and Rogers, S. (2002). Light in the Heart of Darkness: EMDR and the Treatment of War and Terrorism Survivors. New York: Norton.

Silver, S. M., Rogers, S., and Russell, M. C. (2008). Eye movement desensitization and reprocessing (EMDR) in the treatment of war veterans. Journal of Clinical Psychology: In Session, 64, 947–957.

Wesson, M., and Gould, M. (2009). Intervening early with EMDR on military operations: A case study. *Journal of EMDR Practice and Research, 3*, 91–97.

APPENDIX C

EMDR THERAPY: EVALUATED CLINICAL APPLICATIONS

EMDR therapy is now widely recognized as a first-line treatment of trauma (e.g., American Psychiatric Association, 2004; Bisson and Andrew, 2007; Bleich et al., 2002; CREST, 2003; VA/DoD, 2004; Foa et al., 2009; INSERM, 2004; NICE, 2005; SAMHSA, 2010; World Health Organization, 2013). Clinical applications of EMDR are based on the Adaptive Information Processing model (Shapiro, 2001, 2002, 2006, 2007), which posits that the direct reprocessing of the stored memories of etiological events and other experiential contributors can have a positive effect in the treatment of most clinical complaints. This prediction has received support in case studies and other research with a variety of diagnoses. Expanding the standard protocols (Shapiro, 1995, 2001), experts and consultants in various specialty areas have developed additional applications in clinical practice. To date, while numerous randomized controlled studies have supported EMDR therapy's effectiveness in the treatment of trauma and PTSD across the life span, other clinical applications are generally evaluated in case studies or open trials and need further investigation.

Another excellent resource is the Francine Shapiro Library, created by Barbara Hensley and hosted by the EMDR International Association. The library provides information for clinicians, researchers, and laypeople on the efficaciousness of EMDR therapy for a wide range of mental health issues. This compendium of scholarly articles and other important literature related to Adaptive Information Processing and EMDR therapy can be found at this website: http://emdria.omeka.net.

Since the initial efficacy study (Shapiro, 1989a), positive therapeutic results with EMDR therapy have been reported with a wide range of populations and include the following:

1. *Combat veterans from the Iraq Wars, the Afghanistan War, the Vietnam War, the Korean War, and World War II who were formerly treatment resistant and who no longer experience flashbacks, nightmares, and other PTSD sequelae:* Blore, 1997a; Brickell, Russell, and Smith, 2015; Carlson et al., 1996, 1998; Daniels et al., 1992; Lansing, 2013; Lipke, 2000; Lipke and Botkin, 1992; Narimani, Sadeghieh Ahari, and Rajabi, 2008; Niroomandi, 2012; Russell, 2006, 2008a, 2008b; Russell, Silver, Rogers, and Darnell, 2007; Silver and Rogers, 2001; Silver, Rogers, and Russell, 2008; Russell and Figley, 2012; Thomas and Gafner, 1993; Wesson and Gould, 2009; White, 1998; Young, 1995; Zimmermann et al., 2005.

2. *People with phobias, panic disorder, obsessive compulsive disorder, and generalized anxiety disorder who revealed a reduction of fear and symptoms:* Böhm and Voderholzer, 2010; Cook-Vienot and Taylor, 2012; de Castro Lopes, Carvalho, and Barbosa, 2014; de Jongh, 2012; de Jongh et al., 2010; de Jongh and ten Broeke, 1998; de Jongh, ten Broeke, and Renssen, 1999; de Jongh, van den Oord, and ten Broeke, 2002; Doering et al., 2013; de Roos and de Jongh, 2008; Feske and Goldstein, 1997; Farima, Dowlatabadi, and Behzadi, 2015; Fernandez and Faretta, 2007; Faretta, 2013; Goldstein, 1992; Gauvreau and Bouchard, 2008; Gattinara, 2009; Goldstein and Feske, 1994; Grey, 2011; Gupta, Gupta, and Choudhary, 2014; Harada, 2013; Howard and Cox, 2006; Kleinknecht, 1993; Leeds, 2012; Lobenstine and Courtney, 2013; Marr, 2012; Nadler, 1996; Morrissey, 2013; Nazari et al., 2011; Newgent, Paladino, and Reynolds, 2006; O'Brien, 1993; Protinsky, Sparks, and Flemke, 2001a; Rathschlag and Memmert, 2014; de Roos et al., 2010; Rougemont-Bucking and Zimmermann, 2012; Schurmans, 2007. Some controlled studies of people with arachnophobia have revealed comparatively little benefit from EMDR (e.g., Muris and Merckelbach, 1997; Muris et al., 1997, 1998), but evaluations have been confounded by lack of fidelity to the published protocols (de Jongh, ten Broeke, and Renssen, 1999; Shapiro, 1999). One evaluation of panic disorder with agoraphobia (Goldstein et al., 2000) also reported limited results (for comprehensive discussion, see Shapiro, 2001, 2002).

3. *Crime victims, police officers, firefighters, field workers, and caregivers who are no longer disturbed by the aftereffects of violent assaults and/or the stressful nature of their work:* Baker and McBride, 1991; Dyregrov, 1993; Jensma, 1999; Kitchiner, 2004; Kitchiner and Aylard, 2002; Kleinknecht and Morgan, 1992; Koeva, 2012; Lansing et al., 2005; McNally and Solomon, 1999; Page and Crino, 1993; Rost, Hofmann, and Wheeler, 2009; Shapiro and Solomon, 1995; Solomon, 1995, 1998; Solomon and Dyregrov, 2000; Wilson et al., 2001.

4. *People relieved of excessive grief due to the loss of a loved one or to line-of-duty deaths, such as engineers no longer devastated with guilt because their train unavoidably killed pedestrians:* Gattinara, 2009; Lazrove, Triffleman, Kite, McGlasshan, and Rounsaville, 1998; Puk,1991; Shapiro and Solomon, 1995; Solomon, 1995, 1998; Solomon and Kaufman, 2002; Solomon and Rando, 2007; Solomon and Shapiro, 1997; Sprang, 2001.

5. *Children and adolescents healed of the symptoms, including depression, caused by disturbing life experiences:* Ahmad, Larsson, and Sundelin-Wahlsten, 2007; Bae, Kim, and Park, 2008; Beer and Bronner, 2010; Bronner et al., 2009; Chemtob et al., 2002; Cocco and Sharpe, 1993; Datta and Wallace, 1994, 1996; Fernandez, 2007; Fernandez, Gallinari, and Lorenzetti, 2004; Gomez, 2012; Greenwald, 1994, 1998, 1999, 2000, 2002; Hensel, 2006, 2009; Jaberghaderi et al., 2004; Jarero, Artigas, and Hartung, 2006; Korkmazler-Oral and Pamuk, 2002; Lovett, 1999; Maxfield, 2007; Oras, de Ezpeleta, and Ahmad, 2004; Pellicer, 1993; Puffer, Greenwald, and Elrod, 1998; Rodenburg et al., 2009; Russell and O'Connor, 2002; Scheck, Schaeffer, and Gillette, 1998; Shapiro, 1991; Soberman, Greenwald, and Rule, 2002; Stewart and Bramson, 2000; Taylor, 2002; Tinker and Wilson, 1999; Tufnell, 2005; Wadaa, Zaharim, and Alqashan, 2010; Wanders, Serra, and de Jongh, 2008; Zaghrout-Hodali, Alissa, and Dodgson, 2008.

6. *Sexual assault victims who are now able to lead normal lives and have intimate relationships:* Allon, 2015; Edmond, Rubin, and Wambach, 1999; Hyer, 1995; Kowal, 2005; Posmontier, Dovydaitis, and Lipman, 2010; Puk, 1991; Rothbaum, 1997; Rothbaum, Astin, and Marsteller, 2005; Scheck, Schaeffer, and Gillette, 1998; Shapiro, 1989b, 1991, 1994; Tang et al., 2015; Tarquinio, Brennstuhl, Reichenbach, et al., 2012; Tarquinio, Brennstuhl, Rydberg, et al., 2012; Wolpe and Abrams, 1991.

7. *Victims of natural and human-made disasters who are able to resume normal lives:* Chemtob et al., 2002; Colelli and Patterson, 2008; Farrell et al., 2011; Fernandez, 2008; Fernandez,

Gallinari, and Lorenzetti, 2004; Gelbach, 2008; Grainger et al., 1997; Jarero and Artigas, 2010; Jarero et al., 1999; Jarero and Uribe, 2012a, 2012b; Jayatunge, 2008; Konuk et al., 2006; Shapiro and Laub, 2008; Silver et al., 2005.

8. *Accident, surgery, and burn victims who were once emotionally or physically debilitated and who are now able to resume productive lives:* Blore, 1997b; Broad and Wheeler, 2006; Hassard, 1993; McCann, 1992; Moradi, Chatrrooz, Sarichlu, and Alipourheidari, 2015; Softic, 2009; Stramrood et al., 2012.

9. *Victims of family, marital, and sexual dysfunction who are now able to maintain healthy relationships:* Bardin, 2004; Capps, 2006; Errebo and Sommers-Flanagan, 2007; Keenan and Farrell, 2000; Gattinara, 2009; Jarero, Roque-Lopez, Gomez, and Givaudan, 2014; Kaslow, Nurse, and Thompson, 2002; Knudsen, 2007; Koedam, 2007; Madrid, Skolek, and Shapiro, 2006; Moses, 2007; Phillips et al. 2009; Protinsky, Sparks, and Flemke, 2001b; Reicherzer, 2011; Shapiro, Kaslow, and Maxfield, 2007; Stowasser, 2007; Talan, 2007; Wernik, 1993; Tsuchimochi and Sasaki, 2012; Wesselmann et al., 2012; Wesselmann and Potter, 2009; Wesselmann, Schweitzer, and Armstrong, 2014.

10. *Clients at all stages of chemical dependency and sexual deviation/addiction and pathological gamblers who now show stable recovery and a decreased tendency to relapse:* Abel and O'Brien, 2010; Bae, Hahn, and Kim, 2015; Bae and Kim, 2012; Besson et al., 2006; Brown et al., 2015; Cox and Howard, 2007; Hase, Schallmayer, and Sack, 2008; Henry, 1996; Krupnik, 2015; Marich, 2009; Meysami-Bonab et al., 2012; Popky, 2005; Ricci, 2006; Ricci, Clayton, and Shapiro, 2006; Shapiro and Forrest, 1997; Shapiro, Vogelmann-Sine, and Sine, 1994; Vogelmann-Sine et al., 1998; Zweben and Yeary, 2006.

11. *People with dissociative disorders who progress at a rate more rapid than that achieved by traditional treatment:* Amano, Seiyama, and Toichi, 2012; Barol and Seubert, 2010; Cohen, 2009; Dilly, 2014; Fine, 1994; Fine and Berkowitz, 2001; Gonzalez and Mosquera, 2012; Knipe, 2014; Lazrove and Fine, 1996; Paulsen, 1995; Twombly, 2000, 2005; Young, 1994; van der Hart, Groenendijk, Gonzalez, Mosquera, and Solomon, 2014.

12. *People who have performance anxiety or deficits in school, business, performing arts, or sports and who have benefited from EMDR as a tool to help enhance performance:* Barker and Barker, 2007; Crabbe, 1996; Foster and Lendl, 1995, 1996; Graham, 2004; Maxfield and Melnyk, 2000; Silverman, 2011.

13. *People with somatic problems or somatoform disorders, including migraines, chronic pain, phantom limb pain, chronic eczema, gastrointestinal problems, chronic fatigue syndrome, psychogenic seizures, eating disorders, and negative body image, and who have attained relief of suffering:* Amano, Seiyama, and Toichi 2013; Bloomgarden and Calogero, 2008; Brennstuhl and Tarquinio, 2012; Brown, McGoldrick, and Buchanan, 1997; Chemali and Meadows, 2004; de Groot and de Jongh, 2012; de Roos et al., 2010; Dziegielewski and Wolfe, 2000; Gattinara, 2009; Grant, 1999; Grant and Threlfo, 2002; Gupta and Gupta, 2002; Halvgaard, 2015; Hughes, 2014; Janssen, 2012; Kavakci, Semyz, Kaptanoglu, and Ozer, 2012; Kelley and Selim, 2007; Kneff and Krebs, 2004; Konuk et al., 2011; Kowal, 2005; Marcus, 2008; Mazzola et al., 2009; McGoldrick, Begum, and Brown, 2008; Meignant, 2012; Ray and Zbik, 2001; Royle, 2008; Russell, 2008a, 2008b; Schneider et al., 2007, 2008; Silver, Rogers, and Russell, 2008; Tinker and Wilson, 2006; Torun, 2010; Wilensky, 2006; Wilson et al., 2000.

14. *Adults and adolescents successfully treated for diagnosed depression:* Bae, Kim, and Park, 2008; Behnam, Behnam, and Salehian, 2015; Behnammoghadam et al., 2015; Broad and Wheeler, 2006; Grey, 2011; Hase et al., 2015; Lobenstine and Courtney, 2013; Manfield, 1998b; Protinsky, Sparks, and Flemke, 2001a; Srivastava and Mukhopadhyay, 2008; Tanaka and Inoue, 1999; Uribe and Ramirez, 2006.

15. *Clients with acute trauma and a wide variety of PTSD and trauma-based personality issues and who experience substantial benefit from EMDR:* Allen and Lewis, 1996; Barol and Seubert, 2010; Bisson et al., 2007; Brown and Shapiro, 2006; Carbone, 2008; Cohn, 1993; Croes et al., 2014; de Bont et al., 2013; Farrell et al., 2010; Fensterheim, 1996; Forbes, Creamer, and Rycroft, 1994; Gelinas, 2003; George et al., 2014; Mosquera and Gonzalez-Vazquez, 2012; Högberg, Pagani, Sundin, Soares, Åberg-Wistedt, Tärnell, and Hällström, 2007; Inoue, 2009; Kim and Choi, 2004; Kutz, Resnik, and Dekel, 2008; Ironson et al., 2002; Kosatka and Ona, 2014; Kitchiner, 2000; Korn and Leeds, 2002; Landin-Romero et al., 2013; Laub and Weiner, 2011; Lee et al., 2002; Manfield, 1998a; Manfield and Shapiro, 2003; Marcus, Marquis, and Saki, 1997; Marquis, 1991; Maxwell, 2003; McCullough, 2002; McLaughlin et al., 2008; Mevissen and de Jongh, 2010; Mevissen, Lievegoed, and de Jongh, 2010; Mevissen et al., 2011; Mosquera and Gonzalez, 2014; Mosquera and Knipe, 2015; Mosquera, Leeds, and Gonzalez, 2014; Novo et al., 2014; Parnell, 1996; Pollock, 2000; Power et al., 2002; Protinsky, Sparks, and Flemke, 2001a; Raboni, Tufik, and Suchecki, 2006; Renfrey and Spates, 1994; Rittenhouse, 2000; Sandström et al., 2008; Schneider, Nabavi, and Heuft, 2005; Seidler and Wagner, 2006; Shapiro, 2012; Shapiro and Forrest, 1997; Shapiro and Laub, 2008; Spates and Burnette, 1995; Spector and Huthwaite, 1993; Sprang, 2001; van der Kolk et al., 2007; Tofani and Wheeler, 2011; van der Vleugel, van den Berg, and Staring, 2012; van den Berg and van der Gaag, 2012; Vaughan, Armstrong, et al., 1994; Vaughan, Wiese, et al., 1994; Wilson, Becker, and Tinker, 1995, 1997; Wolpe and Abrams, 1991; Zabukovec, Lazrove, and Shapiro, 2000.

References

Abel, N. J., and O'Brien, J. M. (2010). EMDR treatment of comorbid PTSD and alcohol dependence: A case example. *Journal of EMDR Practice and Research, 4,* 50–59.

Adúriz, M. E., Bluthgen, C., and Knopfler, C. (2009). Helping child flood victims using group EMDR intervention in Argentina: Treatment outcome and gender differences. *International Journal of Stress Management, 16,* 138–153.

Ahmad, A., Larsson, B., and Sundelin-Wahlsten, V. (2007). EMDR treatment for children with PTSD: Results of a randomized controlled trial. *Nordic Journal of Psychiatry, 61,* 349–354.

Allen, J. G., and Lewis, L. (1996). A conceptual framework for treating traumatic memories and its application to EMDR. *Bulletin of the Menninger Clinic, 60,* 238–263.

Allon, M. (2015). EMDR group therapy with women who were sexually assaulted in the Congo. *Journal of EMDR Practice and Research, 9,* 28–34.

Amano, T., Seiyama, A., and Toichi, M. (2012). [Activation of the brain cortex measured by near-infrared spectroscopy during ego state therapy with EMDR in dissociative disorder]. xs*Japanese Journal of EMDR Research and Practice, 4,* 18–28. In Japanese.

Amano, T., Seiyama, A., and Toichi, M. (2013). Brain activity measured with near-infrared spectroscopy during EMDR treatment of phantom limb pain. *Journal of EMDR Practice and Research, 7,* 144–153.

American Psychiatric Association (2004). *Practice Guideline for the Treatment of Patients with Acute Stress Disorder and Posttraumatic Stress Disorder.* Arlington, VA: American Psychiatric Association Practice Guidelines.

Bae, H., Han, C., and Kim, D. (2015). Desensitization of triggers and urge reprocessing for pathological gambling: A case series. *Journal of Gambling Studies, 31,* 331–342.

Bae, H., and Kim, D. (2012). Desensitization of triggers and urge reprocessing for an adolescent with internet addiction disorder. *Journal of EMDR Practice and Research, 6,* 73–81.

Bae, H., Kim, D., and Park, Y. C. (2008). Eye movement desensitization and reprocessing for adolescent depression. *Psychiatry Investigation*, 5, 60–65.

Baker, N., and McBride, B. (1991). Clinical applications of EMDR in a law enforcement environment: Observations of the psychological service unit of the LA county sheriff's department. Paper presented at the Police Psychology (Division 18, Police and Public Safety Sub-section) Mini-Convention at the American Psychological Association Annual Convention, San Francisco.

Bardin, A. (2004). EMDR within a family perspective. *Journal of Family Psychotherapy*, 15, 47–61.

Barker, R. T., and Barker, S. B. (2007). The use of EMDR in reducing presentation anxiety. *Journal of EMDR Practice and Research*, 1, 100–108.

Barol, B. I., and Seubert, A. (2010). Stepping stones: EMDR treatment of individuals with intellectual and developmental disabilities and challenging behavior. *Journal of EMDR Practice and Research*, 4, 156–169.

Beer, R., and Bronner, M. B. (2010). EMDR in paediatrics and rehabilitation: An effective tool for reduction of stress reactions? *Developmental Neurorehabilitation*, 13, 307–309.

Behnam, M. M., Behnam, M. A., and Salehian, T. (2015). Efficacy of eye movement desensitization and reprocessing (EMDR) on depression in patients with myocardial infarction (MI) in a 12-month follow up. *Iranian Journal of Critical Care Nursing*, 7, 221–226.

Behnammoghadam, M., Alamdari, A. K., Behnammoghadam, A., and Darban, F. (2015). Effect of eye movement desensitization and reprocessing (EMDR) on depression in patients with myocardial infarction. *Global Journal Health Science*, 7, 258–262.

Besson, J., Eap, C., Rougemont-Buecking, A., Simon, O., Nikolov, C., and Bonsack, C. (2006). [Addictions]. *Revue Médicale Suisse, 2(47),* 9–13. In French.

Bisson, J. I., and Andrew, M. (2007). Psychological treatment of post-traumatic stress disorder (PTSD). *Cochrane Database of Systematic Reviews*, 3, art. no. CD003388.

Bisson, J. I., Ehlers, A., Matthews, R., Pilling, S., Richards, D., and Turner, S. (2007). Psychological treatments for chronic post-traumatic stress disorder. Systematic review and meta-analysis. *British Journal of Psychiatry*, 190, 97–104.

Bleich, A., Kotler, M., Kutz, I., and Shalev, A. (2002). Guidelines for the assessment and professional intervention with terror victims in the hospital and in the community. Position paper of the (Israeli) National Council for Mental Health, Jerusalem.

Bloomgarden, A., and Calogero, R. M. (2008). A randomized experimental test of the efficacy of EMDR treatment on negative body image in eating disorder inpatients. *Eating Disorders*, 16, 418–427.

Blore, D. C. (1997a). Reflections on "a day when the whole world seemed to be darkened." *Changes: An International Journal of Psychology and Psychiatry*, 15, 89–95.

Blore, D. C. (1997b). Use of EMDR to treat morbid jealousy: A case study. *British Journal of Nursing*, 6, 984–988.

Böhm, K., and Voderholzer, U. (2010). [Use of EMDR in the treatment of obsessive-compulsive disorders: A case series]. *Verhaltenstherapie*, 20, 175–181. In German.

Brennstuhl, M.-J., and Tarquinio, C. (2012). [Efficacy of a specific target on the reduction of chronic pain therapy based on eye-movement desensitization and reprocessing (EMDR): Clinical perspectives]. *Douleurs: Evaluation-Diagnostic-Traitement*, 13, A95. In French.

Brickell, M., Russell, M. C., and Smith, R. B. (2015). The effectiveness of evidence-based treatments in treatment of active military personnel and their families. *Journal of EMDR Practice and Research*, 9, 198–208.

Broad, R. D., and Wheeler, K. (2006). An adult with childhood medical trauma treated with Psychoanalytic Psychotherapy and EMDR: A case study. *Perspectives in Psychiatric Care, 42*, 95–105.

Bronner, M. B., Beer, R., Jozine van Zelm van Eldik, M., Grootenhuis, M. A., and Last, B. F. (2009). Reducing acute stress in a 16-year old using trauma-focused cognitive behaviour therapy and eye movement desensitization and reprocessing. *Developmental Neuro-rehabilitation, 12*, 170–174.

Brown, K. W., McGoldrick, T., and Buchanan, R. (1997). Body dysmorphic disorder: Seven cases treated with eye movement desensitization and reprocessing. *Behavioural and Cognitive Psychotherapy, 25*, 203–207.

Brown, S. H., Gilman, S. G., Goodman, E. G., Adler-Tapia, R., and Freng, S. (2015). Integrated trauma treatment in drug court: Combining EMDR and seeking safety. *Journal of EMDR Practice and Research, 9*, 123–136.

Brown, S., and Shapiro, F. (2006). EMDR in the treatment of borderline personality disorder. *Clinical Case Studies, 5*, 403–420.

Capps, F. (2006). Combining eye movement desensitization and reprocessing with Gestalt techniques in couples counseling. *Family Journal: Counseling and Therapy for Couples and Families, 14*, 49.

Carbone, D. J. (2008). Treatment of gay men for post-traumatic stress disorder resulting from social ostracism and ridicule: Cognitive behavior therapy and eye movement desensitization and reprocessing approaches. *Archives of Sexual Behavior, 37*, 305–316.

Carlson, J. G., Chemtob, C. M., Rusnak, K., and Hedlund, N. L. (1996). Eye movement desensitization and reprocessing treatment for combat PTSD. *Psychotherapy, 33*, 104–113.

Carlson, J. G., Chemtob, C. M., Rusnak, K., Hedlund, N. L., and Muraoka, M. Y. (1998). Eye movement desensitization and reprocessing treatment for combat related posttraumatic stress disorder. *Journal of Traumatic Stress, 11*, 3–24.

Chambless, D. L. et al. (1998). Update on empirically validated therapies, II. *Clinical Psychologist, 51*, 3–16.

Chemali, Z., and Meadows, M. (2004). The use of eye movement desensitization and reprocessing in the treatment of psychogenic seizures. *Epilepsy and Behavior, 5*, 784–787.

Chemtob, C. M., Nakashima, J., Hamada, R. S., and Carlson, J. G. (2002). Brief-treatment for elementary school children with disaster-related posttraumatic stress disorder: A field study. *Journal of Clinical Psychology, 58*, 99–112.

Cocco, N., and Sharpe, L. (1993). An auditory variant of eye movement desensitization in a case of childhood post-traumatic stress disorder. *Journal of Behavior Therapy and Experimental Psychiatry, 24*, 373–377.

Cohen, A. (2009). Treatment of dissociation with EMDR when war interrupts the process: The integration of EMDR with e-mail therapy. *Journal of EMDR Practice and Research, 3*, 50–56.

Cohn, L. (1993). Art psychotherapy and the new eye treatment desensitization and reprocessing (EMD/R) method, an integrated approach. In *California Art Therapy Trends*, edited by E. Dishup, 275–290. Chicago: Magnolia Street Publishers.

Colelli, G., and Patterson, B. (2008). Three case reports illustrating the use of the protocol for recent traumatic events following the World Trade Center terrorist attack. *Journal of EMDR Practice and Research, 2*, 114–123.

Cook-Vienot, R., and Taylor, R. J. (2012). Comparison of eye movement desensitization and reprocessing and biofeedback/stress inoculation training in treating test anxiety. *Journal of EMDR Practice and Research, 6*, 62–72.

Cox, R. P., and Howard, M. D. (2007). Utilization of EMDR in the treatment of sexual addiction: A case study. *Sexual Addiction and Compulsivity, 14*, 1.

Crabbe, B. (1996). Can eye-movement therapy improve your riding? *Dressage Today,* 28–33.

CREST (Clinical Resource Efficiency Support Team) (2003). *The Management of Post Traumatic Stress Disorder in Adults.* Belfast: Clinical Resource Efficiency Support Team, Northern Ireland Department of Health, Social Services and Public Safety.

Croes, C. F., van Grunsven, R., Staring, A. B., van den Berg, D. P., de Jongh, A., and van der Gaag, M. (2014). [Imagery in psychosis: EMDR as a new intervention in the treatment of delusions and auditory hallucinations]. *Tijdschrift Voor Psychiatrie, 56*, 568–576. In Dutch.

Daniels, N., Lipke, H., Richardson, R., and Silver, S. (1992). Vietnam veterans' treatment programs using eye movement desensitization and reprocessing. Symposium presented at the International Society for Traumatic Stress Studies annual convention, Los Angeles.

Datta, P. C., and Wallace, J. (1994). Treatment of sexual traumas of sex offenders using eye movement desensitization and reprocessing. Paper presented at the 11th Annual Symposium in Forensic Psychology, San Francisco.

Datta, P. C., and Wallace, J. (1996). Enhancement of victim empathy along with reduction of anxiety and increase of positive cognition of sex offenders after treatment with EMDR. Paper presented at the EMDR Special Interest Group at the Annual Convention of the Association for the Advancement of Behavior Therapy, New York.

de Bont, P. A., van den Berg, D. P., van der Vleugel, B. M., de Roos, C., Mulder, C. L., Becker, E. S., de Jongh, A., van der Gaag, M., and van Minnen, A. (2013). A multi-site single blind clinical study to compare the effects of prolonged exposure, eye movement desensitization and reprocessing and waiting list on patients with a current diagnosis of psychosis and co morbid post traumatic stress disorder: Study protocol for the randomized controlled trial treating trauma in psychosis. *Trials, 14*, 151.

de Castro Lopes, C., Carvalho, S. C., and Barbosa, M. R. (2014). [Treatment of specific phobia through eye movement desensitization and reprocessing]. *Psicologia: Teoria e Prática, 16*, 31–42. In Portuguese.

de Groot, J., and de Jongh, A. (2012). [EMDR treatment for PTSD of a sexually abused woman with vaginismus: A case study]. *Tijdschrift voor Seksuologie, 36*, 197–199. In Dutch.

de Jongh, A. (2012). Treatment of a woman with emetophobia: A trauma focused approach. *Mental Illness, 4*, 10–14.

de Jongh, A., Holmshaw, M., Carswell, W., and van Wijk, A. (2010). Usefulness of a trauma-focused treatment approach for travel phobia. *Clinical Psychology and Psychotherapy, 18*, 124–137.

de Jongh, A., and Ten Broeke, E. (1998). Treatment of choking phobia by targeting traumatic memories with EMDR: A case study. *Clinical Psychology and Psychotherapy, 5*, 264–269.

de Jongh, A., ten Broeke, E., and Renssen, M. R. (1999). Treatment of specific phobias with eye movement desensitization and reprocessing (EMDR): Protocol, empirical status, and conceptual issues. *Journal of Anxiety Disorders, 13*, 69–85.

de Jongh, A., van den Oord, H. J. M., and ten Broeke, E. (2002). Efficacy of eye movement desensitization and reprocessing (EMDR) in the treatment of specific phobias: Four single-case studies on dental phobia. *Journal of Clinical Psychology, 58*, 1489–1503.

de Roos, C., and de Jongh, A. (2008). EMDR treatment of children and adolescents with a choking phobia. *Journal of EMDR Practice and Research, 2*, 201–211.

de Roos, C., Veenstra, A. C., de Jongh, A., den Hollander-Gijsman, M. E., van der Wee, N. J. A., Zitman, F. G., and van Rood, Y. R. (2010). Treatment of chronic phantom limb pain using a trauma-focused psychological approach. *Pain Research and Management, 15*, 65–71.

Dilly, R. (2014). Eye movement desensitisation and reprocessing in the treatment of trauma with mild intellectual disabilities. *Advances in Mental Health and Intellectual Disabilities, 8*, 63–71.

Doering, S., Ohlmeier, M. C., de Jongh, A., Hofmann, A., and Bisping, V. (2013). Efficacy of a trauma-focused treatment approach for dental phobia: a randomized clinical trial. *European Journal of Oral Sciences, 121*, 584–593.

Dyregrov, A. (1993). [EMDR: A new method in the treatment of trauma]. *Tidsskrift for Norsk Psykologforening, 30*, 975–981. In Norwegian.

Dziegielewski, S., and Wolfe, P. (2000). Eye movement desensitization and reprocessing (EMDR) as a time-limited treatment intervention for body image disturbance and self-esteem: A single subject case study design. *Journal of Psychotherapy in Independent Practice, 1*, 1–16.

Edmond, T., Rubin, A., and Wambach, K. G. (1999). The effectiveness of EMDR with adult female survivors of childhood sexual abuse. *Social Work Research, 23*, 103–116.

Errebo, N., and Sommers-Flanagan, R. (2007). EMDR and emotionally focused couple therapy for war veteran couples. In *Handbook of EMDR and Family Therapy Processes*, edited by F. Shapiro, F. W. Kaslow, and L. Maxfield. Hoboken, N.J.: Wiley.

Faretta, E. (2013). EMDR and cognitive behavioral therapy in the treatment of panic disorder: A comparison. *Journal of EMDR Practice and Research, 7*, 121–133.

Farima, R., Dowlatabadi, S., and Behzadi, S. (2015). The effectiveness of eye movement desensitization and reprocessing (EMDR) in reducing pathological worry in patients with generalized anxiety disorder: A preliminary study. *Archives of Psychiatry and Psychotherapy, 1*, 33–43.

Farrell, D. P., Dworkin, M., Keenan, P., and Spierings, J. (2010). Using EMDR with survivors of sexual abuse perpetrated by Roman Catholic priests. *Journal of EMDR Practice and Research, 4*, 124–133.

Farrell, D. P., Keenan, P. S., Wajid Ali, M., Bilal, S. M., Tareen, S. M., Keenan, L., and Rana, M. H. (2011). Training Pakistani mental health workers in EMDR in the aftermath of the 2005 earthquake in Northern Pakistan. *Counselling Psychology Quarterly, 24*, 127–137.

Fensterheim, H. (1996). Eye movement desensitization and reprocessing with complex personality pathology: An integrative therapy. *Journal of Psychotherapy Integration, 6*, 27–38.

Fernandez, I. (2007). EMDR as treatment of post-traumatic reactions: A field study on child victims of an earthquake. *Educational and Child Psychology. Special Issue: Therapy, 24*, 65–72.

Fernandez, I. (2008). EMDR after a critical incident: Treatment of a tsunami survivor with acute posttraumatic stress disorder. *Journal of EMDR Practice and Research, 2*, 156–159.

Fernandez, I., and Faretta, E. (2007). EMDR in the treatment of panic disorder with agoraphobia. *Clinical Case Studies, 6*, 44–63.

Fernandez, I., Gallinari, E., and Lorenzetti, A. (2004). A school-based EMDR intervention for children who witnessed the Pirelli Building airplane crash in Milan, Italy. *Journal of Brief Therapy, 2*, 129–136.

Feske, U., and Goldstein, A. (1997). Eye movement desensitization and reprocessing treatment for panic disorder: A controlled outcome and partial dismantling study. *Journal of Consulting and Clinical Psychology, 36,* 1026–1035.

Fine, C. G. (1994). Eye movement desensitization and reprocessing (EMDR) for dissociative disorders. Presentation at the Eastern Regional Conference on Abuse and Multiple Personality. Alexandria, Va.

Fine, C. G., and Berkowitz, A. (2001). The wreathing protocol: The imbrication of hypnosis and EMDR in the treatment of dissociative identity disorder and other dissociative responses. *American Journal of Clinical Hypnosis, 43,* 275–290.

Foa, E. B., Keane, T. M., Friedman, M. J., and Cohen, J. A. (2009). *Effective Treatments for PTSD: Practice Guidelines of the International Society for Traumatic Stress Studies.* New York: Guilford Press.

Forbes, D., Creamer, M., and Rycroft, P. (1994). Eye movement desensitization and reprocessing in posttraumatic stress disorder: A pilot study using assessment measures. *Journal of Behavior Therapy and Experimental Psychiatry, 25,* 113–120.

Foster, S., and Lendl, J. (1995). Eye movement desensitization and reprocessing: Initial applications for enhancing performance in athletes. *Journal of Applied Sport Psychology, 7,* 63.

Foster, S., and Lendl, J. (1996). Eye movement desensitization and reprocessing: Four case studies of a new tool for executive coaching and restoring employee performance after setbacks. *Consulting Psychology Journal, 48,* 155–161.

Gattinara, P. C. (2009). Working with EMDR in chronic incapacitating diseases: The experience of a neuromuscular diseases center. *Journal of EMDR Practice and Research, 3,* 169–177.

Gauvreau, P., and Bouchard, S. P. (2008). Preliminary evidence for the efficacy of EMDR in treating generalized anxiety disorder. *Journal of EMDR Practice and Research, 2,* 26–40.

Gelbach, R. (2008). Trauma, research, and EMDR: A disaster responder's wish list. *Journal of EMDR Practice and Research, 2,* 146–155.

Gelinas, D. J. (2003). Integrating EMDR into phase-oriented treatment for trauma. *Journal of Trauma and Dissociation, 4,* 91–135.

George, A., Thilly, N., Rydberg, J. A., Luz, R., and Spitz, E. (2013). Effectiveness of EMDR treatment in PTSD after childbirth: A randomized controlled trial protocol. *Acta Obstetrica et Gynecologica Scandinavica, 22,* 866–868.

Goldstein, A. (1992). Treatment of panic and agoraphobia with EMDR: Preliminary data of the Agoraphobia and Anxiety Treatment Center, Temple University. Paper presented at the Fourth World Congress on Behavior Therapy, Queensland, Australia.

Goldstein, A., and Feske, U. (1994). Eye movement desensitization and reprocessing for panic disorder: A case series. *Journal of Anxiety Disorders, 8,* 351–362.

Goldstein, A. J., de Beurs, E., Chambless, D. L., and Wilson, K. A. (2000). EMDR for panic disorder with agoraphobia: comparison with waiting-list and credible attention-placebo control condition. *Journal of Consulting and Clinical Psychology, 68,* 947–956.

Gomez, A. (2012). *EMDR Therapy and Adjunct Approaches with Children: Complex Trauma, Attachment, and Dissociation.* New York: Springer.

Gonzalez, A., and Mosquera, D. (2012). *EMDR and Dissociation: The Progressive Approach.* A.I.

Graham, L. (2004). Traumatic swimming events reprocessed with EMDR. *www.Thesport journal.org, 7,* 1–5.

Grainger, R. D., Levin, C., Allen-Byrd, L., Doctor, R. M., and Lee, H. (1997). An empirical evaluation of eye movement desensitization and reprocessing (EMDR) with survivors of a natural disaster. *Journal of Traumatic Stress, 10,* 665–671.

Grant, M. (1999). *Pain Control with EMDR*. New Hope, PA: EMDR Humanitarian Assistance Program.

Grant, M., and Threlfo, C. (2002). EMDR in the treatment of chronic pain. *Journal of Clinical Psychology*, *58*, 1505–1520.

Greenwald, R. (1994). Applying eye movement desensitization and reprocessing to the treatment of traumatized children: Five case studies. *Anxiety Disorders Practice Journal*, *1*, 83–97.

Greenwald, R. (1998). Eye movement desensitization and reprocessing (EMDR): New hope for children suffering from trauma and loss. *Clinical Child Psychology and Psychiatry*, *3*, 279–287.

Greenwald, R. (1999). *Eye Movement Desensitization and Reprocessing (EMDR) in Child and Adolescent Psychotherapy*. New Milford, NJ: Jason Aronson Press.

Greenwald, R. (2000). A trauma-focused individual therapy approach for adolescents with conduct disorder. *International Journal of Offender Therapy and Comparative Criminology*, *44*, 146–163.

Greenwald, R. (2002). Motivation-adaptive skills-trauma resolution (MASTR) therapy for adolescents with conduct problems: An open trial. *Journal of Aggression, Maltreatment, and Trauma*, *6*, 237–261.

Grey, E. (2011). A pilot study of concentrated EMDR: A brief report. *Journal of EMDR Practice and Research*, *5*, 14–24.

Gupta, D., Gupta, N., and Choudhary, T. (2014). Effectiveness of the EMDR therapy on specific phobia in young children. *Delhi Psychiatry Journal*, *17*, 175–178.

Gupta, M., and Gupta, A. (2002). Use of eye movement desensitization and reprocessing (EMDR) in the treatment of dermatologic disorders. *Journal of Cutaneous Medicine and Surgery*, *6*, 415–421.

Halvgaard, K. (2015). Single case study: Does EMDR psychotherapy work on emotional eating? *Journal of EMDR Practice and Research*, *9*, 188–197.

Harada, N. (2013). [EMDR for stuttering points: From the viewpoint of post-onset trauma as target]. *Japanese Journal of EMDR Research and Practice*, *5*, 37–47. In Japanese.

Hase, M. et al. (2007). On treatment with eye movement desensitization and reprocessing of chronic post-traumatic stress disorder in public transportation workers: A randomized controlled trial. *Nordic Journal of Psychiatry*, *61*, 54–61.

Hase, M., Schallmayer, S., and Sack, M. (2008). EMDR reprocessing of the addiction memory: Pretreatment, posttreatment, and 1-month follow-up. *Journal of EMDR Practice and Research*, *2*, 170–179.

Hase, M. et al. (2015). Eye movement desensitization and reprocessing (EMDR) therapy in the treatment of depression: A matched pairs study in an inpatient setting. *Brain and Behavior*, 5.

Hassard, A. (1993). Eye movement desensitization of body image. *Behavioural Psychotherapy*, *21*, 157–160.

Henry, S. L. (1996). Pathological gambling: Etiological considerations and treatment efficacy of eye movement desensitization/reprocessing. *Journal of Gambling Studies*, *12*, 395–405.

Hensel, T. (2006). [Effectiveness of EMDR with psychologically traumatized children and adolescents.]. *Kindheit und Entwicklung*, *15(2)*, 107. In German.

Hensel, T. (2009). EMDR with children and adolescents after single-incident trauma: An intervention study. *Journal of EMDR Practice and Research*, *3*, 2–9.

Högberg, G., Pagani, M., Sundin, O., Soares, J., Åberg-Wisted, A., Tärnell, B., and Hällström, T. (2007). On treatment with eye movement desensitization and reprocessing of chronic post-traumatic stress disorder in public transportation workers: A randomized controlled study. *Nordic Journal of Psychiatry, 61,* 54–61.

Howard, M. D., and Cox, R. P. (2006). Use of EMDR in the treatment of water phobia at Navy boot camp: A case study. *Traumatology, 12,* 302–313.

Hughes, M. (2014). EMDR as a therapeutic treatment for complex regional pain syndrome: A case report. *Journal of EMDR Practice and Research, 8,* 66–73.

Hyer, L. (1995). Use of EMDR in a "dementing" PTSD survivor. *Clinical Gerontologist, 16,* 70–73.

Inoue, N. (2009). Evaluation of an EMDR treatment outcome using the Rorschach, the TAT, and the IES-R: A case study of a human-caused trauma survivor. *Rorschachiana, 30,* 180–218.

INSERM (2004). *Psychotherapy: An Evaluation of Three Approaches.* Paris: French National Institute of Health and Medical Research.

Ironson, G. I., Freund, B., Strauss, J. L., and Williams, J. (2002). A comparison of two treatments for traumatic stress: A pilot study of EMDR and prolonged exposure. *Journal of Clinical Psychology, 58,* 113–128.

Jaberghaderi, N., Greenwald, R., Rubin, A., Dolatabadim, S., and Zand, S. O. (2004). A comparison of CBT and EMDR for sexually abused Iranian girls. *Clinical Psychology and Psychotherapy, 11,* 358–368.

Janssen, J. (2012). [A special case (series): EMDR treatment of early childhood trauma in a client with an eating disorder]. *Tijdschrift voor Psychotherapie, 38,* 21–37. In Dutch.

Jarero, I., and Artigas, L. (2010). The EMDR integrative group treatment protocol: Application with adults during ongoing geopolitical crisis. *Journal of EMDR Practice and Research, 4,* 148–155.

Jarero, I., Artigas, L., and Hartung, J. (2006). EMDR integrative group treatment protocol: A postdisaster trauma intervention for children and adults. *Traumatology, 12,* 121–129.

Jarero, I., Artigas, L., Mauer, M., Lopez Cano, T., and Alcala, N. (1999). Children's post traumatic stress after natural disasters: Integrative treatment protocols. Poster presented at the annual meeting of the International Society for Traumatic Stress Studies, Miami.

Jarero, I., Roque-Lopez, S., Gomez, J., and Givaudan, M. (2014). [Third research study on the provision of the EMDR integrative group treatment protocol with child victims of severe interpersonal violence]. *Revista Iberoaméricana de Psicotraumatología y Disociación, 6,* 1–23. In Spanish.

Jarero, I., and Uribe, S. (2012a). [Early mental health intervention in human slaughter situation: Mass graves in 2011 Durango]. *Revista Iberoaméricana de Psicotraumatología y Disociación, 4.* In Spanish.

Jarero, I., and Uribe, S. (2012b). The EMDR protocol for recent critical incidents: Follow-up report of an application in a human massacre situation. *Journal of EMDR Practice and Research, 6,* 50–61.

Jayatunge, R. M. (2008). Combating tsunami disaster through EMDR. *Journal of EMDR Practice and Research, 2,* 140–145.

Jensma, J. (1999). Critical incident intervention with missionaries: A comprehensive approach. *Journal of Psychology and Theology, 27,* 130–138.

Kaslow, F. W., Nurse, A. R., and Thompson, P. (2002). EMDR in conjunction with family systems therapy. In *EMDR as an Integrative Psychotherapy Approach: Experts of Diverse*

Orientations Explore the Paradigm Prism, edited by F. Shapiro, 289–318. Washington, DC: American Psychological Association.

Kavakci, O., Semyz, M., Kaptanoglu, E., and Ozer, Z. (2012). [EMDR treatment of fibromyalgia, a study of seven cases]. *Anatolian Journal of Psychiatry/Anadolu Psikiyatri Dergisi, 13*, 75–81. In Turkish.

Keenan, P., and Farrell, D. (2000). Treating morbid jealousy with eye movement desensitization and reprocessing utilizing cognitive inter-weave: A case report. *Counselling Psychology Quarterly, 13*, 175–189.

Kelley, S. D. M., and Selim, B. (2007). Eye movement desensitization and reprocessing in the psychological treatment of trauma-based psychogenic non-epileptic seizures. *Clinical Psychology and Psychotherapy, 14*, 135.

Kim, D., and Choi, J. (2004). Eye movement desensitization and reprocessing for disorder of extreme stress: A case report. *Journal of the Korean Neuropsychiatric Association, 43*, 760–763.

Kitchiner, N. J. (2000). Using eye movement desensitisation reprocessing (EMDR) to treat post-traumatic stress disorder in a prison setting. *British Journal of Community Nursing, 5*, 26–31.

Kitchiner, N. J. (2004). Psychological treatment of three urban fire fighters with post-traumatic stress disorder using eye movement desensitisation reprocessing (EMDR) therapy. *Journal of Complimentary Therapy, 10*, 186–193.

Kitchiner, N., and Aylard, P. (2002). Psychological treatment of post-traumatic stress disorder: A single case study of a UK police office. *Mental Health Practice, 5*, 34–38.

Kleinknecht, R. A. (1993). Rapid treatment of blood and injection phobias with eye movement desensitization. *Journal of Behavior Therapy and Experimental Psychiatry, 24*, 211–217.

Kleinknecht, R. A., and Morgan, M. P. (1992). Treatment of post-traumatic stress disorder with eye movement desensitization and reprocessing. *Journal of Behavior Therapy and Experimental Psychiatry, 23*, 43–50.

Kneff, J. C., and Krebs, K. (2004). Eye movement desensitization and reprocessing (EMDR): Another helpful mind-body technique to treat GI problems. *Gastroenterology Nursing, 27*, 286–287.

Knipe, J. (2014). *EMDR Toolbox: Theory and Treatment of Complex PTSD and Dissociation.* New York: Springer.

Knudsen, N. (2007). Integrating EMDR and Bowen theory in treating chronic relationship dysfunction. In *Handbook of EMDR and Family Therapy Processes*, edited by F. Shapiro, F. W. Kaslow, and L. Maxfield, 169–186. Hoboken, N.J.: Wiley.

Koedam, W. S. (2007). Sexual trauma in dysfunctional marriages: Integrating structural therapy and EMDR. In *Handbook of EMDR and Family Therapy Processes*, edited by F. Shapiro, F. W. Kaslow, and L. Maxfield, 223–242). Hoboken, N.J.: Wiley.

Konuk, E., Epözdemir, H., Atçeken, S. H., Aydın, Y. E., and Yurtsever, A. (2011). EMDR treatment of migraine. *Journal of EMDR Practice and Research, 5*, 166–176.

Konuk, E., Knipe, J., Eke, I., Yuksek, H., Yurtsever, A., and Ostep, S. (2006). The effects of eye movement desensitization and reprocessing (EMDR) therapy on posttraumatic stress disorder in survivors of the 1999 Marmara, Turkey, earthquake. *International Journal of Stress Management, 13*, 291.

Korkmazler-Oral, U., and Pamuk, S. (2002). Group EMDR with child survivors of the earth-quake in Turkey. Association for Child Psychiatry and Psychology, Occasional Paper No. 19, 47–50.

Korn, D. L., and Leeds, A. M. (2002). Preliminary evidence of efficacy for EMDR resource development and installation in the stabilization phase of treatment of complex posttrau-matic stress disorder. *Journal of Clinical Psychology, 58,* 1465–1487.

Kosatka, D., and Ona, C. (2014). Eye movement desensitization and reprocessing in a patient with Asperger's disorder: Case report. *Journal of EMDR Practice and Research, 8,* 13–18.

Kowal, J. A. (2005). QEEG analysis of treating PTSD and bulimia nervosa using EMDR. *Journal of Neurotherapy, 9,* 114–115.

Krupnik, V. (2015). Integrating EMDR into an evolutionary-based therapy for depression: A case study. *Clinical Case Reports, 3,* 301–307.

Kutz, I., Resnik, V., and Dekel, R. (2008). The effect of single-session modified EMDR on acute stress syndromes. *Journal of EMDR Practice and Research, 2,* 190–200.

Landin-Romero, R., Novo, P., Vicens, V., McKenna, P. J., Santed, A., Pomarol-Clotet, E., Salgado-Pineda, P., Shapiro., F., and Amann, B. L. (2013). EMDR therapy modulates the default mode network in a subsyndromal, traumatized bipolar patient. *Neuropsychobiol-ogy, 67,* 181–184.

Lansing, K. (2013). *The Rite of Return: Coming Back from Duty-Induced PTSD.* High Ground Press.

Lansing, K., Amen, D. G., Hanks, C., and Rudy, L. (2005). High-resolution brain SPECT im-aging and eye movement desensitization and reprocessing in police officers with PTSD. *Journal of Neuropsychiatry and Clinical Neurosciences, 17,* 526–532.

Laub, B., and Weiner, N. (2011). A developmental/integrative perspective of the recent traumatic episode protocol. *Journal of EMDR Practice and Research, 5,* 57–72.

Lazrove, S., and Fine, C. G. (1996). The use of EMDR in patients with dissociative identity disorder. *Dissociation, 9,* 289–299.

Lazrove, S., Triffleman, E., Kite, L., McGlasshan, T., and Rounsaville, B. (1998). An open trial of EMDR as treatment for chronic PTSD. *American Journal of Orthopsychiatry, 69,* 601–608.

Lee, C., Gavriel, H., Drummond, P., Richards, J., and Greenwald, R. (2002). Treatment of PTSD: Stress inoculation training with prolonged exposure compared to EMDR. *Journal of Clinical Psychology, 58,* 1071–1089.

Leeds, A. (2012). EMDR treatment of panic disorder and agoraphobia: Two model treatment plans. *Journal of EMDR Practice and Research, 6,* 110–119.

Lipke, H. (2000). *EMDR and Psychotherapy Integration: Theoretical and Clinical Suggestions with Focus on Traumatic Stress.* New York: CRC Press.

Lipke, H., and Botkin, A. (1992). Brief case studies of eye movement desensitization and repro-cessing with chronic post-traumatic stress disorder. *Psychotherapy, 29,* 591–595.

Lobenstine, F., and Courtney, D. (2013). A case study: The integration of intensive EMDR and ego state therapy to treat comorbid posttraumatic stress disorder, depression, and anxi-ety. *Journal of EMDR Practice and Research, 7,* 65–80.

Lovett, J. (1999). *Small Wonders: Healing Childhood Trauma with EMDR.* New York: Free Press.

Madrid, A., Skolek, S., and Shapiro, F. (2006). Repairing failures in bonding through EMDR. *Clinical Case Studies, 5,* 271–286.

Manfield, P., ed. (1998a). *Extending EMDR.* New York: W.W. Norton.

Manfield, P. (1998b). Filling the void: Resolution of a major depression. In *Extending EMDR: A Casebook of Innovative Applications*, edited by P. Manfield, 113–137. New York: W.W. Norton.

Manfield, P., and Shapiro, F. (2003). The application of EMDR to the treatment of personality disorders. In *Handbook of Personality: Theory and Practice*, edited by J. F. Magnavita. New York: Wiley.

Marcus, S. V. (2008). Phase 1 of integrated EMDR: An abortive treatment for migraine headaches. *Journal of EMDR Practice and Research, 2*, 15–25.

Marcus, S. V., Marquis, P., and Saki, C. (1997). Controlled study of treatment of PTSD using EMDR in an HMO setting. *Psychotherapy, 34*, 307–315.

Marich, J. (2009). EMDR in the addiction continuing care process: Case study of a cross-addicted female's treatment and recovery. *Journal of EMDR Practice and Research, 3*, 98–106.

Marquis, J. N. (1991). A report on seventy-eight cases treated by eye movement desensitization. *Journal of Behavior Therapy and Experimental Psychiatry, 22*, 187–192.

Marr, J. (2012). EMDR treatment of obsessive-compulsive disorder: Preliminary research. *Journal of EMDR Practice and Research, 6*, 2–15.

Mate, D., Marazzi, L., and Cavallerio, F. (2013). [Rehabilitate the mind after a sports injury: Apply the EMDR method in sports]. *Giornale Italiano di Psicologia dello Sport, 17*, 23–32. In Italian.

Maxfield, L. (2007). Integrative treatment of intrafamilial child sexual abuse. In *Handbook of EMDR and Family Therapy Processes*, edited by F. Shapiro, F. W. Kaslow, and L. Maxfield, 344–364. Hoboken, NJ: Wiley.

Maxfield, L., and Melnyk, W. T. (2000). Single session treatment of test anxiety with eye movement desensitization and reprocessing (EMDR). *International Journal of Stress Management, 7*, 87–10.

Maxwell, J. P. (2003). The imprint of childhood physical and emotional abuse: A case study on the use of EMDR to address anxiety and lack of self-esteem. *Journal of Family Violence, 18*, 281–293.

Mazzola, A., Calcagno, M. L., Goicochea, M. T., Pueyrredòn, H., Leston, J., and Salvat, F. (2009). EMDR in the treatment of chronic pain. *Journal of EMDR Practice and Research, 3*, 66–79.

McCann, D. L. (1992). Post-traumatic stress disorder due to devastating burns overcome by a single session of eye movement desensitization. *Journal of Behavior Therapy and Experimental Psychiatry, 23*, 319–323.

McCullough, L. (2002). Exploring change mechanisms in EMDR applied to "small t trauma" in short term dynamic psychotherapy: Research questions and speculations. *Journal of Clinical Psychology, 58*, 1465–1487.

McGoldrick, T., Begum, M., and Brown, K. W. (2008). EMDR and olfactory reference syndrome: A case series. *Journal of EMDR Practice and Research, 2*, 63–68.

McLaughlin, D. F., McGowan, I. W., Paterson, M. C., and Miller, P. W. (2008). Cessation of deliberate self-harm following eye movement desensitisation and reprocessing: A case report. *Cases Journal, 1*, 177.

McNally, V. J., and Solomon, R. M. (1999). The FBI's critical incident stress management program. *FBI Law Enforcement Bulletin, 68*, 20–26.

Meignant, I. (2012). [The treatment of limb pain phantom EMDR]. *Annals of Physical and Rehabilitation Medicine, 55*, e85-e86. In French.

Mevissen, L., and de Jongh, A. (2010). PTSD and its treatment in people with intellectual disabilities: A review of the literature. *Clinical Psychology Review, 30*, 308–316.

Mevissen, L., Lievegoed, R., and de Jongh, A. (2010). EMDR treatment in people with mild ID and PTSD: 4 cases. *Psychiatric Quarterly*, 82, 43–57.

Mevissen, L., Lievegoed, R., Seubert, A., and de Jongh, A. (2011). Do persons with intellectual disability and limited verbal capacities respond to trauma treatment? *Journal of Intellectual and Developmental Disability*, 36, 278–283.

Meysami-Bonab, S., Abolghasemi, A., Sheikhian, M., Barahmand, U., and Rasooliazad, M. (2012). The effectiveness of eye movement desensitization and reprocessing therapy on the emotion regulation and emotion recognition of addicted individuals. *Zahedan Journal of Research in Medical Sciences*, 14, 33–37.

Moradi, M., Chatrrooz, M., Sarichlu, M. A., and Alipourheidari, M. (2015). The effect of eye movement with desensitization and reprocessing on anxiety induced by dressing pain in burn patients. *Iranian Journal of Psychiatric Nursing*, 2, 80–88.

Morrissey, M. (2013). EMDR as an integrative therapeutic approach for the treatment of separation anxiety disorder. *Journal of EMDR Practice and Research*, 7, 200–207.

Moses, M. (2007). Enhancing attachments: conjoint couple therapy. In *Handbook of EMDR and Family Therapy Processes*, edited by F. Shapiro, F. W. Kaslow, and L. Maxfield, 146–168. Hoboken, N.J.: Wiley.

Mosquera, D., and Gonzalez, A. (2014). *Borderline Personality Disorder and EMDR Therapy*. United Kingdom: D.M.B.

Mosquera, D., and Gonzalez-Vazquez, A. (2012). [Borderline personality disorder, trauma and EMDR]. *Rivista di Psichiatria*, 47, 26–32. In Italian.

Mosquera, D., and Knipe, J. (2015). Understanding and treating narcissism with EMDR therapy. *Journal of EMDR Practice and Research*, 9, 4663.

Mosquera, D., Leeds, A. M., and Gonzalez, A. (2014). Application of EMDR therapy for borderline personality disorder. *Journal of EMDR Practice and Research*, 8, 74–89.

Muris, P., and Merckelbach, H. (1997). Treating spider phobics with eye movement desensitization and reprocessing: A controlled study. *Behavioral and Cognitive Psychotherapy*, 25, 39–50.

Muris, P., Merkelbach, H., Holdrinet, I., and Sijenaar, M. (1998). Treating phobic children: Effects of EMDR versus exposure. *Journal of Consulting and Clinical Psychology*, 66, 193–198.

Muris, P., Merckelbach, H., van Haaften, H., and Nayer, B. (1997). Eye movement desensitization and reprocessing versus exposure in vivo. *British Journal of Psychiatry 171*, 82–86.

Nadler, W. (1996). EMDR: Rapid treatment of panic disorder. *International Journal of Psychiatry*, 2, 1–8.

Narimani, M., Sadeghieh Ahari, S., and Rajabi, S. (2008). Comparison of efficacy of eye movement desensitization and reprocessing and cognitive behavioral therapy therapeutic methods for reducing anxiety and depression of Iranian combatant afflicted by post traumatic stress disorder. *Journal of Applied Sciences*, 8, 1932–1937.

Nazari, H., Momeni, N., Jariani, M., and Tarrahi, M. J. (2011). Comparison of eye movement desensitization and reprocessing with citalopram in treatment of obsessive-compulsive disorder. *International Journal of Psychiatry in Clinical Practice*, 15, 270–274.

Newgent, R. A., Paladino, D. A., and Reynolds, C. A. (2006). Single session treatment of nontraumatic fear of flying with eye movement desensitization reprocessing: Pre and post-September 11. *Clinical Case Studies*, 5, 25–36.

NICE (National Institute for Clinical Excellence) (2005). *Post Traumatic Stress Disorder (PTSD): The Management of Adults and Children in Primary and Secondary Care*. London: NICE Guidelines.

Niroomandi, R. (2012). Efficacy of eye movement desensitization and reprocessing (EMDR) in the Iranian veterans with chronic posttraumatic stress disorder (PTSD) after Iran/Iraq War. *International Proceedings of Economic Development and Research, 40*, 52–56.

Novo, P., Landin-Romero, R., Radua, J., Vicens, V., Fernandez, I., Garcia, F., . . . Amann, B. L. (2014). Eye movement desensitization and reprocessing therapy in subsyndromal bipolar patients with a history of traumatic events: A randomized, controlled pilot-study. *Psychiatry Research, 219*, 122–128.

O'Brien, E. (1993). Pushing the panic button. *Family Therapy Networker,* 75–83.

Oras, R., de Ezpeleta, S., and Ahmad, A. (2004). Treatment of traumatized refugee children with eye movement desensitization and reprocessing. *Nordic Journal of Psychiatry, 58*, 1999–2203.

Page, A. C., and Crino, R. D. (1993). Eye-movement desensitization: A simple treatment for post-traumatic stress disorder. *Australian and New Zealand Journal of Psychiatry, 27*, 288–293.

Parnell, L. (1996). Eye movement desensitization and reprocessing (EMDR) and spiritual unfolding. *Journal of Transpersonal Psychology, 28*, 129–153.

Paulsen, S. (1995). Eye movement desensitization and reprocessing: Its use in the dissociative disorders. *Dissociation, 8*, 32–44.

Pellicer, X. (1993). Eye movement desensitization treatment of a child's nightmares: A case report. *Journal of Behavior Therapy and Experimental Psychiatry, 24*, 73–75.

Phillips, K. M., Freund, B., Fordiani, J., Kuhn, R., and Ironson, G. (2009). EMDR treatment of past domestic violence: A clinical vignette. *Journal of EMDR Practice and Research, 3*, 192–197.

Pollock, P. (2000). Eye movement desensitization and reprocessing (EMDR) for post-traumatic stress disorder (PTSD) following homicide. *Journal of Forensic Psychiatry, 11*, 176–184.

Popky, A. J. (2005). DeTUR, an urge reduction protocol for addictions and dysfunctional behaviors. *EMDR Solutions: Pathways to Healing,* edited by R. Shapiro, 167–188. New York: W.W. Norton.

Posmontier, B., Dovydaitis, T., and Lipman, K. (2010). Sexual violence: Psychiatric healing with eye movement reprocessing and desensitization. *Health Care for Women International, 31*, 755–768.

Protinsky, H., Sparks, J., and Flemke, K. (2001a). Eye movement desensitization and reprocessing: Innovative clinical applications. *Journal of Contemporary Psychotherapy, 31*, 125–135.

Protinsky, H., Sparks, J., and Flemke, K. (2001b). Using eye movement desensitization and reprocessing to enhance treatment of couples. *Journal of Marital and Family Therapy, 27*, 157–164.

Power, K. G. et al. (2002). A controlled comparison of eye movement desensitization and reprocessing versus exposure plus cognitive restructuring, versus waiting list in the treatment of post-traumatic stress disorder. *Journal of Clinical Psychology and Psychotherapy, 9*, 299–318.

Puffer, M. K., Greenwald, R., and Elrod, D. E. (1998). A single session EMDR study with twenty traumatized children and adolescents. *Traumatology, 3(2)*.

Puk, G. (1991). Treating traumatic memories: A case report on the eye movement desensitization procedure. *Journal of Behavior Therapy and Experimental Psychiatry, 22*, 149–151.

Raboni, M. R., Tufik, S., and Suchecki, D. (2006). Treatment of PTSD by eye movement desensitization reprocessing (EMDR) improves sleep quality, quality of life, and perception of stress. *Annals of the New York Academy of Sciences, 1071*, 508–513.

Rathschlag, M., and Memmert, D. (2014). Reducing anxiety and enhancing physical performance by using an advanced version of EMDR: A pilot study. *Brain and Behavior, 4,* 348–355.

Ray, A. L., and Zbik, A. (2001). Cognitive behavioral therapies and beyond. In *Practical Pain Management,* 3rd ed., edited by C. D. Tollison, J. R. Satterthwaite, and J. W. Tollison, 189–208. Philadelphia: Lippincott.

Reicherzer, S. (2011). Eye movement desensitization and reprocessing in counseling a male couple. *Journal of EMDR Practice and Research, 5,* 111–120.

Renfrey, G., and Spates, C. R. (1994). Eye movement desensitization and reprocessing: A partial dismantling procedure. *Journal of Behavior Therapy and Experimental Psychiatry, 25,* 231–239.

Ribchester, T., Yule, W., and Duncan, A. (2010). EMDR for childhood PTSD after road traffic accidents: Attentional, memory, and attributional processes. *Journal of EMDR Practice and Research, 4,* 138–147.

Ricci, R. J. (2006). Trauma resolution using eye movement desensitization and reprocessing with an incestuous sex offender: An instrumental case study. *Clinical Case Studies, 5,* 248.

Ricci, R. J., Clayton, C. A., and Shapiro, F. (2006). Some effects of EMDR treatment with previously abused child molesters: Theoretical reviews and preliminary findings. *Journal of Forensic Psychiatry and Psychology, 17,* 538–562.

Rittenhouse, J. (2000). Using eye movement desensitization and reprocessing to treat complex PTSD in a biracial client. *Cultural Diversity and Ethnic Minority Psychology, 6,* 399–408.

Rodenburg, R., Benjamin, A., Meijer, A. M., and Jongeneel, R. (2009). Eye movement desensitization and reprocessing in an adolescent with epilepsy and mild intellectual disability. *Epilepsy and Behavior, 16,* 175–180.

Rost, C., Hofmann, A., and Wheeler, K. (2009). EMDR treatment of workplace trauma. *Journal of EMDR Practice and Research, 3,* 80–90.

Rothbaum, B. O. (1997). A controlled study of eye movement desensitization and reprocessing for posttraumatic stress disordered sexual assault victims. *Bulletin of the Menninger Clinic, 61,* 317–334.

Rothbaum, B. O., Astin, M. C., and Marsteller, F. (2005). Prolonged exposure versus eye movement desensitization and reprocessing (EMDR) for PTSD rape victims. *Journal of Traumatic Stress, 18,* 607–616.

Rougemont-Bucking, A., and Zimmermann, E. N. (2012). EMDR-based treatment of psychotraumatic antecedents in illicit drug abusers: A report of two cases. *Swiss Archives of Neurology and Psychiatry, 163,* 107–115.

Royle, L. (2008). EMDR as a therapeutic treatment for chronic fatigue syndrome (CFS). *Journal of EMDR Practice and Research, 2,* 226–232.

Russell, A., and O'Connor, M. (2002). Interventions for recovery: The use of EMDR with children in a community-based project. Association for Child Psychiatry and Psychology, Occasional Paper No. 19, 43–46.

Russell, M. C. (2006). Treating combat-related stress disorders: A multiple case study utilizing eye movement desensitization and reprocessing (EMDR) with battlefield casualties from the Iraqi War. *Military Psychology, 18,* 1.

Russell, M. C. (2008a). War-related medically unexplained symptoms, prevalence, and treatment: Utilizing EMDR within the armed services. *Journal of EMDR Practice and Research, 2,* 212–225.

Russell, M. C. (2008b). Treating traumatic amputation-related phantom limb pain. *Clinical Case Studies, 7,* 136–153.

Russell, M. C., and Figley, C. R. (2012). *Treating Traumatic Stress Injuries in Military Personnel: An EMDR Practitioner's Guide.* New York: Routledge.

Russell, M. C., Silver, S. M., Rogers, S., and Darnell, J. N. (2007). Responding to an identified need: A joint Department of Defense–Department of Veterans Affairs training program in eye movement desensitization and reprocessing (EMDR) for clinicians providing trauma services. *International Journal of Stress Management, 14,* 61.

SAMHSA (Substance Abuse and Mental Health Services Administration). (2010). *Eye Movement Desensitization and Reprocessing.* Rockville, MD: National Registry of Evidence-Based Programs and Practices.

Sandström, M., Wiberg, B., Wikman, M., Willman, A. K., and Högberg, U. (2008). A pilot study of eye movement desensitisation and reprocessing treatment (EMDR) for post-traumatic stress after childbirth. *Midwifery, 24,* 62–73.

Scheck, M. M., Schaeffer, J. A., and Gillette, C. S. (1998). Brief psychological intervention with traumatized young women: The efficacy of eye movement desensitization and reprocessing. *Journal of Traumatic Stress, 11,* 25–44.

Schneider, G., Nabavi, D., and Heuft, G. (2005). Eye movement desensitization and reprocessing in the treatment of posttraumatic stress disorder in a patient with comorbid epilepsy. *Epilepsy and Behavior, 7,* 715–718.

Schneider, J., Hofmann, A., Rost, C., and Shapiro, F. (2007). EMDR and phantom limb pain: Case study, theoretical implications, and treatment guidelines. *Journal of EMDR Science and Practice, 1,* 31–45.

Schneider, J., Hofmann, A., Rost, C., and Shapiro, F. (2008). EMDR in the treatment of chronic phantom limb pain. *Pain Medicine, 9,* 76–82.

Schurmans, K. (2007). EMDR treatment of choking phobia. *Journal of EMDR Practice and Research, 1,* 118–121.

Seidler, G. H., and Wagner, F. E. (2006). Comparing the efficacy of EMDR and trauma-focused cognitive-behavioral therapy in the treatment of PTSD: A meta-analytic study. *Psychological Medicine, 36,* 1515–1522.

Shapiro, E., and Laub, B. (2008). Early EMDR intervention (EEI): A summary, a theoretical model, and the recent traumatic episode protocol (R-TEP). *Journal of EMDR Practice and Research, 2,* 79–96.

Shapiro, F. (1989a). Efficacy of the eye movement desensitization procedure in the treatment of traumatic memories. *Journal of Traumatic Stress. 2,* 199–223.

Shapiro, F. (1989b). Eye movement desensitization: A new treatment for post-traumatic stress disorder. *Journal of Behavior Therapy and Experimental Psychiatry, 20,* 211–217.

Shapiro, F. (1991). Eye movement desensitization and reprocessing procedure: From EMD to EMDR: A new treatment model for anxiety and related traumata. *Behavior Therapist, 14,* 133–135.

Shapiro, F. (1994). Eye movement desensitization and reprocessing: A new treatment for anxiety and related trauma. In *Trauma Victim: Theoretical and Practical Suggestions,* edited by Lee Hyer, 501–521. Muncie, IN: Accelerated Development Publishers.

Shapiro, F. (1995). *Eye Movement Desensitization and Reprocessing: Basic Principles, Protocols and Procedures.* New York: Guilford Press.

Shapiro, F. (1999). Eye movement desensitization and reprocessing (EMDR) and the anxiety disorders: Clinical and research implications of an integrated psychotherapy treatment. *Journal of Anxiety Disorders, 13,* 35–67.

Shapiro, F. (2001). *Eye Movement Desensitization and Reprocessing: Basic Principles, Protocols and Procedures,* 2nd ed. New York: Guilford Press.

Shapiro, F. (2002). *EMDR as an Integrative Psychotherapy Approach: Experts of Diverse Orientations Explore the Paradigm Prism.* Washington, D.C.: American Psychological Association Press.

Shapiro, F. (2006). *EMDR and New Notes on Adaptive Information Processing: Case Formulation Principles, Scripts and Worksheets.* Camden, CT: EMDR Humanitarian Assistance Programs.

Shapiro, F. (2007). EMDR, adaptive information processing, and case conceptualization. *Journal of EMDR Practice and Research, 1,* 68–87.

Shapiro, F. (2012). *Getting Past Your Past: Take Control of Your Life with Self-Help Techniques from EMDR Therapy.* New York: Rodale.

Shapiro, F., and Forrest, M. (1997). *EMDR: The Breakthrough Therapy for Overcoming Anxiety, Stress and Trauma.* New York: Basic Books.

Shapiro, F., Kaslow, F. W., and Maxfield, L. (2007). *Handbook of EMDR and Family Therapy Processes.* Hoboken, NJ: Wiley.

Shapiro, F., and Solomon, R. (1995). Eye movement desensitization and reprocessing: Neurocognitive information processing. In *Innovations in Disaster and Trauma Psychology,* Vol. 1, edited by G. Everly, 216–237. Ellicott City, MD: Chevron Publishing.

Shapiro, F., Vogelmann-Sine, S., and Sine, L. (1994). Eye movement desensitization and reprocessing: Treating trauma and substance abuse. *Journal of Psychoactive Drugs, 26,* 379–391.

Silver, S. M., and Rogers, S. (2001). *Light in the Heart of Darkness: EMDR and the Treatment of War and Terrorism Survivors.* New York: Norton.

Silver, S. M., Rogers, S., Knipe, J., and Colelli, G. (2005). EMDR therapy following the 9/11 terrorist attacks: A community-based intervention project in New York City. *International Journal of Stress Management, 12,* 29–42.

Silver, S. M., Rogers, S., and Russell, M. (2008). Eye movement desensitization and reprocessing (EMDR) in the treatment of war veterans. *Journal of Clinical Psychology, 64,* 947–957.

Silverman, S. (2011). Effecting peak athletic performance with neurofeedback, interactive metronome, and EMDR: A case study. *Biofeedback, 39,* 40–42.

Soberman, G. B., Greenwald, R., and Rule, D. L. (2002). A controlled study of eye movement desensitization and reprocessing (EMDR) for boys with conduct problems. *Journal of Aggression, Maltreatment, and Trauma, 6,* 217–236.

Softic, R. (2009). [Complete symptom's remissions of acute non-combat PTSD after one session]. *Acta Medica Saliniana, 37,* 147–150. In Bosnian.

Solomon, R. M. (1995). Critical incident trauma: Lessons learned at Waco, Texas. Paper presented at the Law Enforcement Psychology Conference, San Mateo, CA.

Solomon, R. M. (1998). Utilization of EMDR in crisis intervention. *Crisis Intervention, 4,* 239–246.

Solomon, R. M., and Dyregrov, A. (2000). Eye movement desensitization and reprocessing (EMDR): Rebuilding assumptive words. *Tidsskrift for Norsk Psykologforening, 37,* 1024–1030.

Solomon, R. M., and Kaufman, T. E. (2002). A peer support workshop for the treatment of traumatic stress of railroad personnel: Contributions of eye movement desensitization and reprocessing (EMDR). *Journal of Brief Therapy*, 2, 27-33.

Solomon, R. M., and Rando, T. A. (2007). Utilization of EMDR in the treatment of grief and mourning. *Journal of EMDR Practice and Research*, 1, 109-117.

Solomon, R. M., and Shapiro, F. (1997). Eye movement desensitization and reprocessing: An effective therapeutic tool for trauma and grief. In *Death and Trauma: The Traumatology of Grieving*, edited by C. R. Figley, B. E. Bride, and N. Mazza, 231-247. Washington, D.C.: Taylor and Francis.

Spates, R. C. and Burnette, M. M. (1995). Eye movement desensitization and reprocessing: Three unusual cases. *Journal of Behavior Therapy and Experimental Psychiatry*, 26, 51-55.

Spector, J., and Huthwaite, M. (1993). Eye-movement desensitisation to overcome post-traumatic stress disorder. *British Journal of Psychiatry*, 163, 106-108.

Sprang, G. (2001). The use of eye movement desensitization and reprocessing (EMDR) in the treatment of traumatic stress and complicated mourning: Psychological and behavioral outcomes. *Research on Social Work Practice*, 11, 300-320.

Srivastava, U., and Mukhopadhyay, A. (2008). Application of EMDR in the treatment of major depressive disorder: A case study. *Indian Journal of Clinical Psychology*, 35, 163-172.

Stewart, K., and Bramson, T. (2000). Incorporating EMDR in residential treatment. *Residential Treatment for Children and Youth*, 17, 83-90.

Stowasser, J. (2007). EMDR and family therapy in the treatment of domestic violence. In *Handbook of EMDR and Family Therapy Processes*, edited by F. Shapiro, F. W. Kaslow, and L. Maxfield, 243-264. Hoboken, NJ: Wiley.

Stramrood C. A. I., van der Velde, J., Doornbos, B., Marieke Paarlberg, K., Weijmar Schultz, W. C. M., and van Pampus, M. G. (2012). The patient observer: Eye-movement desensitization and reprocessing for the treatment of posttraumatic stress following childbirth. *Birth*, 39, 70-76.

Talan, B. S. (2007). Integrating EMDR and imago relationship therapy in treatment of couples. In *Handbook of EMDR and Family Therapy Processes*, edited by F. Shapiro, F. W. Kaslow, and L. Maxfield, 187-201. Hoboken, NJ: Wiley.

Tanaka, K., and Inoue, K. (1999). EMDR treatment for childhood traumatic memories: A case of seasonal depression as an anniversary phenomenon. *Kokoro no Rinsho Arakaruto*, 18, 69-75.

Tang, T. C., Yang, P., Yen, C. F., and Liu, T. L. (2015). Eye movement desensitization and reprocessing for treating psychological disturbances in Taiwanese adolescents who experienced Typhoon Morakot. *Kaohsiung Journal of Medical Sciences*, 31, 363-369.

Tarquinio, C., Brennstuhl, M.-J., Reichenbach, S., Rydberg, J. A., and Tarquinio, P. (2012). [Early treatment of rape victims: Presentation of an emergency EMDR protocol]. *Sexologies*, 21, 147-156. In French.

Tarquinio, C., Brennstuhl, M.-J., Rydberg, J. A., Schmitt, A., Mouda, F., Lourel, M., and Tarquinio, P. (2012). [Eye movement desensitization and reprocessing (EMDR) therapy in the treatment of victims of domestic violence: A pilot study]. *Revue Européenne de Psychologie Appliquée*, 62, 205-212. In French.

Tarquinio C., Schmitt, A., and Tarquinio, P. (2012). [Conjugal violence and eye movement desensitization and reprocessing (EMDR): Case studies]. *L'Evolution Psychiatrique*, 77, 97-108. In French.

Tarquinio, C., Schmitt, A., Tarquinio, P., Rydberg, J.-A., and Spitz, E. (2012). [Benefits of "eye movement desensitization and reprocessing" psychotherapy in the treatment of female victims of intimate partner rape]. *Sexologies, 21*, 92–99. In French.

Taylor, R. (2002). Family unification with reactive attachment disorder: A brief treatment. *Contemporary Family Therapy: An International Journal, 24*, 475–481.

Thomas, R., and Gafner, G. (1993). PTSD in an elderly male: Treatment with eye movement desensitization and reprocessing (EMDR). *Clinical Gerontologist, 14*, 57–59.

Tinker, R. H., and Wilson, S. A. (1999). *Through the Eyes of a Child: EMDR with Children*. New York: Norton.

Tinker, R. H., and Wilson, S. A. (2006). The phantom limb pain protocol. In *EMDR Solutions: Pathways to Healing*, edited by R. Shapiro, 147–159. New York, W.W. Norton.

Tofani, L. R., and Wheeler, K. (2011). The recent-traumatic episode protocol: Outcome evaluation and analysis of three case studies. *Journal of EMDR Practice and Research, 5*, 95–110.

Torun, F. (2010). Treatment of vaginismus with EMDR: A report of two cases. *Türk Psikiyatri Dergisi, 21*, 243–248.

Tsuchimochi, S., and Sasaki, K. (2012). [The possibility of EMDR use to juvenile delinquents: A short-term intervention in the inquiry stage at a family court]. *Japanese Journal of EMDR Research and Practice, 4*, 29–40. In Japanese.

Tufnell, G. (2005). Eye movement desensitization and reprocessing in the treatment of preadolescent children with post-traumatic symptoms. *Clinical Child Psychology and Psychiatry, 10*, 587.

Twombly, J. H. (2000). Incorporating EMDR and EMDR adaptations into the treatment of clients with dissociative identity disorder. *Journal of Trauma and Dissociation, 1*, 61–81.

Twombly, J. H. (2005). EMDR for clients with dissociative identity disorder, DDNOS, and ego states. In *EMDR Solutions: Pathways to Healing*, edited by R. Shapiro, 88–120. New York: W.W. Norton.

Uribe, M. E. R., and Ramirez, E. O. L. (2006). The effect of EMDR therapy on the negative information processing on patients who suffer depression. *Revista Electrónica de Motivación y Emoción (REME), 9*, 23–24.

VA/DoD (U.S. Department of Veterans Affairs and U.S. Department of Defense) (2004). *VA/DoD Clinical Practice Guideline for the Management of Post-Traumatic Stress*. Washington, DC: Veterans Health Administration, Department of Veterans Affairs and Health Affairs, Department of Defense. Office of Quality and Performance publication 10Q-CPG/PTSD-04.

van den Berg, D. P. G., de Bont, P. A. J. M., van der Vleugel, B. M., de Roos, C., de Jongh, A., van Minnen, A., and van der Gaag, M. (2015). Prolonged exposure vs eye movement desensitization and reprocessing vs waiting list for posttraumatic stress disorder in patients with a psychotic disorder: A randomized clinical trial. *JAMA Psychiatry, 72*, 259–267.

van den Berg, D. P. G., and van den Gaag, M. (2012). Treating trauma in psychosis with EMDR: A pilot study. *Journal of Behavior Therapy and Experimental Psychiatry, 43*, 664–671.

van den Berg, D. P. G., van der Vleugel, B. M., Staring, A. B. P., de Bont, P. A. J., and de Jongh, A. (2015). [EMDR in psychosis: Guidelines for conceptualization and treatment]. *Journal of EMDR Practice and Research, 9*, E29-E45. In French.

van der Hart, O., Groenendijk, M., Gonzalez, A., Mosquera, D., and Solomon, R. (2014). Dissociation of the personality and EMDR therapy in complex trauma-related disorders: Applications in phases 2 and 3 treatment. *Journal of EMDR Practice and Research, 8*, 33–48.

van der Kolk, B. A. et al. (2007). A randomized clinical trial of eye movement desensitization and reprocessing (EMDR), fluoxetine, and pill placebo in the treatment of posttraumatic stress disorder: treatment effects and long-term maintenance. *Journal of Clinical Psychiatry, 68*, 37–46.

van der Vleugel, B. M., van den Berg, D. P. G., and Staring, A. B. P. (2012). [Trauma, psychosis, post-traumatic stress disorder and the application of EMDR]. *Rivista di Psichiatria, 47*, 33S–38S. In Italian.

Vaughan, K., Armstrong, M. F., Gold, R., O'Connor, N., Jenneke, W., and Tarrier, N. (1994). A trial of eye movement desensitization compared to image habituation training and applied muscle relaxation in post-traumatic stress disorder. *Journal of Behavior Therapy and Experimental Psychiatry, 25*, 283–291.

Vaughan, K., Wiese, M., Gold, R., and Tarrier, N. (1994). Eye-movement desensitisation: Symptom change in post-traumatic stress disorder. *British Journal of Psychiatry, 164*, 533–541.

Vogelmann-Sinn, S., Sine, L. F., Smyth, N. J., and Popky, A. J. (1998). *EMDR Chemical Dependency Treatment Manual.* New Hope, PA: EMDR Humanitarian Assistance Programs.

Wadaa, N. N., Zaharim, N. M., and Alqashan, H. F. (2010). The use of EMDR in treatment of traumatized Iraqi children. *Digest of Middle East Studies, 19*, 26–36.

Wanders, F., Serra, M., and de Jongh, A. (2008). EMDR versus CBT for children with self-esteem and behavioral problems: A randomized controlled trial. *Journal of EMDR Practice and Research*, 2, 180–189.

Wernik, U. (1993). The role of the traumatic component in the etiology of sexual dysfunctions and its treatment with eye movement desensitization procedure. *Journal of Sex Education and Therapy, 19*, 212–222.

Wesselmann, D., Davidson, M., Armstrong, S., Schweitzer, C., Bruckner, D., and Potter, A. E. (2012). EMDR as a treatment for improving attachment status in adults and children. *Revue Européenne de Psychologie Applique/European Review of Applied Psychology, 62*, 223–230.

Wesselmann, D., and Potter, A. E. (2009). Change in adult attachment status following treatment with EMDR: Three case studies. *Journal of EMDR Practice and Research, 3*, 178–191.

Wesselmann, D., Schweitzer, C., and Armstrong, S. (2014*). Integrative Team Treatment for Attachment Trauma in Children: Family Therapy and EMDR.* New York: W.W. Norton.

Wesson, M., and Gould, M. (2009). Intervening early with EMDR on military operations: A case study. *Journal of EMDR Practice and Research, 3*, 91–97.

White, G. D. (1998). Trauma treatment training for Bosnian and Croatian mental health workers. *American Journal of Orthopsychiatry, 63*, 58–62.

Wilensky, M. (2006). Eye movement desensitization and reprocessing (EMDR) as a treatment for phantom limb pain. *Journal of Brief Therapy, 5*, 31–44.

Wilson, S. A., Becker, L. A., and Tinker, R. H. (1995). Eye movement desensitization and reprocessing (EMDR) treatment for psychologically traumatized individuals. *Journal of Consulting and Clinical Psychology, 63*, 928–937.

Wilson, S. A., Becker, L. A., and Tinker, R. H. (1997). Fifteen-month follow-up of eye movement desensitization and reprocessing (EMDR) treatment for PTSD and psychological trauma. *Journal of Consulting and Clinical Psychology, 65*, 1047–1056.

Wilson, S. A., Becker, L. A., Tinker, R. H., and Logan, C. R. (2001). Stress management with law enforcement personnel: A controlled outcome study of EMDR versus a traditional stress management program. *International Journal of Stress Management, 8,* 179–200.

Wilson, S. A., Tinker, R., Becker, L. A., Hofmann, A., and Cole, J. W. (2000). EMDR treatment of phantom limb pain with brain imaging (MEG). Paper presented at the annual meeting of the EMDR International Association, Toronto, Canada.

Wolpe, J., and Abrams, J. (1991). Post-traumatic stress disorder overcome by eye movement desensitization: A case report. *Journal of Behavior Therapy and Experimental Psychiatry 22,* 39–43.

World Health Organization (2013). *Guidelines for the Management of Conditions That Are Specifically Related to Stress.* Geneva: WHO.

Young, W. (1994). EMDR treatment of phobic symptoms in multiple personality. *Dissociation, 7,* 129–133.

Young, W. (1995). EMDR: Its use in resolving the trauma caused by the loss of a war buddy. *American Journal of Psychotherapy, 49,* 282–291.

Zabukovec, J., Lazrove, S., and Shapiro, F. (2000). Self-healing aspects of EMDR: The therapeutic change process and perspective of integrated psychotherapies. *Journal of Psychotherapy Integration, 10,* 189–206.

Zaghrout-Hodali, M., Alissa, F., and Dodgson, P. W. (2008). Building resilience and dismantling fear: EMDR group protocol with children in an area of ongoing trauma. *Journal of EMDR Practice and Research, 2,* 106–113.

Zimmermann, P., Güse, U., Barre, K., and Biesold, K. H. (2005) [EMDR in the German armed forces: Therapeutic impact of inpatient therapy of posttraumatic stress disorder]. *Krankenhauspsychiatrie, 16,* 57–63. In German.

Zweben, J., and Yeary, J. (2006). EMDR in the treatment of addiction. *Journal of Chemical Dependency Treatment, 8,* 115–127.

NOTES

Introduction, pp. 1–12

1. B. A. van der Kolk, "Beyond the Talking Cure: Somatic Experiences and Subcortical Imprints in the Treatment of Trauma," in *EMDR as an Integrative Psychotherapy Approach: Experts of Diverse Orientations Explore the Paradigm Prism*, ed. F. Shapiro (Washington, DC: American Psychological Association), 57–83.

2. F. Shapiro, *Eye Movement Desensitization and Reprocessing: Basic Principles, Protocols, and Procedures*, 2nd ed. (New York: Guilford Press, 1995; 2001).

3. D. J. Siegel, *The Developing Mind: Toward a Neurobiology of Interpersonal Experience* (New York: Guilford, 1999).

R. Stickgold, "EMDR: A Putative Neurobiological Mechanism of Action," *Journal of Clinical Psychology* 58 (2002): 61–75.

B. A. van der Kolk, "The Body Keeps the Score: Memory and the Evolving Psychobiology of Posttraumatic Stress," *Harvard Review of Psychiatry* 1 (1994): 253–265.

F. Shapiro, "The Role of Eye Movement Desensitization and Reprocessing (EMDR) Therapy in Medicine: Addressing the Psychological and Physical Symptoms Stemming from Adverse Life Experiences," *Permanente Journal* 18 (2014): 71–77.

4. S. D. Gold, B. P. Marx, J. M. Soler-Baillo, and D. M. Sloan, "Is Life Stress More Traumatic Than Traumatic Stress?" *Journal of Anxiety Disorders* 19 (2005): 687–698.

S. S. L. Mol et al., "Symptoms of Post-Traumatic Stress Disorder After Non-Traumatic Events: Evidence from an Open Population Study," *British Journal of Psychiatry* 186 (2005): 494–499.

5. V. J. Felitti et al., "Relationship of Childhood Abuse and Household Dysfunction to Many of the Leading Causes of Death in Adults: The Adverse Childhood Experiences (ACE) Study," *American Journal of Preventive Medicine* 14 (1998): 245–258.

6. E. B. Foa, T. N. Keane, M. J. Friedman, and J. A. Cohen, *Effective Treatments for PTSD: Practice Guidelines from the International Society for Traumatic Stress Studies* (New York: Guilford, 2009).

7. A. Bleich, M. Kotler, E. Kutz, and A. Shaley, "Guidelines for the Assessment and Professional Intervention with Terror Victims in the Hospital and the Community," A Position Paper of the (Israeli) National Council for Mental Health, 2002.

8. VA/DoD (Department of Veterans Affairs, and U.S. Department of Defense), *VA/DoD Clinical Practice Guideline for the Management of Post-Traumatic Stress* (Washington, DC:

Veterans Health Administration, Department of Veterans Affairs and Health Affairs, Department of Defense, 2010).

9. World Health Organization, *Guidelines for the Management of Conditions That Are Specifically Related to Stress* (Geneva: WHO, 2013), 1.

10. S. Marcus, P. Marquis, and C. Sakai, "Controlled Study of Treatment of PTSD Using EMDR in an HMO Setting," *Psychotherapy* 34 (1997): 307–315.

B. O. Rothbaum, "A Controlled Study of Eye Movement Desensitization and Reprocessing in the Treatment of Post-Traumatic Stress Disordered Sexual Assault Victims," *Bulletin of the Menninger Clinic* 61 (1997): 317–334.

S. Wilson., L. A. Becker, and R. H. Tinker, "Fifteen-Month Follow-Up of Eye Movement Desensitization and Reprocessing (EMDR) Treatment of Post-Traumatic Stress Disorder and Psychological Trauma," *Journal of Consulting and Clinical Psychology* 65 (1997): 1047–1056.

11. J. Carlson, C. M. Chemtob, K. Rusnak, N. L. Hedlund, and M. Y. Muraoka, "Eye Movement Desensitization and Reprocessing (EMDR): Treatment for Combat-Related Post-Traumatic Stress Disorder," *Journal of Traumatic Stress* 11 (1998): 3–24.

12. M. C. Russell and C. R. Figley, *Treating Traumatic Stress Injuries in Military Personnel: An EMDR Practitioner's Guide* (New York: Routledge, 2012).

13. M. C. Russell, S. M. Silver, S. Rogers, and J. Darnell, "Responding to an Identified Need: A Joint Department of Defense–Department of Veterans Affairs Training Program in Eye Movement Desensitization and Reprocessing (EMDR) for Clinicians Providing Trauma Services," *International Journal of Stress Management* 14 (2007): 61–71.

14. B. Van der Kolk, J. Spinazzola, M. Blaustein, J. Hopper, E. Hopper, D. Korn, and W. Simpson, "A Randomized Clinical Trial of EMDR, Fluoxetine and Pill Placebo in the Treatment of PTSD: Treatment Effects and Long-Term Maintenance," *Journal of Clinical Psychiatry* 68 (2007): 37–46.

15. G. I. Ironson, B. Freund, J. L. Strauss, and J. Williams, "A Comparison of Two Treatments for Traumatic Stress: A Pilot Study of EMDR and Prolonged Exposure," *Journal of Clinical Psychology* 58 (2002): 113–128.

S. Rogers, S. Silver, J. Goss, J. Obenchain, A. Willis, and R. Whitney, "A Single Session, Controlled Group Study of Flooding and Eye Movement Desensitization and Reprocessing in Treating Posttraumatic Stress Disorder Among Vietnam War Veterans: Preliminary Data," *Journal of Anxiety Disorders* 13 (1999): 119–130.

16. R. Stickgold, "Neurobiological Concomitants of EMDR: Speculations and Proposed Research," *Journal of Clinical Psychology* 58 (2002): 61–75.

17. See, for example, two references:

M. Hersen and W. Sledge, eds., *Encyclopedia of Psychotherapy* (New York: Elsevier Science, 2002), 1:777–785.

I. Weiner and W. E. Craighead, eds., *The Corsini Encyclopedia of Psychology*, 4th ed. (Hoboken, NJ: Wiley, 2010).

18. R. Stickgold, "Neurobiological Concomitants of EMDR: Speculations and Proposed Research," *Journal of Clinical Psychology* 58 (2002): 61–75.

19. See references in Appendix B.

20. C. M. Chemtob, D. F. Tolin, B. A. van der Kolk, and R. K. Pitman, "Eye Movement Desensitization and Reprocessing," in *Effective Treatments for PTSD: Practice Guidelines from the International Society for Traumatic Stress Studies*, eds. E. A. Foa, T. M. Keane, and M. J. Friedman (New York: Guilford, 2000).

21. C. W. Lee and P. Cuijpers "A Meta-Analysis of the Contribution of Eye Movements in Processing Emotional Memories," *Journal of Behavior Therapy and Experimental Psychiatry* 44 (2013): 231–239.

22. R. Stickgold, "EMDR: A Putative Neurobiological Mechanism of Action," *Journal of Clinical Psychology* 58 (2002): 61–75.

23. See list of research in Appendix B.

24. K. W. Brown, T. McGoldrick, and R. Buchanan, "Body Dysmorphic Disorder: Seven Cases Treated with Eye Movement Desensitization and Reprocessing," *Behavioural and Cognitive Psychotherapy* 25 (1997): 203–207.

25. F. Shapiro, *Getting Past Your Past: Take Control of Your Life with Self-Help Techniques from EMDR Therapy* (New York: Rodale, 2012).

26. F. Shapiro, *Eye Movement Desensitization and Reprocessing: Basic Principles, Protocols, and Procedures*, 2nd ed. (New York: Guilford Press, 2001).

27. B. Van der Kolk, J. Spinazzola, M. Blaustein, J. Hopper, E. Hopper, D. Korn, and W. Simpson, "A Randomized Clinical Trial of EMDR, Fluoxetine and Pill Placebo in the Treatment of PTSD: Treatment Effects and Long-Term Maintenance," *Journal of Clinical Psychiatry* 68 (2007): 37–46.

28. F. Shapiro, "EMDR Therapy Humanitarian Assistance Programs: Treating the Psychological, Physical, and Societal Effects of Adverse Experiences Worldwide," *Journal of EMDR Practice and Research* 8 (2014): 181–186.

Chapter 1, pp. 13–24
The Journey of Discovery

1. S. Rogers, "EMDR Reviews," Veterans Affairs Internet Forum, 1996.

2. F. Ryan, *The Forgotten Plague* (Boston: Little Brown, 1992).

3. See Appendix C. Surprisingly, most well-known psychological treatments have come into the consulting room with no research at all to sanction them and sometimes no expectation of any research in the future. In fact, when I began developing EMDR in 1987, I conducted a literature review of all the publications on trauma. There was only one controlled study on the clinical treatment of PTSD (comparing forty-five sessions of desensitization to no therapy) even though it had been identified and categorized in the diagnostic manuals seven years before. The more than one hundred published studies I did find, which were done since 1980, when PTSD was formally recognized as a psychological disorder, focused on the causes, demographics, and theory of PTSD. In 1992 (thirteen years after PTSD had been categorized), a review article reported that only eleven controlled studies had been completed and five of them involved the use of psychotropic drugs; the authors of these studies reported widely conflicting results (see S. D. Solomon, E. T. Gerrity, and A. M. Muff, "Efficacy of Treatments for Posttraumatic Stress Disorder," *Journal of the American Medical Association* 268 [1992]: 633–638).

4. S. Marcus, P. Marquis, and C. Sakai, "Controlled Study of Treatment of PTSD Using EMDR in an HMO Setting," *Psychotherapy* 34 (1997): 307–315.

S. Marcus, P. Marquis, and C. Sakai, "Three-and 6-Month Follow-Up of EMDR Treatment of PTSD in an HMO Setting," *International Journal of Stress Management* 11 (2004): 195–208.

B. O. Rothbaum, "A Controlled Study of Eye Movement Desensitization and Reprocessing in the Treatment of Posttraumatic Stress Disordered Sexual Assault Victims," *Bulletin of the Menninger Clinic* 61 (1997): 317–334.

M. M. Scheck, J. A. Schaeffer, and C. S. Gillette, "Brief Psychological Intervention with Traumatized Young Women: The Efficacy of Eye Movement Desensitization and Reprocessing," *Journal of Traumatic Stress* 11 (1998): 25–44.

S. A. Wilson, L. A. Becker, and R. H. Tinker, "Eye Movement Desensitization and Reprocessing (EMDR) Treatment for Psychologically Traumatized Individuals," *Journal of Consulting and Clinical Psychology* 63 (1995): 928–937.

S. A. Wilson, L. A. Becker, and R. H. Tinker, "15-Month Follow-Up of Eye Movement Desensitization and Reprocessing (EMDR) Treatment for Psychological Trauma," *Journal of Consulting and Clinical Psychology* 65 (1997): 1047–1056. See also F. Shapiro, "The Role of Eye Movement Desensitization and Reprocessing (EMDR) Therapy in Medicine: Addressing the Psychological and Physical Symptoms Stemming from Adverse Life Experiences," *Permanente Journal* 18: 71–77 (2014).

5. M. Cloitre and U. Schnyder, eds., *Evidence Based Treatments for Trauma-Related Psychological Disorders: A Practical Guide for Clinicians* (New York: Springer, 2015).

6. When the popular media joined the debate, their coverage fueled both sides of the controversy. *New York Magazine* ran a headline hailing it as "a miracle cure" but in small print asked if it was "hand jive." A reporter for *Psychology Today* called EMDR "a quick psychiatric fix for those unwilling to do the hard everyday work necessary for mental health in a complex world." *Newsweek* asked whether EMDR was "the new Prozac or the old snake oil?" A 1994 article in the *Washington Post* included remarks from psychologists who called it a major breakthrough and one who likened believing in EMDR to believing in UFOs. A sign of the changing times, however, was a follow-up article a year later that reported the use of EMDR in Oklahoma City and was universally positive about the results. The more recent newspaper articles talk about its positive effects but wonder *how* it works.

7. See Appendix A.

8. N. Cousins, *Anatomy of an Illness* (New York: Norton, 1979).

9. O. C. Simonton and J. Creighton, *Getting Well Again* (New York: Bantam Books, 1982).

Chapter 2, pp. 25–42
Laying the Foundation

1. In fact it is now recognized that general adverse life experiences can cause even more PTSD symptoms than major trauma: S. S. L. Mol, A. Arntz, J. F. M. Metsemakers, G. Dinant, P. A. P. Van Montfort, and A. Knottnerus, "Symptoms of Post-Traumatic Stress Disorder After Non-Traumatic Events: Evidence from an Open Population Study," *British Journal of Psychiatry* 186 (2005): 494–499.

Adverse experiences are also correlated with a wide range of problems: V. J. Felitti, "Relationship of Childhood Abuse and Household Dysfunction to Many of the Leading Causes of Death in Adults: The Adverse Childhood Experiences (ACE) Study," *American Journal of Preventive Medicine* 14 (1998): 245–258.

2. J. Wolpe, *Psychotherapy by Reciprocal Inhibition* (Stanford, CA: Stanford University Press, 1958).

3. The SUD Scale may seem simple, but it provides more information about the immediate effects of treatment on a single memory than any other measurement. Most of the so-called global measures of mental health are designed to evaluate the subject's overall psychological state: his personality and his general way of being and behaving in the world. They are not much use in measuring whether a one-session EMDR treatment with someone who has experienced

many disturbing events has had any effect. Treating a single traumatic incident (such as seeing your best buddy take a bullet meant for you) in a person who experienced multiple trauma (booby traps, interrogation, the loss of a leg) and then measuring overall mental health would be like yanking one log out of a roaring fire and measuring to see whether the blaze was still giving off heat. The SUD Scale lets us measure the temperature of the single log, and practitioners still use it today for that purpose when doing EMDR therapy. It lets both the therapist and the client see how successful a single treatment of a single event has been. Later, we use global measures to judge the effectiveness of the overall treatment plan, including the whole succession of EMDR sessions.

4. F. Shapiro, "Efficacy of the Eye Movement Desensitization Procedure in the Treatment of Traumatic Memories," *Journal of Traumatic Stress Studies* 2 (1989): 199–223.

F. Shapiro, "Eye Movement Desensitization: A New Treatment for Post-Traumatic Stress Disorder," *Journal of Behavior Therapy and Experimental Psychiatry* 20 (1989): 211–217.

One of the things I hoped for was that other psychologists would read the articles and want to do their own studies on the effectiveness of EMDR. This was important because my study had a weakness: I was both the originator of the treatment and the person who administered it to the subjects during the study, which might have influenced their responses. My results needed independent verification for credibility. Although I had expected a deluge of interest from researchers, it didn't come immediately. Studies confirming the positive effects of EMDR were years away. However, clinicians needed something to treat the pain here and now. Because no other methods were showing comparable results, I began teaching EMDR to clinicians as an "experimental procedure" until research was completed.

5. See Appendix B.

6. I. P. Pavlov, *Conditioned Reflexes* (New York: Liveright, 1927).

7. A. N. Goldstein and M. P. Walker, "The Role of Sleep in Emotional Brain Function," *Annual Review of Clinical Psychology* 10 (2014): 679–708.

E. J. Wamsley and R. Stickgold, "Dreaming and Offline Memory Processing," *Current Biology* 20, no. 23 (2010): R1010–1013.

E. J. Wamsley, M. Tucker, J. D. Payne, J. A. Benavides, and R. Stickgold, "Dreaming of a Learning Task Is Associated with Enhanced Sleep-Dependent Memory Consolidation," *Current Biology* 20, no. 9 (2010): 850–855.

8. J. Wolpe, *The Practice of Behavior Therapy*, 4th ed. (New York: Pergamon Press, 1991).

9. S. J. Ellman and J. S. Antrobus, *The Mind in Sleep* (New York: Wiley, 1991).

10. C. Hong, C. Gillin, G. A. Callaghan, and S. Potkin, "Correlation of Rapid Eye Movement Density with Dream Report Length and Not with Movements in the Dream: Evidence Against the Scanning Hypothesis," *Annual Meeting Abstracts*, Association of Professional Sleep Societies, Poster 12, 1992.

11. M. S. Armstrong and K. Vaughan, "An Orienting Response Model of Eye Movement Desensitization," *Journal of Behavior Therapy and Experimental Psychiatry* 27 (1996): 21–32.

M. J. MacCulloch, M. P. Feldman, and G. Wilkinson, "Eye Movement Desensitization Treatment Utilizes the Positive Visceral Element of the Investigatory Reflex to Inhibit the Memories of Post Traumatic Stress Disorder: A Theoretical Analysis," *British Journal of Psychiatry* 169 (1996): 571–579.

In addition, many researchers believe that the eye movements "tax working memory," resulting in a decrease of memory vividness and negative emotions. A recent meta-analysis of more than twenty randomized studies has demonstrated the positive effects of the eye movement component: C. W. Lee and P. Cuijpers, "A Meta-Analysis of the Contribution of Eye Movements in Processing Emotional Memories," *Journal of Behavior Therapy and Experimental Psychiatry* 44 (2013): 231–239.

For an annotated list of more than thirty studies evaluating the eye movement component of EMDR therapy, see Appendix B.

12. A. Arai and G. Lynch, "Factors Regulating the Magnitude of Long-Term Potentiation Induced by Theta Pattern Stimulation," *Brain Research* 598 (1992): 173–184.

G. Barrionuevo, F. Schottler, and G. Lynch, "The Effects of Repetitive Low-Frequency Stimulation on Control and 'Potentiated' Synaptic Responses in the Hippocampus," *Life Sciences* 27 (1980): 2385–2391.

13. F. Shapiro, *Eye Movement Desensitization and Reprocessing: Basic Principles, Protocols, and Procedures* (New York: Guilford Press, 2001).

F. Shapiro, "EMDR, Adaptive Information Processing, and Case Conceptualization," *Journal of EMDR Practice and Research* 1 (2007): 68–87.

F. Shapiro, "The Role of Eye Movement Desensitization and Reprocessing (EMDR) Therapy in Medicine: Addressing the Psychological and Physical Symptoms Stemming from Adverse Life Experiences," *Permanente Journal* 18 (2014): 71–77.

Chapter 3, pp. 43–62
The Spirit and the Sword: Combat's Tragic Legacy

1. R. A. Kulka,W. E. Schlenger, J. A. Fairbank, B. K. Jordan, R. L. Hough, C. R. Marmar, and D. S. Weiss, *Trauma and the Vietnam War Generation* (New York: Brunner/Mazel, 1990).

2. J. D. Kinzie and R. R. Goetz, "A Century of Controversy Surrounding Posttraumatic Stress-Spectrum Syndromes: The Impact on DSM-III and DSM-IV," *Journal of Traumatic Stress* 9 (1996): 159–179.

3. Z. Solomon, "Oscillating Between Denial and Recognition of PTSD," *Journal of Traumatic Stress* 8 (1995): 271–281.

4. R. A. Kulka,W. E. Schlenger, J. A. Fairbank, B. K. Jordan, R. L. Hough, C. R. Marmar, and D. S. Weiss, *Trauma and the Vietnam War Generation* (New York: Brunner/Mazel, 1990).

5. S. D. Solomon, E. T. Gerrity, and A. M. Muff, "Efficacy of Treatments for Posttraumatic Stress Disorder," *Journal of the American Medical Association* 268 (1992): 633–638.

6. The most recent meta-analysis of psychotherapy for military-related PTSD reports that "the most frequently studied psychotherapies for military-related PTSD" result in positive changes, but that most of those treated "retained their PTSD diagnosis after treatment (range, 60%–72%)": M. M. Steenkamp, B. T. Litz, C. W. Hoge, and C. R. Marmar, "Psychotherapy for Military-related PTSD: A Review of Randomized Clinical Trials," *Journal of the American Medical Association* 314, no. 5 (2015): 489–500.

In contrast, the one rigorous randomized study of EMDR therapy with Vietnam veterans (according to the 2000 *Practice Guidelines of the International Society for Traumatic Stress Studies*) reported a 78 percent elimination of PTSD and a zero drop-out rate: J. Carlson, C. M. Chemtob, K. Rusnak, N. L. Hedlund, and M. Y. Muraoka, "Eye Movement Desensitization and Reprocessing (EMDR): Treatment for Combat-Related Post-Traumatic Stress Disorder," *Journal of Traumatic Stress* 11 (1998): 3–24.

Similarly positive results were reported with EMDR treatment of recent war veterans and active military: M. C. Russell, S. M. Silver, S. Rogers, and J. Darnell, "Responding to an Identified Need: A Joint Department of Defense–Department of Veterans Affairs Training Program in Eye Movement Desensitization and Reprocessing (EMDR) for Clinicians Providing Trauma Services," *International Journal of Stress Management* 14 (2007): 61–71.

7. E. W. McCranie, L. A. Hyer, P. A. Boudewyns, and M. G. Woods, "Negative Parenting Behavior, Combat Exposure, and PTSD Symptom Severity," *Journal of Nervous and Mental Disease* 180 (1992): 431–438.

8. Earlier in this session, Eric had reported a moderate level of fear around his recollection of calling in the artillery, just as he had the very first time we worked on it. However, the fear had changed. This fear was about his inability to remember many of the details of that night. It was linked to yet another fear: that he might have done something else, something that he didn't remember. When Eric and I next targeted his memory of being blown up by the grenade, it carried the same fear because Eric could not remember exactly what had happened; there was intense fear locked into the experience because he couldn't foresee the results. Once he had resolved his fear from the grenade memory, we went back and retargeted his memory about calling in the artillery. What we found was another generalization effect: The artillery memory had dropped from a 6 to "a 1 or a 2"; then it appeared to be completely resolved. The intricate association between different memories and emotions and between memories and behavior is also illustrated by the fact that Eric's nightmares stopped after the first session of EMDR treatment. This was because his two major memories of having been the cause of "unnecessary" death had been processed.

Chapter 4, pp. 63–79
The Fabric of Treatment: Uncovering the Hidden Depths of Pain

1. F. Shapiro, *Eye Movement Desensitization and Reprocessing: Basic Principles, Protocols, and Procedures* (New York: Guilford Press, 2001).

2. On the other hand, the presence of these conditions does not automatically rule out the use of EMDR therapy. One woman I worked with was pregnant but terrified of giving birth. When we discussed her history, we discovered that her fear stemmed from her childhood. She was the eldest of eight children, and having her own baby was connected in her mind with becoming prematurely old like her mother. In two EMDR processing sessions, we resolved this woman's fear, and she proceeded to have a peaceful pregnancy and uneventful birth. Likewise, cardiac patients who live with the constant stress of unresolved trauma might be better off using EMDR at the risk of temporarily increasing their stress rather than continuing to live with the daily strain that unhealed trauma can put on the heart. In fact, EMDR therapy was used to treat the negative psychological effects of those undergoing cardiac rehabilitation: E. Arabia, M. L. Manca, and R. M. Solomon, "EMDR for Survivors of Life-Threatening Cardiac Events: Results of a Pilot Study," *Journal of EMDR Practice and Research* 5 (2011): 2–13.

3. R. Stickgold, "EMDR: A Putative Neurobiological Mechanism of Action," *Journal of Clinical Psychology* 58 (2002): 61–75.

4. How do therapists know when someone has a damaging belief locked in his nervous system? We evaluate the behavior. We search the person's history and notice which past events still provoke strong emotional or physical reactions. For instance, take a moment and bring up a memory from more than ten years ago that still causes you distress. Do you feel some of the emotions and sensations that were there at the time? What thoughts come up about yourself? If you examine them closely, you may find that these thoughts incorporate negative self-beliefs that will explain the negative responses you may be having in similar situations in the present. This memory and its resulting negative beliefs have not yet been effectively processed.

Chapter 5, pp. 81–104
The Many Faces of Fear: Phobias and Panic Attacks

1. I. P. Pavlov, *Conditioned Reflexes* (New York: Liveright, 1927).

2. J. Wolpe, *The Practice of Behavior Therapy* (New York: Pergamon Press, 1990).

3. D. Wilson, S. M. Silver, W. Covi, and S. Foster, "Eye Movement Desensitization and Reprocessing: Effectiveness and Autonomic Correlates," *Journal of Behavior Therapy and Experimental Psychiatry* 27 (1996): 219–229. See Appendix B for a long list of comparable studies reporting a decrease in physical and/or emotional arousal.

4. American Psychiatric Association, *Diagnostic and Statistical Manual of Mental Disorders* (Washington, DC: American Psychiatric Association, 2013). Social phobias constitute 10 to 20 percent of anxiety disorders. However, for a diagnosis of social phobia, such as fear of public speaking, the fear must interfere with the person's normal routine. Many people do not have their lives interrupted sufficiently for the problem to be designated as a phobia. For instance, one community-based study found that although 20 percent of participants reported an excessive fear of performance or public speaking, only 2 percent suffered enough life impairment to be diagnosed as phobic. Nonetheless, as we have seen, the absence of a diagnosis does not make the symptoms any less intense.

5. S. Doering, M. C. Ohlmeier, A. de Jongh, A. Hofmann, and V. Bisping, "Efficacy of a Trauma-Focused Treatment Approach for Dental Phobia: A Randomized Clinical Trial," *European Journal of Oral Sciences* 121 (2013): 584–593.

6. "Wiped Right Off the Map," *Time*, 18 June 1984, 30.

7. C. Tamarkin, "Tornado," *People Weekly*, 9 July 1984, 24–31.

8. For instructions on self-use of a wide range of relaxation techniques, see F. Shapiro, *Getting Past Your Past: Take Control of Your Life with Self-Help Techniques from EMDR Therapy* (New York: Rodale, 2012).

Chapter 6, pp. 105–125
When Terror Stalks the Night:
Sleep Disorders and Childhood Trauma

1. R. J. Ross, W. A. Ball, N. B. Kribbs, A. R. Morrison, S. M. Silver, and F. D. Mulvanye, "Rapid Eye Movement Sleep Disturbance in Posttraumatic Stress Disorder," *Biological Psychiatry* 35 (1994): 195–202.

R. J. Ross, W. A. Ball, K. A. Sullivan, and S. N. Caroff, "Sleep Disturbance as the Hallmark of Posttraumatic Stress Disorder," *American Journal of Psychiatry* 146 (1989): 697–707.

As a matter a fact, Pierre Janet, a contemporary of Freud, described intrusive PTSD phenomena as "somnambulistic crises": See B. S. van der Kolk and O. van der Hart, "Pierre Janet and the Breakdown of Adaptation in Psychological Trauma," *American Journal of Psychiatry* 146 (1989): 1530–1540.

2. E. Aserinsky and N. Kleitman, "Regularly Occurring Periods of Eye Motility and Concomitant Phenomena During Sleep," *Science* 118 (1953): 273–274.

O. Van Reeth, L. Weibel, K. Spiegel, R. Leproult, C. Dugovic, and S. Maccari, "Physiology of Sleep (Review)–Interactions Between Stress and Sleep: From Basic Research to Clinical Situations," *Sleep Medicine Reviews* 4, no. 2 (2000): 201–219.

3. E. Aserinsky and N. Kleitman, "Regularly Occurring Periods of Eye Motility and Concomitant Phenomena During Sleep," *Science* 118 (1953): 273–274.

4. See M. L. Perlis and T. A. Nielsen, "Mood Regulation, Dreaming and Nightmares: Evaluation of a Desensitization Function for REM Sleep," *Dreaming* 3 (1993): 243–257.

5. D. Wilson, S. M. Silver, W. Covi, and S. Foster, "Eye Movement Desensitization and Reprocessing: Effectiveness and Autonomic Correlates," *Journal of Behavior Therapy and Experimental Psychiatry* 27 (1996): 219–229.

U. O. E. Elofsson, B. von Scheele, T. Theorell, and H. P. Sondergaard, "Physiological Correlates of Eye Movement Desensitization and Reprocessing," *Journal of Anxiety Disorders* 22 (2008): 622–634.

6. A. N. Goldstein and M. P. Walker, "The Role of Sleep in Emotional Brain Function," *Annual Review of Clinical Psychology* 10 (2014): 679–708.

R. Benca, W. Obermeyer, R. Thisled, and J. Gillin, "Sleep and Psychiatric Disorders: Meta-Analysis," *Archives of General Psychiatry* 49 (1992): 651–668. The increase in anxiety is particularly interesting, as is the apparent effect on memory consolidation. See also A. Karni, D. Tanne, B. S. Rubenstein, J. J. Askenasi, and D. Sagi, "No Dreams, No Memory: The Effect of REM Sleep Deprivation on Learning a New Perceptual Skill," *Society for Neuroscience Abstracts* 18 (1992): 387; M. J. McGrath and D. B. Cohen, "REM Sleep Facilitation of Adaptive Waking Behavior: A Review of the Literature," *Psychological Bulletin* 85 (1978): 24–57. However, REM deprivation does not generally cause psychosis, as popular myth would have it.

7. S. Freud, *The Interpretation of Dreams* (New York: Penguin Books, 1900/1953).

8. J. A. Hobson and R. W. McCarley, "The Brain as a Dream State Generator: An Activation-Synthesis Hypothesis of the Dream Process," *American Journal of Psychiatry* 134 (1977): 1334–1338.

9. J. A. Hobson, *Sleep* (San Francisco: Freeman, 1989).

10. J. Winson, "The Meaning of Dreams," *Scientific American* 262 (1990): 86–96.

J. Winson, "The Biology and Function of Rapid Eye Movement Sleep," *Current Opinion in Neurobiology* 3 (1993): 243–248.

11. M. Nishida, J. Pearsall, R. L. Buckner, and M. P. Walker, "REM Sleep, Prefrontal Theta, and the Consolidation of Human Emotional Memory," *Cerebral Cortex* 19, no. 5 (2009): 1158–1166.

Winson noted that the rapid eye movements in both the waking state and during REM may reflect complementary information processing functions. See J. Winson, "The Meaning of Dreams," *Scientific American* 262 (1990): 86–96.

12. A. N. Goldstein and M. P. Walker, "The Role of Sleep in Emotional Brain Function," *Annual Review of Clinical Psychology* 10 (2014): 679–708.

M. Nishida, J. Pearsall, R. L. Buckner, and M. P. Walker, "REM Sleep, Prefrontal Theta, and the Consolidation of Human Emotional Memory," *Cerebral Cortex* 19, no. 5 (2009): 1158–1166.

13. A. Karni, D. Tanne, B. S. Rubenstein, J. J. Askenasi, and D. Sagi, "No Dreams, No Memory: The Effect of REM Sleep Deprivation on Learning a New Perceptual Skill," *Society for Neuroscience Abstracts* 18 (1992): 387.

M. J. McGrath and D. B. Cohen, "REM Sleep Facilitation of Adaptive Waking Behavior: A Review of the Literature," *Psychological Bulletin* 85 (1978): 24–57.

14. E. J. Wamsley and R. Stickgold, "Dreaming and Offline Memory Processing," *Current Biology* 20, no. 23 (2010): R1010–1013.

E. J. Wamsley, M. Tucker, J. D. Payne, J. A. Benavides, and R. Stickgold, "Dreaming of a Learning Task Is Associated with Enhanced Sleep-Dependent Memory Consolidation," *Current Biology* 20, no. 9 (2010): 850–855.

15. B. A. van der Kolk, "The Body Keeps the Score: Memory and the Evolving Psychobiology of Posttraumatic Stress Disorder," *Harvard Review of Psychiatry* 1 (1994): 253–265.

It is also interesting to note that spontaneous saccadic eye movements have been found to cause significant activation in the hippocampus in monkeys. See J. L. Ringo, S. Sobotka, M. D. Diltz, and C. M. Bunce, "Eye Movements Modulate Activity in Hippocampal, Parahippocampal, and Inferotemporal Neurons," *Journal of Neurophysiology* 71 (1994): 1285–1288.

16. P. Roffwarg, J. N. Muzio, and W. C. Dement, "Ontogenic Development of the Human Sleep-Dream Cycle," *Science* 152 (1966): 604–619.

17. B. A. van der Kolk and R. E. Fisler, "Childhood Abuse and Neglect and Loss of Self-Regulation," *Bulletin of the Menninger Clinic* 58 (1994): 145–168.

18. J. E. LeDoux, "Emotion, Memory, and the Brain," *Scientific American*, June 1994, 50–57. There is no doubt that children need to be taught the skills of "self-soothing." However, this is not the same as simply ignoring the baby's cries.

J. E. LeDoux, *The Emotional Brain: The Mysterious Underpinnings of Emotional Life* (New York: Simon and Schuster, 1998).

A whole generation of baby boomers was raised by mothers who were told to feed their children at certain hours and not respond to their cries. I find the image of thousands of children crying alone in the dark particularly haunting, and I wonder about the possible psychological and sociological effects. Certainly many people I have known through the years have evoked the image of "crying alone in the dark" to describe their most traumatic losses and fears. Sometimes it has helped to point out that we are all there together, feeling alone in the dark.

19. P. D. MacLean, *A Triune Concept of the Brain and Behavior* (Toronto, Canada: University of Toronto Press, 1978).

B. A. van der Kolk, *The Body Keeps the Score: Brain, Mind, and Body in the Healing of Trauma* (New York: Viking, 2014).

20. J. C. Pearce, *Evolution's End* (San Francisco: HarperCollins, 1993).

21. M. Kramer, "The Nightmare: A Failure in Dream Function," *Dreaming* 1 (1991): 277–285.

22. See M. L. Perlis and T. A. Nielsen, "Mood Regulation, Dreaming and Nightmares: Evaluation of a Desensitization Function for REM Sleep," *Dreaming* 3 (1993): 243–257.

23. J. Gibson, "Nightmares and Night Terrors," *Parents* 66 (1991): 159.

J. Rosemond, "Night Terrors," *Better Homes and Gardens* 71 (1991): 38.

M. Sacks, "In Dread of Night," *San Jose Mercury News*, 23 January 1966, 1461D–1462D.

24. See B. A. van der Kolk and R. E. Fisler, "Childhood Abuse and Neglect and Loss of Self-Regulation," *Bulletin of the Menninger Clinic* 58 (1994): 145–168.

25. After reading the earlier section in this chapter on REM sleep, the reader must be saying, "So, if you can use tones and taps, the REM hypothesis must be wrong." However, that is not necessarily the case. A variety of studies have supported the REM-EMDR connection (see Appendix B). Additionally, the fact that other kinds of stimuli can be used does not necessarily mean that the same processes that occur in REM are not being stimulated. In other words, the body in sleep is incapable of generating external tones or taps. Because of motor neuron inhibition, the eye movements are all that can be freely generated physiologically. Clearly, we have other choices in the waking state. The task is to stimulate the cortical functions that are necessary to process the disturbing material. Numerous research studies (see Appendix B) have now indicated that the cortical functions are activated by the process of dual attention, regardless of

the nature of the alternate stimuli. It appears that both the orienting response and the taxing of working memory come into play with bilateral eye movements, taps, or tones. The research indicates that the eye movements are most effective and should be the first choice. However, it is good to have the taps or tones as alternatives in cases such as Davy's.

26. See F. Shapiro, *Eye Movement Desensitization and Reprocessing: Basic Principles, Protocols and Procedures* (New York: Guilford Press, 2001).

27. See R. A. Drake, "Processing Persuasive Arguments: Recall and Recognition as a Function of Agreement and Manipulated Activation Asymmetry," *Brain and Cognition* 15 (1993): 83–94.

28. Split-brain research over the years has pointed out differences in function, memory processing, and storage relegated to the different hemispheres. See R. Joseph, *The Right Brain and the Unconscious* (New York: Plenum Press, 1992). The alternating attention used in EMDR may allow for the accelerated integration of function, memory, and adaptive effects.

Chapter 7, pp. 127–149
The Ties That Bind: Disorders of Attachment

1. A. Anastasi, "Heredity, Environment, and the Question 'How?'" *Psychological Review* 65 (1958): 197–208.

L. Eisenberg, "The Social Construction of the Human Brain," *American Journal of Psychiatry* 152 (1995): 1563–1575.

2. F. J. Kallmann, *The Genetics of Schizophrenia* (New York: Augustin, 1938). F. J. Kallmann, "The Genetic Theory of Schizophrenia: An Analysis of 691 Schizophrenic Twin Index Families," *American Journal of Psychiatry* 103 (1946): 309–322.

3. The majority of people who develop schizophrenia have no close family member with the disorder. Additionally, if genetics were completely responsible for schizophrenia, we would find a high concordance rate in monozygotic twins (that is, if one twin had it, the other would, too). Although the concordance rate is higher than in the average population or in dizygotic twins, it is less than 30 percent. Factors other than heredity are clearly involved.

M. L. Kohn, "Social Class and Schizophrenia: A Critical Review and a Reformulation," *Schizophrenia Bulletin* 7 (1973): 60–79.

D. Rosenthal, "The Heredity-Environment Issue in Schizophrenia: Summary of the Conference and Present State of Our Knowledge," in *The Transmission of Schizophrenia*, ed. D. Rosenthal and S. S. Kety (Oxford, England: Pergamon Press, 1968).

Schizophrenia in psychosis is not only hereditary:

J. van Os, G. Kenis, and B. P. Rutten, "The Environment and Schizophrenia," *Nature* 468, no. 7321(2010): 203–212, doi:10.1038/nature0956.

Trauma is highly prevalent in patients with psychotic disorders:

S. L. Matheson, A. M. Shepherd, R. M. Pinchbeck, K. R. Laurens, and V. J. Carr, "Childhood Adversity in Schizophrenia: A Systematic Meta-Analysis," *Psychological Medicine* 43, no. 2 (2013): 225–238, doi:10.1017/S0033291712000785.

Trauma is associated with an increased risk of developing psychotic disorders:

T. Kraan, E. Velthorst, F. Smit, L. de Haan, and M. van der Gaag, "Trauma and Recent Life Events in Individuals at Ultra High Risk for Psychosis: Review and Meta-Analysis," *Schizophrenia Research* (2014), doi:10.1016/j.schres.2014.11.026.

Trauma was found to be an important cause of psychosis. If we eliminated childhood trauma, there would be 33 percent fewer people with psychotic disorders:

F. Varese et al., "Childhood Adversities Increase the Risk of Psychosis: A Meta-Analysis of Patient-Control, Prospective-and Cross-Sectional Cohort Studies," *Schizophrenia Bulletin* 38, no. 4 (2012): 661–671, doi:10.1093/schbul/sbs05.

4. A. J. Sameroff, R. Seifer, and M. Zax, "Early Development of Children at Risk for Emotional Disorder," in *Monographs of the Society for Research in Child Development*, vol. 47, no. 7 (Chicago: University of Chicago Press, 1982).

Childhood trauma was found to be a cause of psychosis, independent of genetic liability, in a sample of people with a genetic risk for psychosis:

J. A. Husted, R. Ahmed, E. W. Chow, L. M. Brzustowicz, and A. S. Bassett, "Childhood Trauma and Genetic Factors in Familial Schizophrenia Associated with the NOS1AP Gene," *Schizophrenia Research* 121, no. 1–3 (2010): 187–192, doi:10.1016/j.schres.2010.05.021.

PTSD is one of the most common co-morbidities in psychosis:

A. M. Achim, M. Maziade, E. Raymond, D. Olivier, C. Mérette, and M. A. Roy, "How Prevalent Are Anxiety Disorders in Schizophrenia? A Meta-Analysis and Critical Review on a Significant Association," *Schizophrenia Bulletin* 37, no. 4 (2011): 811–821, doi:10.1093/schbul /sbp148.

5. D. P. G. van den Berg and M. van den Gaag, "Treating Trauma in Psychosis with EMDR: A Pilot Study," *Journal of Behavior Therapy and Experimental Psychiatry* 43 (2012): 664–671.

6. A. J. DeCasper and M. J. Spence, "Prenatal Maternal Speech Influences Newborns' Perceptions of Speech Sounds," *Infant Behavior and Development* 9 (1986): 133–150. Uterine environment can also have a direct effect on motivation and behavior; for instance, it has been found that newborn French babies suck harder to hear French than another language. J. Mehler, P. W. Jusczyk, and G. Lambertz, "A Precursor to Language Development in Young Infants," *Cognition* 291 (1988): 143–178.

7. Some of his susceptibility to stress might have been caused by an acute sensitivity to certain conditions because of the fetal alcohol effect.

8. S. H. Dinwiddie and C. R. Cloninger, "Family and Adoption Studies in Alcoholism and Drug Addiction," *Psychiatric Annals* 21 (1991): 206–214.

K. S. Kendler, A. C. Heath, M. C. Neale, R. C. Kessler, and L. J. Eaves, "A Population-Based Twin Study of Alcoholism in Women," *Journal of the American Medical Association* 268 (1992): 1877–1882.

M. Potenza, "Biological Contributions to Addictions in Adolescents and Adults: Prevention, Treatment and Policy Implications," *Journal of Adolescent Health* 52, no. 202 (2013): S22–S32.

9. R. F. Anda et al., "The Enduring Effects of Abuse and Related Adverse Experiences in Childhood: A Convergence of Evidence from Neurobiology and Epidemiology," *European Archives of Psychiatry and Clinical Neuroscience* 256 (2006): 174–186.

10. D. M. Bullard, H. H. Glaser, M. C. Heagarty, and E. C. Pivcheck, "Failure to Thrive in the Neglected Child," *American Journal of Orthopsychiatry* 37 (1967): 680–690.

L. Lander, J. Howsare, and M. Byrne, "The Impact of Substance Use Disorders on Family and Children: From Theory to Practice," *Social Work Public Health* 28 (2013): 194–205.

11. S. Boon, K. Steele, and O. van der Hart, *Coping with Trauma-Related Dissociation* (New York: W.W. Norton, 2011).

12. Although in this case Joan is directing a statement at Ashley at the same time that she is leading the eye movements, this is not the same as using hypnosis. During hypnosis, EEG readings indicate that there is an increase in beta and theta waves, which have been associated with an increase in suggestibility: M. E. Sabourin, S. D. Cutcomb, H. J. Crawford, and K. Pribram, "EEG Correlates of Hypnotic Susceptibility and Hypnotic Trance: Spectral Analysis

and Coherence," *International Journal of Psychophysiology* 10, no. 2 (1990): 125–142. Stage hypnotists can make people bark like a dog or act like a chicken. However, EEG readings of people during EMDR therapy do not show that brain wave pattern. EMDR clients show brain waves that are within normal waking parameters. In EMDR processing, the person remains completely conscious and is actually less suggestible than usual to information that is not correct. The statement that Joan made was true. Had it been otherwise, Ashley would have gotten upset and rejected it. Reports from clinicians using EMDR with thousands of clients over the decades continue to indicate that this is true. EMDR therapy will not interfere with appropriate beliefs or feelings, and it will not cause the person to believe anything that is not true.

Chapter 8, pp. 151–167
Healing the Ravages of Rape

1. M. Amir, *Patterns in Forcible Rape* (Chicago: University of Chicago Press, 1971).

J. V. Becker and G. G. Abel, "The Treatment of Victims of Sexual Assault," *Quarterly Journal of Corrections* 1 (1977): 38–42.

A. W. Burgess, "Rape Trauma Syndrome," *Behavioral Science and the Law* 1 (1983): 97–113.

D. Chappell, G. Geis, and F. Fogarty, "Forcible Rape: Bibliography," *Journal of Criminal Law and Criminology* 65 (1974): 248–263.

E. Midlarsky, *Women, Psychopathology, and Psychotherapy: A Partially Annotated Bibliography* (Journal Supplement Abstract Service, ms. 1472, American Psychological Association, 1977).

S. Schafer, *The Victim and His Criminal* (New York: Random House, 1968).

H. von Hentig, *The Criminal and His Victim* (New Haven, Conn.: Yale University Press, 1948).

2. A. W. Burgess and L. L. Holmstrom, "Rape Trauma Syndrome," *Archives of General Psychiatry* 13 (1974): 981–986.

M. A. Largen, "History of the Women's Movement in Changing Attitudes, Laws, and Treatment Toward Rape Victims," in *Sexual Assault*, eds. M. J. Walker and S. L. Brodsky (Lexington, MA: Heath, 1976).

3. American Psychiatric Association, *Diagnostic and Statistical Manual of Mental Disorders*, 3rd ed., rev. (Washington, DC: American Psychiatric Association, 1987).

4. S. D. Solomon, E. T. Gerrity, and A. M. Muff, "Efficacy of Treatments for Posttraumatic Stress Disorder," *Journal of the American Medical Association* 268 (1992): 633–638.

5. D. G. Kilpatrick, L. J. Veronen, and C. L. Best, "Factors Predicting Psychological Distress Among Rape Victims," in *Trauma and Its Wake*, ed. C. R. Figley (New York: Brunner/Mazel, 1985).

M. P. Koss, "Implications for the Clinical Treatment of Victims," *Clinical Psychologist* 36 (1983): 88–91.

6. D. G. Kilpatrick and H. S. Resnick, "PTSD Associated with Exposure to Criminal Victimization in Clinical and Community Populations," in *Posttraumatic Stress Disorder: DSM IV and Beyond*, ed. J. R. T. Davidson and E. B. Foa (Washington, DC: American Psychiatric Press, 1993).

7. M. Black et al., *The National Intimate Partner and Sexual Violence Survey (NISVS): 2010 Summary Report* (Atlanta: National Center for Injury Prevention and Control, Centers for Disease Control and Prevention, 2011).

8. C. Krebs et al., *Campus Climate Survey Validation Study: Final Technical Report*, Bureau of Justice Statistics Research and Development Series R&DP-2015:04 (Washington, DC: Bureau of Justice Statistics, 2016).

9. A. W. Burgess and L. L. Holmstrom, "Adaptive Strategies and Recovery from Rape," *American Journal of Psychiatry* 136 (1979): 1278–1282.

B. L. Green, "Psychosocial Research in Traumatic Stress: An Update," *Journal of Traumatic Stress* 7 (1994): 341–362.

T. W. McCahill, L. C. Meyer, and A. M. Fishman, *The Aftermath of Rape* (Lexington, MA: Heath, 1979).

10. Spontaneous remission is recovery that occurs without treatment, usually within one to three months after the trauma.

D. G. Kilpatrick, L. J. Veronen, and P. A. Resick, "The Aftermath of Rape: Recent Empirical Findings," *American Journal of Orthopsychiatry* 49 (1979): 658–659.

11. B. O. Rothbaum, "A Controlled Study of Eye Movement Desensitization and Reprocessing in the Treatment of Post-Traumatic Stress Disordered Sexual Assault Victims," *Bulletin of the Menninger Clinic* 61 (1997): 317–334.

When multiple traumatized rape victims were treated, EMDR therapy did equally as well as exposure therapy, with less exposure to the memory and no homework:

B. O. Rothbaum, M. C. Astin, and F. Marsteller, "Prolonged Exposure Versus Eye Movement Desensitization (EMDR) for PTSD Rape Victims," *Journal of Traumatic Stress* 18 (2005): 607–616.

12. R. Janoff-Bulman, *Shattered Assumptions* (New York: Free Press, 1992).

13. J. L. Krupnick and M. J. Horowitz, "Stress Response Syndromes: Recurrent Themes," *Archives of General Psychiatry* 38 (1981): 428–435.

14. B. A. van der Kolk, "The Body Keeps the Score: Memory and the Evolving Psychobiology of Posttraumatic Stress," *Harvard Review of Psychiatry* 1 (1994): 253–265.

15. S. A. Wilson, L. A. Becker, and R. H. Tinker, "Eye Movement Desensitization and Reprocessing (EMDR) Treatment for Psychologically Traumatized Individuals," *Journal of Consulting and Clinical Psychology* 63 (1995): 928–937.

S. A. Wilson, L. A. Becker, and R. H. Tinker, "15-Month Follow-Up of Eye Movement Desensitization and Reprocessing (EMDR) Treatment for Psychological Trauma," *Journal of Consulting and Clinical Psychology*, 65 (1997): 1047–1056.

Chapter 9, pp. 169–197
Laying Grief to Rest

1. G. Everley, ed., *Innovations in Disaster and Trauma Psychology* (Elliot City, MD: Chevron Publishing, 1995).

2. EMDR is now being employed by many police department psychologists in the United States. However, it is often not used immediately after a homicide because EMDR treatment sometimes causes the image of the event to fade or permanently disappear. Although the client knows what happened, this dimming or changing of the traumatic image can conflict with the need for the police officers to testify in court and give a detailed description of the original crime scene. Even though emotional resolution may be available to the police through EMDR, they may have to continue to suffer until the trial process is complete. The possibility of the picture fading and the emotions resolving as a result of EMDR treatment also needs to be taken into account concerning potential court witnesses.

3. The problems of emergency personnel and frontline providers are often dramatically increased when the deceased or injured person resembles a loved one.

4. S. Zisook and R. DeVaul, "Grief, Unresolved Grief, and Depression," *Psychosomatics* 24 (1983): 247–256.

5. T. Rando, *Treatment of Complicated Mourning* (Champaign, IL: Research Press, 2000). This excellent volume gives a comprehensive overview of both complicated and uncomplicated bereavement and the phases of healing. The use of EMDR does not take away anything the bereaved needs to remember or go through. The phases of healing and six major processes of mourning described by Dr. Rando unfold fully and naturally, as seen in the transcript presented in this chapter.

6. Mia has verbalized a very profound realization. It should be emphasized, however, that it has been found, both clinically and empirically, that the death of one's child is the most difficult of losses with which one can cope—greater than the loss of any other family member. There is no doubt that it presents the highest risk for complicated bereavement. However, the accommodation of the loss can be achieved. After Mia was healed and connected with her spiritual resources, she could see that all the connections were there and could be at peace with the "why" of it. EMDR therapy does not merely "desensitize" the pain—it reprocesses the experience. I have heard another mother verbalize her realization by saying, "I feel him in my heart. I'm so grateful for the time we had together. He's in a better place."

Chapter 10, pp. 199–223
Breaking the Iron Grasp of Addiction

1. J. Davidson, D. Hughes, D. Blazer, and L. George, "Post-Traumatic Stress Disorder in the Community: An Epidemiological Study," *Psychological Medicine* 21 (1991): 713–721.

S. R. Dube, R. F. Anda, V. J. Felitti, D. P. Chapman, D. F. Williamson, and W. H. Giles, "Childhood Abuse, Household Dysfunction, and the Risk of Attempted Suicide Throughout the Life Span: Findings from the Adverse Childhood Experiences Study," *Journal of the American Medical Association* 286 (2001): 3089–3096.

M. Ystgaard, I. Hestetun, M. Loeb, and L. Mehlum, "Is There a Specific Relationship Between Childhood Sexual and Physical Abuse and Repeated Suicidal Behavior?" *Child Abuse and Neglect* 28, no. 8(2004): 863–875.

2. For instance, studies indicate that approximately 75 percent of combat PTSD victims are also serious substance abusers. Different populations of PTSD victims have varying rates. However, according to several studies, 50 percent of combat and sexual assault victims who have developed PTSD continue to suffer from the disorder. In fact, there is a 9-percent lifetime prevalence of PTSD in the general population of the United States. Victims often try to cope by self-administering substances, such as alcohol, cocaine, amphetamines, heroin, or even food, to try to quiet the pain. For a discussion of pertinent studies, see B. L. Green, "Psychosocial Research in Traumatic Stress: An Update," *Journal of Traumatic Stress* 7 (1994): 341–362. In addition, an examination of the relationship between illicit drug use and ten categories of adverse childhood experiences (ACEs) revealed that each ACE reported increased the likelihood for early initiation (of illicit drug use) two- to fourfold. Compared with people with no ACEs, people with five or more ACEs were seven to ten times more likely to report illicit drug use problems: S. R. Dube, V. J. Felitti, M. Dong, D. P. Chapman, W. H. Giles, and R. F. Anda, "Childhood Abuse, Neglect, and Household Dysfunction and the Risk of Illicit Drug Use: The Adverse Childhood Experiences Study," *Pediatrics* 111 (2003): 564–572.

R. C. Kessler, C. B. Nelson, K. A. McGonagle, M. J. Edlund, R. G. Frank, and P. J. Leaf, "The Epidemiology of Co-occurring Addictive and Mental Disorders: Implications for Prevention and Service Utilization," *American Journal of Orthopsychiatry* 66, no. 1 (2010): 17–31.

For an excellent overview of the relationship between trauma and substance abuse, see J. E. Zweben, W. Clark, and D. E. Smith, "Traumatic Experiences and Substance Abuse: Mapping the Territory," *Journal of Psychoactive Drugs* 26 (1994): 327–344.

3. S. Brown, "Alcoholism and Trauma: A Theoretical Overview and Comparison," *Journal of Psychoactive Drugs* 26 (1994): 345–355.

R. F. Anda, V. J. Felitti, J. Walker, C. L. Whitfield, J. D. Bremner, B. D. Perry, S. R. Dube, and W. H. Giles, "The Enduring Effects of Abuse and Related Adverse Experiences in Childhood: A Convergence of Evidence from Neurobiology and Epidemiology," *European Archives of Psychiatry and Clinical Neurosciences* 256 (2006): 174–186.

V. J. Felitti, R. F. Anda, D. Nordenberg, D. F. Williamson, A. M. Spitz, V. Edwards, and M. P. Koss, "The Relationship of Adult Health Status to Childhood Abuse and Household Dysfunction," *American Journal of Preventive Medicine* 14, no. 4 (1998): 245–258.

4. D. Goodwin, "Is Alcoholism Hereditary?" *Archives of General Psychiatry* 25 (1971): 545–549.

M. A. Schuckit and J. Duby, "Alcohol-Related Flushing and the Risk for Alcoholism in the Sons of Alcoholics," *Journal of Clinical Psychiatry* 43 (1982): 415–518.

M. A. Schuckit, "Genetics of the Risk for Alcoholism," *American Journal on Addictions* 2 (2000): 103–112.

5. C. R. Cloninger, "Genetic and Environmental Factors in the Development of Alcoholism," *Journal of Psychiatric Treatment Evaluation* (special issue on alcoholism, ed. S. Blume, 1983).

H. J. Shaffer, D. A. La Plante, R. A. LaBrie, R. C. Kidman, A. N. Donato, and M. V. Stanton, "Toward a Syndrome Model of Addiction: Multiple Expressions, Common Etiology," *Harvard Review of Psychiatry* 12 (2004): 367–374.

6. Silke had formally diagnosed Amy as having avoidant personality disorder. A personality disorder is a condition in which a person has developed long-standing dysfunctional traits or patterns of behavior to minimize pain. For instance, although everyone fears rejection, Amy's severe sensitivity prevented her from entering into any relationship until she was one hundred percent sure she would not be rebuffed. Amy's long history of depression is also an aspect of avoidant personality disorder and one of the usual handmaidens to substance abuse.

7. Adaptive information processing means that accelerated learning is taking place. We use EMDR processing to help teach people new skills and behaviors to prepare them for the future. After the clinician makes sure the client intellectually understands the concepts and reasons for the behavior, the client imagines taking the needed steps during successive sets of eye movements. When the situation occurs in real life, the client is better prepared to handle it.

8. D. Finklehor and D. Dziuba-Leatherman, "Victimization of Children," *American Psychologist* 49 (1994): 173–183.

B. E. Molnar, S. L. Buka, and R. C. Kessler, "Child Sexual Abuse and Subsequent Psychopathology: Results from the National Comorbidity Survey," *American Journal of Public Health* 91, no. 5 (2001): 753.

D. Finklehor, G. Hotaling, I. A. Lewis, and C. Smith, "Sexual Abuse in a National Survey of Adult Men and Women: Prevalence, Characteristics, and Risk Factors," *Child Abuse and Neglect* 14 (1990): 191–228. This national survey indicated that 16 percent of adult men and 27 percent of adult women experienced child sexual abuse. The prevalence of sexual abuse has been complicated by the current debate raging over the reliability of memory. It is true that clients can be misled by clinicians who give them inaccurate information about the infallibility of their memories. In fact, no emerging "memory" or image of a previously forgotten, long-past abuse can be considered historically accurate without external corroboration. However, clients can also be misled by perpetrators who deny that the abuse occurred. Sometimes the denial is sincere, because the abuse occurred during an alcoholic blackout or other dissociated state. When completely sober, the perpetrator can't imagine having done it and reacts to the accusation with righteous indignation. Substance abuse is often a cause of violence, and it can easily become an effect. A continued chain of violence and assault can develop, which sets up the next generation for the same problems. Fortunately, in EMDR therapy it is not necessary to know whether a memory is historically accurate or not. It is only necessary to reprocess images that are disturbing to the client. The memory may be accurate, or the product of vicarious traumatization, or outright error. Regardless of the validity, the goal is to remove its negative influence on the client.

9. C. Downing, "Surrender to Powerlessness and Its Relationship to Relapse in Recovering Alcoholics" (PhD diss., Saybrook Institute, San Francisco, 1991). Cited in R. H. Kitchen, "Relapse Therapy," *EMDR Newsletter* 1 (1991): 4–6.

M. Farley, J. M. Golding, G. Young, M. Mulligan, and J. R. Minkoff, "Trauma History and Relapse Probability Among Patients Seeking Substance Abuse Treatment," *Journal of Substance Abuse Treatment*, 27, no. 2 (2004):161–167.

10. R. Z. Goldstein and N. D. Volkow, "Dysfunction of the Prefrontal Cortex in Addiction: Neuroimaging Findings and Clinical Implications," *Nature Reviews Neuroscience* 12, no. 11 (2011):652–669.

A. Parsegian and R. E. See, "Dysregulation of Dopamine and Glutamate Release in the Prefrontal Cortex and Nucleus Accumbens Following Methamphetamine Self-Administration and During Reinstatement in Rats," *Neuropsychopharmacology* 39, no. 4 (2013): 811–822.

11. Processing pivotal "addiction memories" with EMDR therapy is also showing excellent results: M. Hase, S. Schallmayer, and M. Sack, "EMDR Reprocessing of the Addiction Memory: Pretreatment, Post-Treatment, and 1-month Follow Up," *Journal of EMDR Practice and Research* 2, no. 3 (2008): 170–179.

Chapter 11, pp. 225–246
The Final Doorway: Facing Disease, Disability, and Death

1. At the heart of every traumatic experience is a sense of horror and even a fear of death. Regardless of the obvious reasons for many of our most disturbing reactions of anxiety, anger, or distress, from an evolutionary point of view it all seems to boil down to a primal fear that somehow our very survival is at stake. This fear appears to be operating even in situations that objectively don't threaten our lives. How else can we explain the intense reactions we felt being humiliated in grade school or being left at summer camp? If we lose a job, why do we see ourselves starving under a bridge? If we lose a relationship, why do we assume that we will die alone and unloved? Could it be that built into our physiology is a survival alarm that goes off anytime our well-being is threatened? Once, being cut out of the herd meant death; perhaps any parallel experience sets off an equivalent emotional response. This is all highly speculative; however, nothing brings up fear of death more clearly than severe physical injury and disease. Although technically disease sufferers cannot be clinically diagnosed with PTSD unless the physical situation is life-threatening, the

psychological consequences may be no less devastating. Often, the condition is compounded by the person viewing his or her own body as an inescapable perpetrator!

2. An interaction of factors seems evident. Genetics may cause a susceptibility to certain diseases. One person may be more prone to heart attacks and another to lung problems or cancer. There are also environmental factors, such as toxins or radiation, that can have an impact. Clinical evidence makes it seem clear that there are also psychological factors involved. A healthy immune system can generally ward off diseases; however, when the immune system is suppressed owing to any number of factors, including some kinds of chronic or acute psychological stress, the person may not be able to avoid disease. Research is ongoing; see, for example, J. H. Nassau, K. Tien, and G. K. Fritz, "Review of the Literature: Integrating Psychoneuroimmunology into Pediatric Chronic Illness Interventions," *Journal of Pediatric Psychology* 33, no. 2 (2008):195–207.However, many classic works are still relevant to readers interested in the field of psychoneuroimmunology:

N. Cousins, *Anatomy of an Illness* (New York: Norton, 1979).

N. Cousins, *Head First: The Biology of Hope* (New York: Norton, 1989).

K. R. Pelletier, *Mind as Healer, Mind as Slayer* (New York: Delacorte, 1977).

E. L. Rossi, *The Psychobiology of Mind-Body Healing* (New York: Norton, 1986).

B. Siegel, *Peace, Love and Healing* (New York: Harper and Row, 1989).

3. Also called Stage IV.

4. Anxiety, depression, intrusive thoughts, and the tendency to become easily upset are all part of the clinical picture when facing a life-threatening disease. In addition to feeling helpless, many people are haunted by intrusive images of the moment of diagnosis. Sometimes physicians, through insensitivity or presenting a sorrowful demeanor, can make people feel as though they have been given a death sentence. When these images exist, they often become the first target of an EMDR processing session. Because disease can be an ongoing trauma, EMDR may be used on the disturbances that remain from previous medical procedures or to prepare for future ones. In addition, for many people with disease, the interactions with family or friends can be a problem. Sometimes, the people we count on most to support us simply cannot cope with the situation and make matters worse. It is important that patients with cancer learn to put themselves high on the priority list. This might not be easy, because it might be the first time they've stopped taking care of others.

5. O. C. Simonton and J. Creighton, *Getting Well Again* (New York: Bantam Books, 1992).

6. T cells provide defense against viruses; a normal count is 800–1,300. AIDS symptoms usually don't crop up until the T-cell count has dropped below 200.

Chapter 12, pp. 247–267
Visions of the Future: The Global Reach of EMDR

1. F. Shapiro, "The Role of Eye Movement Desensitization and Reprocessing (EMDR) Therapy in Medicine: Addressing the Psychological and Physical Symptoms Stemming from Adverse Life Experiences," *Permanente Journal* 18 (2014): 71–77.

2. T. Amano, A. Seiyama, and M. Toichi, "Brain Activity Measured with Near-Infrared Spectroscopy During EMDR Treatment of Phantom Limb Pain," *Journal of EMDR Practice and Research* 7 (2013): 144–153.

C. de Roos, A. C. Veenstra, A. de Jongh, M. E. den Hollander-Gijsman, N. J. A. van der Wee, F. G. Zitman, and Y. R. van Rood, "Treatment of Chronic Phantom Limb Pain Using a Trauma-Focused Psychological Approach," *Pain Research and Management* 15 (2010): 65–71.

M. C. Russell, "Treating Traumatic Amputation-Related Phantom Limb Pain," *Clinical Case Studies* 7 (2008): 136–153.

J. Schneider, A. Hofmann, C. Rost, and F. Shapiro, "EMDR in the Treatment of Chronic Phantom Limb Pain," *Pain Medicine* 9 (2008): 76–82.

M. Wilensky, "Eye Movement Desensitization and Reprocessing (EMDR) as a Treatment for Phantom Limb Pain," *Journal of Brief Therapy* 5 (2006): 31–44.

3. F. Shapiro, "The Role of Eye Movement Desensitization and Reprocessing (EMDR) Therapy in Medicine: Addressing the Psychological and Physical Symptoms Stemming from Adverse Life Experiences," *Permanente Journal* 18 (2014): 71–77.

4. In June 1996, five studies appeared in the *Archives of General Psychiatry* indicating a link between mental health and criminality. For instance, 80 percent of almost thirteen hundred women awaiting trial had a history of mental illness, and 70 percent had shown signs of psychological disorder within the past six months. The studies also noted the high incidence of exposure to trauma, including a documented history of sexual abuse in a large percentage of these people. The editorial cautioned that "a link between violence, crime and mental illness . . . cannot be dismissed." Can the treatment of traumatic memories in crime prevention programs demonstrate a significant impact on the incidence of violence and criminality? One of the goals of some EMDR researchers is to inaugurate large-scale studies to investigate the possibility of using EMDR in the prison systems and in crime prevention programs in the inner cities. This is a special project under the auspices of the EMDR Humanitarian Assistance Programs, a nonprofit organization dedicated to providing EMDR relief services globally (see Appendix A).

5. R. Carriere, "Scaling Up What Works: Using EMDR to Help Confront the World's Burden of Traumatic Stress," *Journal of EMDR Practice and Research* 8, no. 4 (2014): 187–195.

F. Shapiro, "EMDR Therapy Humanitarian Assistance Programs: Treating the Psychological, Physical, and Societal Effects of Adverse Experiences Worldwide," *Journal of EMDR Practice and Research* 8 (2014): 181–186, describes some of the negative effects of unhealed trauma and how they can be treated: "The negative effects of trauma and other adverse life experiences have been shown to interfere with individual, family, and societal functioning. Eye movement desensitization and reprocessing (EMDR) therapy is empirically supported and recommended as a frontline treatment for psychological trauma in numerous practice guidelines. It provides both effective and efficient treatment without the need for detailed descriptions of the disturbing event or homework. This allows field teams to provide culturally sensitive therapy on consecutive days for those in remote areas and in crisis situations."

6. See the following articles from *Journal of EMDR Practice and Research* 8, no. 4 (2014):

K. Alter-Reid, G. Colelli, and N. Simons, "When Disaster Strikes Our Local Communities: U.S. EMDR Trauma Recovery Network Coordinators Reflect on Lessons Learned," pp. 205–214.

D. Farrell, "Developing EMDR Therapy in Pakistan as Part of a Humanitarian Endeavour," pp. 233–239.

I. Fernandez, C. Callerame, G. Maslovaric, and K. Wheeler, "EMDR Europe Humanitarian Programs: Development, Current Status, and Future Challenges," pp. 215–224.

R. Gelbach, "EMDR Humanitarian Assistance Programs: Twenty Years and Counting," pp. 196–204.

I. Jarero, L. Artigas, S. Uribe, and A. Miranda, "EMDR Therapy Humanitarian Trauma Recovery Interventions in Latin America and the Caribbean," pp. 260–268.

H. Mattheß and U. Sodemann, "Trauma-Aid, Humanitarian Assistance Program Germany," pp. 225–232.

S. Mehrotra, "Humanitarian Projects and Growth of EMDR Therapy in Asia," p., 252–259.

M. Zaghrout-Hodali, "Humanitarian Work Using EMDR in Palestine and the Arab World," pp. 240–247.

E. Zimmermann, "EMDR Humanitarian Work: Providing Trainings in EMDR Therapy to African Clinicians," pp. 248–251.

7. R. J. Ricci, C. A. Clayton, and F. Shapiro, "Some Effects of EMDR Treatment with Previously Abused Child Molesters: Theoretical Reviews and Preliminary Findings," *Journal of Forensic Psychiatry and Psychology* 17 (2006): 538–562.

As predicted by the Adaptive Information Processing model, the EMDR therapy treatment of the molesters' own childhood victimization resulted in a decrease in deviant arousal as measured by the plethysmograph, a decrease in sexual thoughts, and increased victim empathy. The effects were maintained at one-year follow-up.

INDEX

The originator and developer of EMDR therapy, **Francine Shapiro, PhD,** currently serves as the Director of the EMDR Institute and is a Senior Research Fellow, Emeritus, at the Mental Research Institute in Palo Alto, California. She is the founder and President Emeritus of the Trauma Recovery, EMDR Humanitarian Assistance Programs, a nonprofit organization that coordinates disaster response and pro bono training worldwide. Internationally recognized in the field of psychology, she has won awards such as the International Sigmund Freud Award for Psychotherapy of the City of Vienna. Her work has enabled thousands of clinicians to treat millions of patients over the last twenty-five years. Dr. Shapiro lives in northern California.

Photograph by Bill Apton

Margot Silk Forrest is a writer and an independent book editor living in Morro Bay, California.